Re-reading the Monstrous-Feminine

'Re-reading the Monstrous-Feminine offers a welcome, far-reaching and much-overdue re-appraisal of one of the most influential pieces of scholarship on women, horror, and psychoanalytic film theory.'

—Erin Harrington, University of Canterbury, New Zealand

'It is long past time for an extended appraisal of Barbara Creed's ground-breaking conception of the "monstrous-feminine," and this collection makes clear the continued relevance of Creed's theory to a proliferating array of bodies and texts.'

—Dawn Keetley, Lehigh University, USA

This book provides a critical reappraisal of Barbara Creed's groundbreaking work of feminist psychoanalytic film scholarship, *The Monstrous-Feminine*, which was first published in 1993. The Monstrous-Feminine married psychoanalytic thinking with film analysis in radically new ways to provide an invaluable corrective to conventional approaches to the study of women in horror films, with their narrow emphasis on woman's victimhood. This volume, which will mark 25 years since the publication of *The Monstrous-Feminine*, brings together essays by international scholars working across a variety of disciplines who take up Creed's ideas in new ways and fresh contexts or, more broadly, explore possible futures for feminist and/or psychoanalytically informed art history and film theory.

Nicholas Chare is Associate Professor in the Department of History of Art and Film Studies at the Université de Montréal, Canada. He is the author of *After Francis Bacon* (2012) and *Sportswomen in Cinema* (2015) and the co-editor with Liz Watkins of *Gesture and Film* (2017) and with Katharina Bonzel of *Representations of Sports Coaches in Film* (2017).

Jeanette Hoorn is Honorary Professorial Fellow and a former Director of Gender Studies and Associate- Dean EO in the Faculty of Arts at the University of Melbourne, Australia. In 2014 she designed *Sexing the Canvas*, filmed and taught at National Gallery of Victoria, Museum of Modern Art New York, and Huntington Library in Pasadena on the Coursera platform https://www.coursera.org/course/sexingthecanvas. Her books include *Australian Pastoral: The Making of a White Landscape*, 2007; *Reframing Darwin: Evolution and Art in Australia*, 2009; *Body Trade: Captivity, Cannibalism and Colonialism in the Pacific*, 2001; *Idylle Marocaine, Hilda Rix Nicholas et Elsie Rix en Maroc*, due October 2019 with Afrique Orient. Her essays have appeared in *Art and Australia, Screen, Third Text, Continuum, Transnational Cinemas, Hecate, Australian Historical Studies; Photofile.*

Audrey Yue is Professor in Media, Culture and Critical Theory, Head of Communications and New Media, and Convenor of the Cultural Studies in Asia PhD Programme at the National University of Singapore. She is author, co-author and co-editor of *Sinophone Cinemas* (2014), *Transnational Australian Cinema* (2013), *Queer Singapore* (2012), *Ann Hui's Song of the Exile* (2010), *AsiaPacifiQueer* (2008) and *Mobile Cultures: New Media in Queer Asia* (2003). Her recent essays appear in *Media and Communication*; *International Journal of Communication*; *Inter-Asia Cultural Studies* and *Urban Studies.*

Routledge Advances in Film Studies

Emotion in Animated Films
Edited by Meike Uhrig

Post-Production and the Invisible Revolution of Filmmaking
From the Silent Era to Synchronized Sound
George Larkin

New Approaches to Cinematic Space
Edited by Filipa Rosário and Iván Villarmea Álvarez

Melancholy in Contemporary Cinema
A Spinozian Analysis of Film Experience
Francesco Sticchi

Found Footage Horror Films
A Cognitive Approach
Peter Turner

Affect and Embodied Meaning in Animation
Becoming-Animated
Sylvie Bissonnette

Classical Hollywood Film Cycles
Zoë Wallin

Re-reading the Monstrous-Feminine
Art, Film, Feminism and Psychoanalysis
Edited by Nicholas Chare, Jeanette Hoorn and Audrey Yue

Ethics of Cinematic Experience
Screens of Alterity
Orna Raviv

For more information about this series, please visit: https://www.routledge.com

Re-reading the Monstrous-Feminine

Art, Film, Feminism and Psychoanalysis

Edited by
Nicholas Chare, Jeanette Hoorn
and Audrey Yue

Routledge
Taylor & Francis Group
LONDON AND NEW YORK

First published 2020 by Routledge

2 Park Square, Milton Park, Abingdon, Oxon OX14 4RN
605 Third Avenue, New York, NY 10017

Routledge is an imprint of the Taylor & Francis Group, an informa business

First issued in paperback 2021

Publisher's Note

The publisher has gone to great lengths to ensure the quality of this reprint but points out that some imperfections in the original copies may be apparent.

Library of Congress Cataloging-in-Publication Data
Library of Congress Control Number: 2019949347

ISBN: 978-1-138-60294-6 (hbk)
ISBN: 978-1-03-217732-8 (pbk)
DOI: 10.4324/9780429469367

Typeset in Sabon
by codeMantra

Contents

Acknowledgments

We would like to thank Michelle Gewurtz, Wilson Koh and Silvestra Mariniello for their help and practical support at various stages of the preparation of this manuscript. We are also indebted to Jane Brown at the Visual Cultures Resource Centre in the School of Culture and Communications at the University of Melbourne for her help in sourcing images and permissions.

Additionally we would like to thank the anonymous reviewers for their helpful comments and insights regarding an earlier draft of the volume. We are also grateful to Suzanne Richardson, Karthikeyan Subramaniam, Felisa Salvago-Keyes, Richa Kohli, Eleanor Catchpole Simmons and Isabella Vitti at Routledge who have been a pleasure to work with throughout.

1 Re-reading *The Monstrous-Feminine*

New Approaches to Psychoanalytic Theory, Affect, Film, and Art

Nicholas Chare, Jeanette Hoorn, and Audrey Yue

> The argument that women's genitals terrify because they might castrate challenges the Freudian and Lacanian view and its association of the symbolic order with the masculine.
>
> (Barbara Creed, *The Monstrous-Feminine*)

In 2008, the comedy horror film *Teeth* (Dir. Mitchell Lichtenstein, USA, 2007) was released in cinemas. The film centres upon a high school student, Dawn O'Keefe, who has a vagina with hidden teeth. Early in the narrative, Dawn is forced to have sex by a young man, Tobey, and the teeth emerge cutting of his penis. Researching her condition, Dawn learns about the legend of the *vagina dentata* or toothed vagina. She seems literally to embody a physical condition previously taken for myth. *Teeth* is a film that exploits anxieties about female sexuality as a means to shock and amuse its audience. The fear of castration that undergirds the plot resonates with some of the themes that Barbara Creed (1993) examines in her groundbreaking analysis of the horror film genre, *The Monstrous-Feminine*. Creed devotes an entire chapter to the *vagina dentata* as it appears in myth and as it relates to Freudian theory. She suggests that the *vagina dentata* is 'particularly relevant to the iconography of the horror film, which abounds with images that play on the fear of castration and dismemberment' (1993, p. 107). *Teeth* manifests imagery of this kind. Dawn's actions are akin to those of the *femme castratrice*, of woman as a castrator (although her vagina practises penectomy). Creed analyses the figure of the *femme castratrice* in the context of rape revenge films such as *I Spit on Your Grave* (Dir. Meir Zarchi, USA, 1978). *Teeth* does not begin as a rape revenge film – in that Dawn's initial acts of dismembering seem instinctive rather than intended – but she does later consciously exploit her toothed vagina to seek vengeance on those who wrong her or those close to her. In the final scene, she is held hostage by an old man who appears willing to trade her freedom for sexual favours. She looks at him, giving a tight-lipped smile, concealing her teeth. In imprisoning Dawn, the sexual predator is clearly shown to have bitten off more than he can chew.

Teeth was released 14 years after the publication of *The Monstrous-Feminine*, and demonstrates that the kinds of anxieties regarding genders and sexualities that Creed examines in her book are remarkably enduring in horror films. It is now over 25 years since Creed's landmark feminist contribution to scholarship on the horror genre. A new, expanded edition of *The Monstrous-Feminine* is currently in preparation to mark the occasion. As the essays in this volume demonstrate, many of the themes and issues examined in *The Monstrous-Feminine* continue to manifest in contemporary art and cinema. Creed's book developed and elaborated upon ideas first considered in her 1986 *Screen* article 'Horror and the Monstrous-Feminine'. *The Monstrous-Feminine* takes representations of 'woman-as-monster' as its subject, analysing case studies including *Alien* (Dir. Ridley Scott, UK, 1979), *Carrie* (Dir. Brian de Palma, USA, 1976), *The Brood* (Dir. David Cronenberg, Canada, 1979), *The Exorcist* (Dir. William Friedkin, USA, 1973), and *The Hunger* (Dir. Tony Scott, USA, 1983). The examples Creed focusses on mainly derive from American and British cinema yet other scholars such as Brown (2018), Meraj Ahmed Mubarki (2014) and Audrey Yue (2000) have taken up the idea of the monstrous-feminine in relation to different geographical and cinematic contexts. Creed's approach is psychoanalytic throughout, building on earlier pioneer texts such as Raymond Bellour's (1979) *L'analyse du film*, Christian Metz's (1975) 'Le signifiant imaginaire', and Laura Mulvey's (1975) 'Visual Pleasure and Narrative Cinema'. Bellour, Metz, and Mulvey are all heavily influenced, in their different ways, by the psychoanalytic theories of Jacques Lacan. Specularity plays an important role in the emergence of subjectivity in Lacanian thought, and as Annette Kuhn (1982, p. 47) has suggested, its pertinence to the study of cinema is therefore easy to comprehend.

Creed critically engages with ideas from both Sigmund Freud and Lacan. Her close readings of Freud's research, including the case history of 'Little Hans', and of excerpts from *The Interpretation of Dreams*, tease out how the analyst's own repressions and displacements influence the kinds of interpretations he provides (Harrington 2016, p. 4). Karen Horney (1967) explains in her 1926 essay 'The Flight from Womanhood', that psychoanalysis was created by a man and predominantly developed by men such that they evolved 'more easily a masculine psychology and [understood] more of the development of men than of women' (p. 54). She goes on to suggest that the psychic development of women as represented within psychoanalysis has 'been measured by masculine standards' (p. 57). Creed's attentive readings of Freud enable the influence of these standards to be recognised and overcome.[1] She notes, for instance, that Freud's justification for identifying the phallus as the primary signifier is not his clinical material but rather social observation (Creed 1993, p. 160). His understanding of sexual difference is influenced by the social norms of Vienna at the time he was writing. Creed repeatedly demonstrates how Freud neglects feminine agency, privileging, for instance, the role of the father as a potential source of castration in his discussion of the Oedipus complex. As Creed (1993, p. 103) observes of both 'Little Hans' and 'The Wolf Man', '[a]t no point in either case study did Freud consider that the child might also fear the *mother's genitals* as an agent of castration'.[2]

In *The Monstrous-Feminine*, Creed draws not solely on Freud's ideas but also on those of Lacan, particularly as they have been taken up and developed by Julia Kristeva in her work on abjection, most notably through her 1980 essay, *Pouvoirs de l'horreur*, published in English translation as *Powers of Horror* in 1982. Kristeva's potential importance for the study of film had been remarked since the late 1970s and her work was regularly debated in journals such as *m/f*, *Screen*, and *Wide Angle*. *The Monstrous-Feminine*, however, provides what is still one of the most sustained and inspiring engagements with Kristeva in the context of film analysis. Other film theorists have made reference to Kristeva's thinking yet very few have placed her work at the heart of their interpretive framework.[3] The centrality of *Powers of Horror* to *The Monstrous-Feminine* cannot be underestimated. Kristeva's exploration of the nascent subject's establishment of its fragile borders through a rejection of the Mother as psychic figure is coupled with a consideration of how these archaic events continue to influence behaviour in adulthood, particularly through anxieties about the breaching of borders. This makes Kristeva an important thinker of the border as a structuring force in society and culture.[4] To best understand the innovativeness of Creed's uptake of Kristeva's thinking, a brief overview of *Powers of Horror* is useful.

Approaching Abjection

In *Powers of Horror*, Kristeva draws on anthropology and psychoanalysis to examine the role of abjection in subject-formation and subjectivity. Abjection, for Kristeva, describes the process by which an infant is able to forge provisional, transitory boundaries between itself and the figure of the Mother. Once these fragile, tentative boundaries are in place, the infant can progress to the mirror-stage of psychic development. Kristeva (1982, p. 13) notes: 'Even before being *like*, "I" am not but do *separate*, *reject*, *ab-ject*'.[5] Prior to being capable of recognising its *likeness* in the mirror, the child must first split from the all-encompassing Mother. These early beginnings of subjectivity, in which the boundary between the nascent subject and the mother are uncertain, are repressed in adulthood but continue to haunt the subject through encounters with abject phenomena. Kristeva (1982, p. 2) lists 'filth, waste and dung' as examples of such phenomena, substances that remind the subject of their precarious origins. Bodily excreta, materials the traverse the body from inside to outside, that cross its putative boundaries, call to mind the fragile boundary that came into being between Mother and infant in early psychic life. For Kristeva (1982, p. 4), the corpse, 'seen without God and outside of science, is the utmost of abjection'.

Kristeva explains that in Jewish and Christian cultures, religion has functioned to protect subjects from encounters with the abject. In an increasingly secular and rationalist society, however, religion no longer performs this task. For Kristeva, this means that art and literature now have an important role to play in policing and processing contemporary encounters with the abject. Her preferred example for unpacking how artistic forms can fulfil the role of religion in modern society, providing controlled encounters with the abject or impure, is the novelist Louis-Ferdinand Céline, whose writings she analyses at length in *Powers of Horror.*[6] In an interview with Charles Penwarden, 'Of Word and Flesh', which discusses Kristeva's (1995) responses to the 1995 Tate Gallery exhibition *Rites of Passage*, she also views contemporary art as offering catharsis in the face of the abject. Kristeva describes 'objects that purify abjection in the work of certain artists' (Kristeva 1995, p. 24). For Kristeva, works by artists such as Louise Bourgeois, Mona Hatoum, and Jana Sterbak embody a language that 'attempts to come as close as possible, almost to accompany [the] state of abjection, [the] permanent oscillation between subject and object' (pp. 22–23). This lends the works a cathartic value. Artworks, in Kristeva's terms, are not passive objects of contemplation. They rouse those who encounter them and act upon them.

Kristeva's emphasis on avant-garde art and literature as media in which sanctioned transgressions of notions of purity are made possible seems to render catharsis through cultural forms the reserve of a relatively small audience. Creed counters this tendency, providing a compelling demonstration of how Kristeva's ideas about abjection can also be illuminating in the context of popular culture. In *The Monstrous-Feminine*, she demonstrates how media such as the horror film also potentially have a therapeutic role.[7] For Creed (1986, p. 53), the horror film can operate as 'a form of modern defilement rite' that 'works to separate out the symbolic order from all that threatens its stability, particularly the mother and all that her universe signifies'. She suggests that the central project of the popular horror film is 'purification of the abject' (Creed 1993, p. 14). Cinema then provides another means by which to speak and thereby assuage individual malaise (and, by extension, social malaise) regarding psychic identity. Creed's reading of horror films as modes of encounter with the abject provides a crucial extension of Kristeva's aesthetics, revealing their pertinence for analyses of popular culture.[8]

Her Body, Himself

In *The Monstrous-Feminine*, Creed acknowledges the important work performed by Carol J. Clover (1987) in relation to depictions of women in horror films. Clover's notion of the Final Girl, the last woman standing who confronts the villain/monster, has become highly influential for the study of slasher films. Creed particularly appreciates Clover's recognition of the different ways in which the deaths of men and women are treated in the horror genre. Clover (1987, p. 212) suggests that women are permitted a greater emotional range in extreme situations, a range that is fully exploited in horror films: 'crying, cowering, screaming, fainting, trembling, begging for mercy belong to the female'. This means that '[a]bject terror [...] is gendered feminine' (ibid.). Creed's and Clover's differing outlooks on horror films, which are both informed by psychoanalysis, have been paired in edited collections such as *Fantasy and the Cinema* (1989) and *The Dread of Difference* (1996). Comparing the two approaches is illuminating in terms of significant differences regarding their conception of sex and gender.

Clover provides a complex reading of the processes of identification that potentially occur when viewing slasher films, the horror genre that forms her primary focus. For Clover, identification in the male audience (which she focusses on as forming the main consumers of the slasher genre) shifts from the often male (or seemingly male) villain to the female victim-hero. For Clover (1987, p. 208), these shifting identifications show that 'gender is less a wall than a permeable membrane'. She does not believe a seamless relation exists between point of view shot (henceforth POV shot) and viewer identification. She does, however, believe it is important that in slasher films, as the narrative unfolds, the POV shot shifts from being predominantly that of the villain to being increasingly that of the Final Girl. There is a complex waxing and waning in operation that ostensibly crosses gender divides (Clover 1987, p. 208). Clover's nuanced reading of processes of identification, however, is somewhat undercut by the seeming essentialism of her arguments. Clover (1987, p. 215), for example, asks that the Final Girl not be simply viewed as a figurative male yet shortly afterwards in a discussion of uncertainty about gender cultivated by the use of POV shot in slasher films her argument relies heavily on taking the anatomical sex of the protagonist as the yardstick against which perceived gender deviations can be measured. The body is thus rendered the truth of the sex of a person. In *Psycho*, for example, 'the dame we glimpse holding the knife [...] is later revealed, after additional gender teasing, to be Norman in his mother's clothes' (Clover 1987, p. 216). In this reading, Norman masquerades as female (through clothing and voice) but is ultimately shown to be male.

For Clover, sex and gender are categorically distinct. This perceived split between sex and gender enables her to observe of slasher films that '[i]t is not that these show us gender and sex in free variation; it is that they fix on the irregular combinations, of which the combination masculine female prevails over the combination feminine male' (Clover 1987, p. 221). Gender is communicated through appearance and/or behaviour and forms a kind of theatre (p. 217). In this context, she reads the gesture of the character Stretch in the denouement to *Texas Chainsaw Massacre 2* as 'a moment of high drag' (p. 217). The film ends with Stretch wielding a chainsaw above her head, triumphant, after despatching her last aggressor, Chop Top. For Clover, the chainsaw figures what Stretch *seems* to be (masculine) rather than what she *is* (feminine). The chainsaw as phallic signifier grants Stretch a measure of masculinity, but her '"tits and scream"' signal her biological sex (p. 217). The male audience is able to identify with characters such as Stretch because of Stretch's ability to proffer simultaneous signifiers of masculinity and femininity. Clover's reading has understandably met with resistance. Judith Jack Halberstam (1995, p. 157), for example, argues compellingly that the notion of audience reception underpinning this logic is one that 'avoids the possibility of a more radical and possible queer gaze'.

Clover hears Stretch's scream over-simplistically as signalling her 'Scream Queen' credentials, positioning her as another in a long line of women giving voice to their terror. Michel Chion (1999) has examined how many films go to extreme lengths to reach what he calls the 'screaming point', the moment of a woman's scream. He suggests that the motivation for cultivating this scream is both sadistic and symptomatic of male anxieties about female sexuality and orgasm (Chion 1999, pp. 77–78). Chion gives examples such as *Psycho* and *King Kong*. He usefully contrasts the scream with the cry or shout. For Chion (1999, p. 79), women in cinema are often portrayed screaming, whereas men are shown shouting, the latter vocalisation understood as '[delimiting] a territory'. For us, Stretch's scream is of this kind. As Halberstam (1995, p. 158) remarks, it is closer to a 'rebel yell' than an expression of terror, forming an aggressively triumphant vocalisation. The clifftop cry marks Stretch's territory, audibly affirming that now Crop Top has been seen off Stretch is 'king' of the hill. As the yell demonstrates, their success is not solely or simply communicated through possessing the chainsaw (as phallic substitute). It manifests by way of the voice, a voice which refuses to scream in terror any longer.

We agree with Clover that Stretch cannot be securely gendered in the masculine yet place less emphasis on the role of screaming in this troubling of gender binaries. For us, it is the twirling Stretch enacts, while brandishing the chainsaw that invites making links with woman as spectacle. This action is visually reminiscent of Diana Prince spinning to transform into Wonder Woman in Lynda Carter's portrayal of the superhero. Wonder Woman, as T.J. Demos (2010, pp. 54–55) notes, displays a complex identity, 'on the one hand the embodiment of physical strength, mental agility and superhero stature – all attributes normally belonging to the male superhero – and on the other hand an object of sexual desire constructed to-be-looked-at'. In *Wonder Woman*, the spin at once indexes a transformation from average Jane to superhero and from plain Jane to glamorous princess. In *Texas Chainsaw Massacre 2* the spin embodies the transformation from Final Girl to a figure refusing any finality, resisting the ready imposition of gender categories. Halberstam (1995, pp. 157–158) is clearly attuned to this queer potential in the closing scene, viewing Stretch as resisting coding as 'tits and ass' and becoming instead 'tits and chainsaw', with the saw standing for 'the chain of signifiers that has become scrambled' in the film.

Creed's interpretative framework, contra Clover's, is able to open valuable spaces for the recognition of identities within horror cinema that are gender variant. This openness is rendered possible by Creed's employment of a psychoanalytic framework that resists essentialising. As Jacqueline Rose (1985, p. 41) explains, for Lacan 'sexual difference is a legislative divide which creates and reproduces its categories'. Sexual difference is therefore not descriptive of a pre-existing biological reality but rather operates prescriptively. Rose suggests that in Lacan's schema:

> Sexual difference is [...] assigned according to whether individual subjects do or do not possess the phallus, which means not that anatomical difference *is* sexual difference (the one as strictly deducible from the other), but that anatomical difference comes to *figure* sexual difference, that is, it becomes the sole representative of what that difference is allowed to be. It thus covers over the complexity of the child's early sexual life with a crude oppression in which that very complexity is refused or repressed. The phallus thus indicates the reduction of difference to an instance of visible perception, a *seeming* value.
>
> (Rose 1985, p. 42)

In this conception of sexual difference, as against Clover's investment in the sexed body, anatomy is very much not destiny. Many of Creed's readings of horror films demonstrate the radical potential of the genre as a means of exposing the value accorded the phallus as a *seeming*. Creed teases out how Woman as a psychic category not only figures as castrated, as not in possession of the phallus, but also as castrating. In this sense, Creed foregrounds the body as signifier of a sex, of sexual difference, as a contested site of meaning. The vagina is open to being figured not only as a signifier of lack but also as a substantial force, a castrating entity.

Creed's analyses enable a more complex understanding of femininity within psychoanalysis to emerge. For Creed (1993, pp. 126–127), in contrast to Clover, characters such as Stretch (who Creed namechecks) are not phallicised and pseudo men. They are rather manifestations of a dimension to femininity that is disavowed by Freud and, by extension, Lacan. Stretch's appropriation of the chainsaw is, in this sense, not a symptom of penis envy but an affirmation of vaginal pride, the teeth of the saw figuring the toothed vagina rather than substituting for the absent phallus.[9] Lacan foreclosed the idea of a symbolic equivalent or alternative to the phallus. For him, hysteria was symptomatic of (failed) efforts to 'symbolize the female organ' (Lacan 1993, p. 178). Creed, however, identifies another sexual signifier, the monstrous-feminine, as in operation within the Symbolic.

Creed does more than simply reveal the monstrous-feminine as an alternative to the feminine as lack. Through building on a Kristevan framework, she is able to gesture towards moments in horror films – encounters with the abject – in which the ways in which anatomical difference has come to figure within patriarchy are troubled and potentially undone. The drive-invested memories of early psychic life that are triggered through encounters with the abject draw the subject back to a period pre-*seeming*, prior to the valorisation of anatomical difference as a figure for sexual difference. Abjection as a psychic process, as already discussed, unfolds in advance of the mirror-phase. It is therefore also prior to the Oedipus complex and the imposition of paternal law. For Lacan, the father as a third term is not absent from the pre-oedipal in that the phallus as an imaginary object registers for the Mother but it is only through the Oedipus complex that the Father becomes a locus of symbolic identification for the child. It is through the Oedipus complex that a child comes to assume a sex and make a sexual object choice: '[i]t is insofar as the function of man and woman is symbolized, it is insofar as it's literally uprooted from the domain of the imaginary and situated in the domain of the symbolic, that any normal, completed sexual position is realized' (Lacan 1993, p. 177). Abjection as psychic experience serves to remind the child of a time prior to this sexing and finding of sexuality, therefore potentially signalling the contingency of these processes. For Creed, as Shohini Chaudhuri (2006, p. 95) discusses, the mother associated with abjection is 'the primeval mother of everything – a parthenogenetic mother, creating all by herself, without the need for a father; she is a pre-phallic mother, existing prior to knowledge of the phallus'. Creed reveals that encounters with abjection such as those that occur in horror films hold the potential to enable the subject to revisit sexual difference, conceivably returning to the Symbolic on changed terms.

The Monstrous Flesh

Halberstam's (1995) critique of Clover is, in part, a critique of her conception of reception, one in which the audience is straightforwardly gendered as masculine (with masculinity singularised). Clover (1987,

p. 205) does, however, productively foreground the importance of expressions of disgust and revulsion by audiences during the viewing of slasher films. She writes of instances of 'uproarious disgust' in audience members, of complex combining of amusement and aversion condensed in the utterance 'Gross!' She also emphasises the intricate vocalisations, or lack thereof, of audiences, the moments of silence, the screams, the 'loud noises of revulsion' (p. 205). Creed is similarly attuned to such phenomena. She draws attention not only to the perverse pleasure audiences take in horror films but also to how that pleasure combines with a desire to reject the horrific spectacle being played out on screen, a desire 'to throw up, throw out, eject the abject' (Creed 1993, p. 10). In both these readings, the body of the spectator becomes an important measure of the impact of horror films. Such films are not simply viewed and reflected upon; they are also keenly felt registered in the pit of the stomach.

As part of her sustained critique of psychoanalytic approaches to the horror genre in *Deleuze and the Horror Film*, Anna Powell (2005, p. 2) foregrounds the incapacity of psychoanalytic frameworks to account for certain phenomena in viewing experiences. For her, psychoanalytic readings focus on narrative and representation at the expense of corporeal affect, reducing films to allegories for pre-existing ideas.[10] Her notion of psychoanalysis is essentially Lacanian. She argues Lacanian-inspired approaches leave no space for 'visual and aural experience or other sensory stimuli that an aesthetics of sensation might afford' (p. 17). Her critique of psychoanalysis is indebted to the ideas of Gilles Deleuze and Félix Guattari. For Deleuze and Guattari, clinical psychoanalysis forms a highly socially repressive activity. Their understanding of psychoanalysis is also primarily influenced by Lacanian approaches. This is unsurprising, given that Guattari attended Lacan's seminars for a period of time and was also Lacan's patient (Roudinesco and Plon 1997, p. 412). Deleuze (2006a, p. 80) described psychoanalysis as leading to 'the reduction and abolition of desire'. In the analytic setting, '[i]t is impossible to produce an utterance without having it reduced to a prefabricated and predetermined grid of interpretation' (Deleuze 2006b, p. 89). Powell transposes this interpretation of the analytic process to the study of cinema, believing a similarly reductive grid operates when psychoanalytic readings of film are undertaken.

The negative perception Deleuze and Guattari possess of psychoanalysis requires historical contextualisation. It is, to a large extent, influenced by and also addressed at the dominant forms of psychoanalysis practised in France in the late 1960s and early 1970s. Powell takes the critique out of context and applies it in blanket form to all psychoanalysis and also to most film theory that is psychoanalytically informed (what she refers to as 'cinepsychoanalysis'). Creed's work as it is discussed in *Deleuze and Horror Film* is aligned with Lacanian theory by Powell despite an acknowledgment of its indebtedness to Kristeva.

For Powell, it seems Kristeva is a rigid Lacanian and her work can be readily subject to the same critiques that Deleuze and Guattari levelled at Lacan. At the time Deleuze and Guattari (1972) were writing *Capitalisme et schizophrénie: L'anti-Œdipe*, however, Kristeva was working on her doctoral thesis which would subsequently be published as *La Révolution du langage poétique* [Revolution in Poetic Language] (Kristeva 1974). Her work in *Powers of Horror*, which inspired Creed, is of a different time and although broadly Lacanian in outlook is also clearly implicitly critical of dimensions of Lacan's thinking. Like other psychoanalytic thinkers such as Nicolas Abraham and Maria Torok (with their embrace of deconstruction) and Bracha Ettinger (who is partly influenced by the anti-Oedipal stance of Deleuze and Guattari), Kristeva is expanding psychoanalysis in ways that cannot and should not be conflated with Lacanian analysis as it is critiqued by Deleuze and Guattari.[11]

Powell (2005, p. 16) does recognise potential in Kristeva's 'suggestive exploration of the fluid nature of abjection' yet does not engage in a meaningful way with *Powers of Horror* or how Creed takes up the idea of abjection. Had she done so, she would have had to revisit her claim that Lacanian-inspired analyses of film leave no space for 'visual and aural experience or other sensory stimuli' in contrast with an 'aesthetics of sensation' inspired by Deleuze (p. 17). Powell's conceptualisation of psychoanalysis is overly reductive, ignoring the importance of recognising non-narrative-based and non-representational phenomena within clinical settings. In this context, Melanie Klein's (1997) notion of 'memories in feelings' as they manifest in analysis is particularly noteworthy.[12] Powell's (2005, p. 5) idea of becoming infected by a film bears some affinities with transference as it occurs in the analytic situation. Kristeva's idea of the semiotic, the drive-invested underside to language, is also noteworthy here as is André Green's theorising of the drives and affect as Kristeva (2010, pp. 178–179) interprets it. Throughout *The Monstrous-Feminine* Creed pays careful heed to moments of semiotic intensity in horror films as they manifest by way of, for example, sound, gesture, and chromatics. The richness of a Kristevan approach of the kind adopted by Creed is precisely that it does permit sensation – the drives as the semiotic underside to signification – to be appreciated and described.

Creed is highly attentive to what might now be referred to as the affective dimension to the horror film experience. Her groundbreaking idea of the *fifth* look, the look that is not, the moment of looking away or of covering the eyes, a look that occurs sometimes when watching horror films, describes experiences that register foremost as feeling rather than sign (Creed 1986, p. 64; 1993, p. 29). In conceiving the *fifth* look, Creed is striving to find a vocabulary capable of describing encounters with film that will subsequently be explained in Anglophone film scholarship through recourse to the ideas of, for example, Gilles Deleuze. In a section of her book *The Matrix of Visual Culture* entitled 'Psychoanalysis and the Monstrous Flesh', Patricia Pisters (2003) provides a thoughtful, if critical, reading of *The Monstrous-Feminine* as part of a general reproach of psychoanalysis. For Pisters (2003, p. 52), psychoanalysis fails to address multiplicity and affect as important dimensions of subjectivity. The *fifth* look, however, can be understood to index reactions to upsurges of affect, of intensity, within a given film. During such upsurges, matter independent of form makes itself manifest, matter freed from any fashioning into objects or entities, presenting anew its ductility, its complexity, and it multiplicity. Creed's framework of understanding is psychoanalytic yet her readings are nonetheless seeking to account for affective experiences that share some of the qualities of the asignifier as it is understood by Deleuze and Guattari (1986, p. 22), a force that strips signification of its capacity for enunciation, transforming it instead into a manifestation of intensity.[13]

Here Kristeva's notion of the abject as that which *shows* itself to those who encounter it is crucial. She clearly accords abject materials a kind of agency, an intensity, which is not dependent upon decoding, upon being read. The corpse, she is at pains to point out, does not *signify* death, it is not a representation, a thing transformed into sign. It is registered as a message without a code, an intense troubling of the separation of subject and object, of the mediating gap required for a sign system or a system of representation to operate. Brought to the brink of psychosis by this boundary troubling, Kristeva (1982, p. 4) describes the subject as falling in faint. This physical response causes the subject, in turn, to become a kind of cadaver (from *cadere*, to fall), a kind of living-dead. In *The Monstrous-Feminine*, Creed examines the corpse as abject abomination as it features in films such as *The Evil Dead* (Dir. Sam Raimi, USA, 1981) and *Zombie Flesh Eaters* (Dir. Lucio Fulci, Italy, 1979). For her the visceral reaction to abject materials in horror film registers abjection at work 'almost in a literal sense' (Creed 1993, p. 10). This seeming literalness, what Kristeva (2010, p. 178) refers to in relation to affect as the 'degree zero of symbolism', forms a symptom of the collapsing of signification that characterises audience responses to horror films at certain moments, a psychic regression. During such moments, difference, including sexual difference, is prospectively rendered abeyant.

In this sense, the violence reduction of sexual potential that Deleuze associates with the imposition of sexual difference is, at least temporarily, undone. Deleuze (2006b, p. 92) suggests that '[t]here are not two sexes, there are *n* sexes; there are as many sexes as there are assemblages'. For him, reducing sexuality 'to the difference between the sexes' is 'a fatal error whether this difference is interpreted organically or structurally, in relation to the penis-organ or in relation to the phallus-signifier' (p. 93). The best way to misunderstand sexuality is to reduce 'everything to the difference between the sexes' (p. 93).

Moments of abjection, however, enact a de-differentiation at the level of sex. In this sense, they open a space for sidestepping existing signifying regimes and embracing sexual creativity. It is this potential in horror cinema that Halberstam, operating within a different theoretical framework, clearly identifies in *Skin Shows*. Through her engagement with abjection in horror films, Creed offers a crucial vocabulary for identifying and describing that potential at work. It is a potential that also registers through abject art practices.

The Art of Abjection

In *The Monstrous-Feminine* although Creed's main focus is the horror film, she also briefly discusses the importance of depictions of the *vagina dentata* in Surrealist art, signalling the potential significance of the monstrous-feminine for art history. In *The Monstrous-Feminine*, there are reproductions of a photograph of Salvador Dali peering out from behind a nude woman who has a lobster covering her genitals and of René Magritte's *The Rape* (1934) in which a woman's torso is transposed on her face such that her eyes are her breasts, her nose is her navel and her mouth is her vulva. The Dali photograph, which is by George Platt Lynes, featured in 'The Dream of Venus' show for the 1939 New York World's Fair.[14] In it, Dali's right hand emerges from a gaping wound in the woman's right thigh. The show included semi-nude models who were adorned with various kinds of seafood including lobsters. Horst P. Horst photographed one of these models seated with a lobster on her crotch. She is holding aloft what appear to be oysters and wears a pearl necklace from which dangle hooks threaded with what seem to be shelled mussels. In another photograph by Horst, the lobster has been transposed to the woman's head.

For Creed, the lobster with its claws figures the *vagina dentata*. This connection is lent credence by the name given to a sexual technique practised by Wallis Simpson on King Edward VIII, later known as the Duke of Windsor. Called the 'lobster grip', the technique involved tightening the vaginal muscles to constrict blood flow to the erect penis.[15] In 1937, Wallis Simpson famously wore a 'lobster dress' that had been designed by Elsa Schiaparelli in collaboration with Dali. The artist painted a large lobster on the sheer A-line skirt of the dress. In Cecil Beaton's photographs for *Vogue* of Wallis Simpson wearing the dress, the tail is positioned roughly above her groin. This positioning encourages linking the lobster with the vulva, intimating some kind of equivalence between the two. The sexual connotations of the lobster would have been enhanced yet further if Wallis Simpson had followed Dali's request to smear it with mayonnaise (Thurman 2012, p. 28).

The lobster as a visual reference has also been identified in a film, *Alien*, which forms a major case study in *The Monstrous-Feminine*.

Creed's reading of *Alien* is much celebrated and has been highly influential. The film narrative is about the crew of a space-freighter, the Nostromo, who investigate a derelict alien spacecraft. During their survey of the vessel, one of the crewmembers, Kane, finds a cargo hold filled with giant, leathery eggs. Peering into one of the eggs, he is attacked by an alien creature which attaches itself to his face and, unbeknownst to the other crew members, impregnates him. The alien, referred to in commentary as a facehugger, possesses a bony carapace and what David Thomson (2000, p. 41) calls 'lobster legs'. The stricken Kane is transported back to the Nostromo where he remains comatose for a period of time, the alien fixed to his face. Eventually the creature falls off, appearing to die. In the scene in *Alien* during which the science officer Ash autopsies the facehugger, the special effects team fabricated the alien's fleshy insides from out of shellfish and a sheep's kidney. In an abject scene, the insides of organisms were brought outside, exposed to view. Kane seems to recover from his ordeal yet at a group meal he begins to retch and convulse. An alien that was growing inside him bursts out of his chest, killing him.

This creature, known in commentary as the 'chestburster', like the others in *Alien*, was designed by the Swiss artist H.R. (Hans Rudolph) Giger. Giger's works have been described as surrealist in nature. Stanislav Grof (2002, pp. 15–16), for example, links Giger with Surrealism and has suggested Dali as a key influence. Dali is identified by David Lomas (2000) as an artist for whom abjection is a key theme. Both Dali and Giger seem to have derived artistic inspiration from anxieties about female sexualities and reproductive capacities. Artworks by Giger such as *Birthmachine* (1967), *Mother with child* (1962) and *Mother with child* (1968) make reference to reproduction and motherhood in their titles. These anxieties, Creed demonstrates, also pervade *Alien* at multiple levels. Although never appearing directly, the film revolves around the figure of the archaic mother, 'the parthenogenetic mother, the mother as primordial abyss' (Creed 1993, p. 17). For Creed, the archaic mother forms 'a vast backdrop for the enactment of all the events' of the film (p. 19). This includes the birth of the alien. It is a birth which 'recalls Freud's description of a common misunderstanding that many children have about birth, that is, that the mother is somehow "impregnated" through the mouth [...] and the baby grows in her stomach, from which it is also born' (p. 19).

The 'chestburster' was designed by Giger but with input from the director Ridley Scott who wanted the creature to resemble Francis Bacon's depictions of the Eumenides or Furies in *Three Studies for Figures at the Base of a Crucifixion* (Giger 1989, p. 56). Bacon is another artist who has been linked with Surrealism, particularly by Dawn Ades who perceives him to be a dissident surrealist, kindred in spirit to Georges Bataille. For Ades, Bacon's surrealism manifests not through technique (such as the painter's use of accident and chance), but by way of his repeated fixation on the mouth and use of it as a motif. Bataille also had an interest in the mouth. He wrote a short text that accompanied Jacques-Andre Boiffard's photograph *Bouche* which was published in *Documents* in 1929. The text, Ades (1985, p. 13) explains, 'focuses on the fact that it is through the mouth that our most concentrated expressions of agony or ecstasy are physiologically expressed, and also that in this expression the human draws particularly close to the animal'. Bataille's 'violent pulling together of man/beast [sic] in such a way that the traditional distinction between them is brought into question was part of Bataille's continual attack on the "idealist deception" that man practices on himself' (Ades 1985, p. 14). The theme of human and non-human animal relations is one Ades (1985, p. 13) sees as shared by Bacon in works such as *Three Studies for Figures at the Base of a Crucifixion*, a painting in which the figures 'have no eyes, but only mouths'. Barbara Creed and Jeanette Hoorn (2016, p. 201) have explored the links between Kristeva's conception of abjection and the figure of the animal in their essay 'Animals, Art, Abjection'. Creed also explores Kristeva's linking of abjection with animality in *Stray* (2017, pp. 21–27).

For Ades, however, the impetus for Bacon's repeated portrayals of mouths is overdetermined and not solely linked to a desire to trouble human-animal differentiation. She also turns to Freudian psychoanalysis to explain the artist's fascination with mouths, discussing 'explicit sexual symbolism connected with the mouth' (Ades 1985, p. 15). Ades recalls Freud's recognition in *The Interpretation of Dreams* that dreams often transpose from a lower to an upper part of the body (such as from genitals to mouth) (p. 16). This is a phenomenon Creed (1993, p. 118) also examines, drawing on Freud's transposition hypothesis to show how teeth dreams represent the *vagina dentata*. Expanding on Creed's interpretation, the Eumenides as they are interpreted by Bacon become incarnations of *femmes castratrices*, toothed vaginas seeking vengeance (although in the paintings why this vengeance is being sought and against whom is unclear). Ades disavows psychoanalytically motivated links between Bacon and the Surrealist movement in which anxieties about female sexualities manifest through vaginal iconography of a particular kind. Building on Creed's discussion of teeth dreams it becomes possible, however, to trace a shared psychic undercurrent across artists such as Bacon and Dali. If the gaping maw in *Three Studies for Figures at the Base of a Crucifixion* is read, on one level, as a *vagina dentata*, then its influence upon the chestburster in *Alien* forms yet another example of the strength of Creed's interpretation of the film.

Art is an inspiration for the physical appearance of the extraterrestrials in *Alien* yet no artworks are shown in the film. The only images the crew seem to be in possession of are pornographic. In *Alien: Covenant*, however, art plays a significant role within the narrative.[16]

Covenant is the second prequel to *Alien* directed by Scott, forming the sequel to *Prometheus*. In *Covenant*, which we will go on to discuss in more depth, a synthetic human, David, who has been marooned on an alien planet for a decade, is shown to have built a 'cabinet of curiosities' and to have made a number of drawings. The drawings are in the style of eighteenth-century anatomical, botanical, and zoological works.[17] Many of them appear to portray marine life, molluscs, and crustaceans. As contributions to David's broader project of conceiving the perfect organism, the origins of the lobster-like facehugger are to be found here. Through a gradual, selective revealing of the corpus of drawings in different scenes and settings, the artworks are employed as a means by which to reveal David's perturbed state of mind. The drawings are clearly linked with David's scientific work. He seems to have been engaged in cataloguing new species on the alien planet and producing biological illustrations. Later it becomes clear that the drawings are also a means for David to record the results of his genetic experiments. The drawings of the results of experimentation frequently leave less blank paper or negative space around the specimens. There is black or grey smudge or an abundance of tuberous forms serving as the ground against which David's nightmarish figures are crafted. Here science as it is practised by David is shown to be an activity that also betrays fascination with 'the mysterious black hole that signifies female genitalia' (Creed 1993, p. 27). The monstrous-feminine manifests in these exquisitely detailed records of experiments in genetic engineering gone drastically awry.

In Femmage to the Monstrous-Feminine[18]

The psychic underpinnings of *Covenant* and its earlier companion film *Prometheus* unsurprisingly resonate strongly with those of *Alien*. For that reason, it is enlightening to bring Creed's ideas about *Alien* in *The Monstrous-Feminine* into dialogue with these more recent films. Annette Kuhn (1990, p. 94) has foregrounded the political importance of Creed's work on *Alien*, seeing it as a vital contribution to a tradition of feminist psychoanalytically informed film theory that provides 'readings of films [which] may be regarded as oppositional in the degree that, in excavating patriarchal meanings, they constitute a resistive practice of reading popular films "against the grain" of hegemonic meanings'. Through such readings, Kuhn suggests that the operations of capitalism and patriarchy can be laid bare. In this spirit, we here take up Creed's ideas to examine the values and beliefs subtending *Prometheus* and *Covenant* and also their repressions. Ridley Scott has endeavoured to present these films as comprising a significant departure from *Alien* but as our analyses demonstrate, at the level of a fascination with the monstrous-feminine, this is not the case in any simple sense.

Scott has framed *Prometheus* and *Covenant* as a new departure intended to reinvigorate the *Alien* franchise, leaving behind what he perceived to be the B-movie heritage of the 1979 film (Ward 2017, p. 9). For Scott, *Covenant* explores the 'a future of interplanetary colonization' and the 'morality of creating life forms' (Scott 2017, p. 7). He has described it as resurrecting *Alien* after too many tiresome sequels (Ward 2017, p. 9). The reference to resurrection suggests that the franchise was dead on its feet and casts the director as akin to Victor Frankenstein, bringing the dead back to life. Mary Shelley's 1818 novel *Frankenstein* was subtitled 'The Modern Prometheus' and, in some ways, the two prequels to *Alien* can be read as transplanting *Frankenstein* to space. Men who attempt to create new life forms occupy a special place in the pantheon of male monsters of horror.

In *The Monstrous-Feminine* Creed explores questions of spectatorship and the nature of the male monster in relation to woman:

> The male spectator is frequently asked to identify with a male monster that is feminized. He is feminized via the body: he bleeds, gives birth, is penetrated, and generally undergoes abject bodily changes associated with the feminine.
>
> (p. 156)

Expanding on this proposition in *Phallic Panic*, Creed (2005) explores six 'faces' of the male monster, in the context of male monstrosity, which are highly pertinent to this analysis of the *Alien* prequels. Creed argues that: 'The male monster is made monstrous when he enters the domain of woman, animal and nature' (p. 17). He is aligned to the monstrous-feminine because the male symbolic defines his monstrosity in relation to the wider context of female monstrosity. Upright, moral men are not monstrous in and of themselves; they do not oppose the male symbolic order from which they derive their authority and power. When patriarchal ideology depicts men as monsters, in the form of mad scientists, ape-men, werewolves, and vampires, it does so by aligning them with woman, death, and the animal. Creed defines this realm as the primal uncanny. The primal uncanny represents a state of extreme 'otherness' (p. 26). It is a kind of inevitable 'beneath' of the patriarchal order – it is the state of being related to the monstrous-feminine, a state of being where borders collapse and where in Kristeva's terms identity, system and order are undermined. As with the monstrous-feminine, the male monster is therefore also an 'other', one who does not 'respect, borders, positions, rules' (Creed 1993, p. 8). The male monster, figures such as Frankenstein's creature, King Kong and the wolf man, is also a sympathetic figure. In contrast to the monstrous-feminine, the male monster is not a parental figure, caught up in a dyadic relationship with its offspring. His monstrousness does not spring from his male reproductive or paternal functions, but rather from his alignment with the sexual and reproductive nature of the monstrous-feminine – hence he is hairy, bleeds, gives birth, creates life forms and changes shape as he metamorphoses from human to animal.

> He transforms into a menstrual monster or blood monster (vampire), a womb monster (male doctor), a cannibalistic monster (werewolf), a blood beast (slasher) or a woman (transgendered monster).
>
> (Creed 2005, p. 17)

The exception is the ripper or slasher, the 'human' male monster who is not aligned closely enough with woman and animal, who is not 'other' enough' (p. 40) who in his savage assault on women expresses the extremes of misogyny, which underpin the symbolic order.

Creed's argument that the male scientist, who tries to create new life forms, is a womb monster, is illuminating in relation to our discussion of *Prometheus* and *Covenant*. For what is possibly most interesting about these uncanny male mothers is that their ultimate goal appears to be to replace the primeval mother herself. She writes of the 1931 film adaptation of *Frankenstein*, that it 'explores the primal uncanny through the illicit activities of its male mothers, presenting a disturbing picture of couvade practices' (p. 51). Male mothers also figure prominently in the two prequels to *Alien*. The films seek to provide the backstory to the earlier effort. In *Alien*, the origins of the eggs being transported on the crashed spacecraft are left unexplained, enigmatic. *Prometheus* and *Covenant* resolve much that was hitherto left mysterious.

The plot of *Prometheus* involves billionaire Peter Weyland funding a deep space venture to the moon LV-223 in search of alien beings. These beings, dubbed the Engineers, have been found by archaeologists to feature in ancient pictograms produced across the visual cultures of diverse civilisations on Earth including those of Babylonia, Egypt, Mesopotamia, Prehistoric Northern Europe, and Sumeria.[19] In each pictogram, the same constellation of stars is depicted. The scientific exploratory vessel Prometheus is despatched to this constellation. It has a crew of 17, including Meredith Vickers who is the overseer, a pilot, Janek, two archaeologists, Charlie Holloway and Elizabeth Shaw, a biologist, Millburn, a geologist, Fifield, a synthetic human, David, and, unknown to most of the others, the ageing Weyland. He hopes the Engineers will give him the key to more life. On LV-223, the team find an alien construction which they investigate.

The archaeologists expect the Engineers to be benevolent but it transpires they are hostile. The team learns that humankind was a genetic experiment which the aliens were set to terminate. They were prevented from destroying humanity by a fatal bioweapons accident that left all but one of them dead. The bioweapons comprise organisms that gestate in their hosts before hatching, fatally killing them. David intentionally surreptitiously infects Holloway with the organism. Shaw is, in turn, unwittingly infected through intercourse with Holloway. Holloway becomes ill while exploring the alien ruins and is killed by Vickers to prevent the Prometheus becoming contaminated. Shaw learns she has an alien organism inside her and has it surgically removed using an automated procedure. The surviving Engineer, a giant pale-skinned biped who has been in stasis, is revived and kills Weyland and beheads David. It then powers up a spacecraft with the intention of completing the mission to destroy humankind. Shaw, however, persuades Janek to crash the Prometheus into the alien vessel, crippling it. The Engineer survives the collision but is incapacitated shortly afterwards by the organism Shaw had incubated. Shaw then rescues David from the wreck of the alien spacecraft and departs the planet on another such craft, her intention to travel to the Engineers' home-world.

Covenant is set roughly a decade after *Prometheus*. It tells the story of what happened to David and Shaw after their exploits in *Prometheus*. The film begins aboard the Covenant, a colonisation ship carrying roughly 2,000 colonists and 1,000 embryos to the planet Origae-6. When the ship is damaged while recharging its power banks, the synthetic human Walter (an almost identical replica of David) who has been overseeing it seeks to rouse the crew of 14, comprising seven couples, although one member, the ship's captain Branson, dies because of a faulty sleep-pod. The crew include Daniels, who is in command of terraforming, Oram, the ship's first mate who now assumes command, two pilots, Tennessee and Maggie, a navigator, Ricks, a communications officer, Upworth, a biologist, Karine, and a security team composed of Ankor, Cole, Hallett, Ledward, Lope, and Rosenthal. While repairing the ship, the crew intercept a transmission of seemingly human origin (a few distorted bars from John Denver's Country Roads) from a nearby planet, known simply as Planet Number 4, which they decide to investigate. All but three of the crew descend to the planet in a lander. Planet Number 4 initially seems prelapsarian, a veritable paradise, verdant with an abundance of freshwater. Soon, however, two crewmembers become infected by fungal spores and rapidly gestate alien creatures which burst from their bodies, killing them. A number of fatalities occur before the remaining crew of the expedition are rescued by David who leads them to what appears to be a vast necropolis, filled with blackened, contorted corpses. He has made his home in a massive, temple-like complex. David gives a version of his arrival on the planet in which the ship he travelled in accidentally transmitted a fatal pathogen that caused the deaths of the Engineers whose city the crew are now in.

The complex proves unsafe. Rosenthal is killed by an alien shortly after their arrival. The survivors seek to make contact with the three remaining crew on the Covenant but their efforts are hampered by an ion storm that disrupts communications. Oram is then lured by David to a cave filled with giant eggs where he is impregnated by a facehugger. He dies when the alien that has been growing inside him bursts from his chest. This alien, designed by David, is qualitatively different from the others that had attacked the crew. Walter learns that David deliberately annihilated the Engineers with a biological weapon. He also discovers that David killed Shaw through experimenting on her. David has spent his time on the alien planet perfecting highly hostile organisms designed to destroy humanity, he has become intent on genocide. Now the Covenant has arrived, he sees a way to continue his research using the colonists as human guinea-pigs. David realises Walter is suspicious of him and attacks him, believing he has killed him. He then pursues Daniels. Meanwhile, Cole and Lope have been searching for Oram. Lope is attacked by a facehugger but Cole is able to rescue him. Cole is then killed by the alien that slew Oram. Walter saves Daniels from David and she leaves the two androids fighting each other, finding Lope. They make their way to a lander that Tennessee has piloted from the Covenant. Someone they take to be Walter joins them and it is inferred that David is dead. Daniels does battle with an alien as the lander takes off and is able to despatch it. The lander then returns to the Covenant and Lope is placed in the medical unit. The next day, Daniels and Tennessee discover Lope dead, killed by an alien that he had unknowingly nurtured. The alien goes on to kill Ricks and Upworth but Daniels and Tennessee are able to defeat it. As Daniels and Tennessee return to their sleep-pods to continue the journey to Origae-6, Daniels realises too late that it is David who they have brought back to the Covenant. As the others sleep, he regurgitates two facehugger embryos he has smuggled on board and carefully places them in cryopreservation.

Prometheus and *Covenant* explore themes that link not solely to *Alien* but also to another of Scott's early films, *Blade Runner.* Weyland's quest for longevity, for instance, echoes that of the bio-engineered synthetic human Roy Batty in *Blade Runner* who also sets out to find his creator and secure more life (Mulhall 2015, p. 226). In that film, synthetic humans known as replicants are marketed as being 'more human than human'. As the plot of *Blade Runner* unfolds, this humanness is shown not simply to manifest in terms of physical resemblance but also in terms of humanity, by way of emerging compassion and tenderness and a capacity for artistic creativity. The exploration of the nature of humanness that is prominent in *Blade Runner* is also key to *Prometheus* and *Covenant* in which the android David, like the replicants, is shown to be capable of developing emotions. Although supposedly incapable of feeling, it is clear David possesses an emotional palette. In *Covenant,* he claims to have been in love with Elizabeth Shaw. He shows pleasure and disappointment, frustration and loss. He is also vain and arrogant.

One of David's favourite films is *Lawrence of Arabia* (Dir. David Lean, UK, 1962) in which Lawrence, as played by Peter O'Toole, is shown to be highly egotistical. The android's vanity, which manifests through him repeatedly slicking his coif, seems influenced by O'Toole's portrayal of Lawrence. *Lawrence of Arabia* also gives indications that Lawrence is gay and possesses masochistic tendencies.[20] Lawrence's sexuality as presented by O'Toole in the film is not inconsequential when explaining David's identification with him. There are a number of instances that encourage a queer reading of the android.[21] *Covenant*, for example, begins with David meeting his creator, his self-professed father, Weyland, for the first time. As the android is admiring Michelangelo's *David*, he is asked what his name is by Weyland and responds "David!" The sculpture of David has often served as shorthand for homosexuality (Butt 2005, p. 61).[22] Later in *Covenant*, David will advise another android Walter, his mirror-image, that 'no one will ever love you like I do' before tenderly kissing him. This kiss could be read as further evidence of David's narcissism yet the suggestive role of flute-playing in David's relationship with Walter indicates otherwise.[23]

Shortly after kissing Walter, a kiss that formed the precursor to stabbing him in the neck, David will assault Daniels, seemingly set on raping her, kissing her, and asking 'Is that how it's done?' He is uncertain about sexuality. Watching the bloody birth of an alien from Oram's quivering body, David smiles, a proud father, as the alien extricates itself from the biologist's chest. The smile, emerging as it does against the backdrop of Oram's death spasms, also implies a sadistic streak in the android. [24] In this, his sadism, David is the inverse of O'Toole's masochistic Lawrence. David's sadism carries through to his progeny which also seem to take pleasure in the pain and fear of others. Creed (1993, p. 16) has previously emphasised the sadism of the monster in *Alien* (p. 16). The origins of this sadism are signalled in these earlier versions of the creature, David's prototypes, which sometimes appear to pause before killing their victims. In the scene in which the security team member Rosenthal is killed, the alien watches her bathe before creeping up behind her and attacking and killing her. It seems capable of taking voyeuristic pleasure. David's voyeurism was indicated in *Prometheus* when he was shown spying on the unconscious of Shaw, on her dreams, as she was in hypersleep. Voyeurism and sadism are connected (Mulvey 1975).[25] Charles Socarides (1974) links voyeurism as a defence against sadism with fear of fusion with the Mother, with fear of a loss of boundaries. He suggests that the 'paramount desire' of the sadist is to have a woman be powerless so that he [sic] can fulfil his basic aim which is 'to gain control of the fearful demonic mother' (p. 194).[26] The monsters mimic David's voyeuristic comportment. In a sense, the android is their precursor. He is the Ur-monster. Through David, as an embodiment of the male monster, *Prometheus* and *Covenant* can be read as speaking to us 'about the nature of masculinity and man's ambiguous relationship with the realms of woman, the animal and death, and the symbolic order of law, civilisation and language' (Creed 2005, p. xix).

The vision of the future offered by *Prometheus* and *Covenant* appears stubbornly patriarchal. The gender of the Engineers is never explored but they seem to be masculine and their moniker may also imply that they are men (engineering along with science, technology, and mathematics has traditionally, stereotypically been cast as a male profession).[27] Towards the end of *Prometheus*, David refers to the Engineer that seeks to kill Shaw using a masculine pronoun. The feminist message of *Alien* as embodied by the character of Ellen Ripley is also absent from the prequels. Shaw and Daniels as Final Girls end up being manipulated by David and therefore do not triumph over their adversaries in the way Ripley does. In this context, a third woman also merits mention as being offered as a possible successor to Ripley, Vickers. She is shown as tough and uncompromising, killing Holloway to protect Prometheus from contamination. *Prometheus* contrives a race between Shaw and Vickers for the role of Final Girl. Both struggle to outrun the crash wreckage of a spacecraft but Vickers is ultimately crushed by it. Shaw, who is left the last woman standing, provides a softer vision of femininity than Vickers. Like Ripley, she is tough but also tender. Vickers, as an embodiment of female masculinity, is ultimately too hard to survive.[28] In this way, Scott rewrites the narrative of *Alien* so Ripley no longer comes out on top. Vickers is punished for her masculinity by death, Daniels and Shaw enjoy only hollow victories. Shaw will be subject to genetic experimentation and, using a ruse, David will put Daniels to sleep. Through the fates of these three women, Scott seems to be rewriting Ripley's success as failure, intent on reining in and containing the positive role model he helped create.

The patriarchal ideology underpinning *Prometheus* and *Covenant* manifests not solely through narrative and dialogue, but also by way of mise-en-scène. The giant sculpted heads in *Prometheus* and *Covenant*, for instance, appear to be of male countenances. In this, the culture of the Engineers is seen to mirror that of Earth as it is presented in the film in that it is a celebration of the masculine. In the opening to *Covenant*, David is shown identifying various cultural artefacts visible in Weyland's countryside retreat, which are all produced by men. He recognises Piero della Francesca's *The Nativity* (c1470), which shows the Virgin Mary kneeling in adoration before a newly born Christ, the child's immaculate conception prefiguring that of his own. He also notes a Carlo Bugatti throne chair (c1900) and a Steinway piano. Additionally, as already mentioned, he sees and names Michelangelo's *David* (1501–1504), simultaneously styling himself after a sculpture that has been celebrated as the epitome of male physical perfection. He fails to identify the Eileen Grey E1027 side table that is beside the Bugatti chair. Female creativity is clearly not, at that point, part of the knowledge gifted to David through his programming or gleaned by way of his learning.

The objects on display in Weyland's residence reflect what he values, providing a selective cultural history that privileges American and European achievements. The blond David, fashioned by Weyland, is superficially figured as part of this cultural lineage. In fact, however, David circulates as a complex Other in the film. This is, in part, because he is uncanny. In *Phallic Panic*, Creed (2005, p. 11) foregrounds how artificial life signifies 'the fragility of the boundary between animate and inanimate'. Freud lists dolls and automata as potentially frightening, as familiar objects that come to unnerve become uncanny (ibid., p. 3). David, in his not being android enough, in his being too similar to his non-synthetic companions, causes anxiety. Jessica Balanzategui (2018, p. 23), writing in the context of the child as uncanny, suggests that the cognitive dissonance caused by oscillations between the familiar and unfamiliar can cause a horror film's spectators to become profound unnerved. David is similarly at once a familiar (seen to be human in appearance albeit known not to be) and a discomfiting stranger. This strangeness manifests through his being frequently alienated, presented at different times as Mother and othered through his class and, possibly, by racial references.

Because of her focus on the feminine in her reading of *Alien*, Creed does not engage with its problematic racial politics which coalesce in the figure of the full-grown alien that terrorises the Nostromo. The alien was not produced using Computer-generated imagery (CGI) but was a man, Bolaji Badejo, in a latex suit. H.R. Giger suggest that the inspiration for casting a tall, thin man as the monster was a photograph by Leni Riefenstahl of her standing next to a Nuba man from Northern Africa.[29] In Giger's (1989, p. 60) account, the photograph of the 'huge Nubian' only indicated that Scott wanted 'a man of that size for the Alien'. The decision to cast Badejo, a Nigerian, another man from Africa, albeit Western Africa, as the monster cannot, however, be ignored. In *Prometheus* and *Covenant*, the aliens are often the product of CGI yet these digital xenomorphs are strangely familiar, intertextually indissociable from Badejo's earlier incarnation of the alien.[30] David's racial alterity is referred to in terms which imply ethnic difference. In *Prometheus*, the archaeologist Holloway says to David at one point: 'You, boy, you're coming with us!' Referring to David as 'boy' echoes the kind of derogatory language adopted by slave owners in the US to address black adult males.

Casting David as a slave reinforces links with Scott's *Blade Runner* in which the replicant Roy Batty uses the term slave to describe those, such as himself, who live in fear. Synthetic humans are cast in both films as chattels. They form an underclass regarded as sub-human. Although Weyland identifies David as his son, he treats him as his servant.

Weyland's sadism manifests when he is invited by David to confront his own mortality, and responds by ordering the android to pour him tea, to perform the role of manservant, menial. Weyland asserts difference and thereby distance from his purported kin.[31] David is othered in this moment in terms of class and, possibly, ethnicity. Like the alien in *Alien*, as Other he serves as cover for the archaic Mother. The theme of motherhood is explicitly referred to in relation to David when he leads Oram into the egg cave he has built. As David stands to one side in the cave, Oram asks the android what he is waiting for, to which he responds "Mother!" Mother in this context is, on one level, Oram as it is he who will ingest an alien organism and incubate it to term. In a sense, however, David is also waiting to fulfil the role of Mother himself, the eggs are his, produced by him. David represents at once the male monster and the monstrous-feminine, he is both castrated (he is decapitated by an Engineer in *Prometheus*) and castrating (he cuts off his own arm in *Covenant*).

The Engineers, giant pale-skinned bipeds, also serve as displaced references to the archaic mother. They are the mysterious point of genesis, a portrayal of the primordial abyss. Their castrating potential is evident through one decapitating David. The biological weapons they create also seem to embody 'the fascinating and abject inside of the maternal body' (Kristeva 1982, p. 54; cited in Creed 1993, p. 51). In *Prometheus*, Fifield and Millburn are confronted by a snake-like creature which emerges from some black ooze. The biologist identifies the entity as female. It is a monstrous femme fatale. Enchanted by the organism, Millburn approaches it with mortal consequences. It attacks him, eventually breaching his spacesuit and forcing its way down his throat. Here, like Kane in *Alien*, Milburn becomes part of the primal scene, taking the place of the mother, becoming the one who is penetrated (Creed 1993, p. 19). Although serpents are traditionally phallic symbols, the head of this creature bears some resemblance to a vulva. *Covenant* also includes a womb-like chamber filled with eggs reminiscent of the one that appears in *Alien*. There is therefore crossover between the three films in terms of the archaic mother functioning as backdrop.

This dimension is, however, unconscious. Scott largely wants to erase the Mother, to render the alien patrilineal, providing a backstory in which the creature is designed by an android, David, who was engineered by a man, Weyland. There are also important textural difference between *Alien* and the prequels. Something of the vapourousness and viscidity of the alien craft in *Alien* is absent from the tunnels and chambers of the alien structure the crew explore in *Prometheus*. The alien biological weapons are stored not in leathery eggs but in black canisters, inorganic-looking cylinders. The alien universe is more ordered here, more reasoned, even if it is still subject to seepage, to leaking. Similarly on Planet Number 4, the alien civilisation builds its monuments out of stone. The temple interior is rocky rather than slimy. The industrial patina of parts of the Nostromo, its dirt and grime, has also been replaced by the clean, clinical-looking decks of the Prometheus and the Covenant. We would suggest these differences are not insignificant. They are symptomatic of efforts by Scott to gradually sanitise the universe he helped to manufacture. He is paring the semiotic (in Kristeva's sense of the term) register of meaning, muffling affect and drive, excising the rhythms of glisten and gloom at play in *Alien* (Chare 2012). If our reading here focusses primarily on narrative and symbolism, this is because much of semiotic richness of *Alien* is absent in the two prequels. It is as if the psychic forces unintentionally revealed and released by Scott in *Alien*, the monstrous power of the feminine so eloquently teased out by Creed in her reading of the film, must now be suppressed. Scott opened Pandora's Box with *Alien* and seeks to close it with *Prometheus* and its sequel. As Creed discusses in the interview she gives for this volume, the origin of life narrative offered by Scott through the films is dull in its insistence on creation as a masculine prerogative.

Scott's efforts to disavow the monstrous-feminine, however, carry considerable risk. The hazards of not confronting anxieties towards the feminine manifest through the underlying theme of genocide in both *Prometheus* and *Covenant*. In *Prometheus* when Fifield is confronted by a pile of corpses of dead Engineers he remarks: 'It's like a scene out of some sort of Holocaust painting!' The sight is reminiscent of documentary film and photographs taken at liberation of piles of corpses at concentration camps or of descriptions (Chare and Williams 2019, pp. 151–152) of the interior of the gas chambers at Birkenau immediately after a gassing. Association with the Shoah is therefore encouraged in the audience. One of the characters in *Covenant*, Rosenthal, is also revealed to be Jewish. When she removes her shirt to bathe her face and tend her injured arm, a gold Star of David on a neck chain that she has been wearing becomes visible. In a part of this scene that was subsequently deleted, she was also portrayed reciting the Shema Yisrael. The Shema is sometimes recited by Jews who believe they are about to die. It was pronounced by Jews on occasion on the way to their deaths in the crematoria at Auschwitz-Birkenau. David literally exterminates all Indigenous animal life on Planet Number 4, his genocidal project commencing with the carpet-bombing with bioweapons of the city complex of the Engineers. This destructivity is symptomatic of fear of the Other, of the psychic figure of the Mother and also all Others that this fear is mapped onto.[32]

David not only enacts violence against the Other, he also functions as a manifestation of Otherness in the film, forming its central monster. In this, he is somewhat like Kurtz in Joseph Conrad's 1899 novella *Heart of Darkness*. The character of Kurtz, as Hannah Arendt (1968, p. 189) notes, may have been inspired by Carl Peters, the brutal Reichkommisar of East Africa (others have suggested Léon Rom as a template). Arendt observes that Peters engaged in 'wild murdering' (p. 185). She (p. 189) also draws attention to Peters' stated wish to cease being a pariah and instead join a master race. David seems comparably motivated, seeking to leave behind his pariah status as android by exterminating all humans, replacing them with a master race of aliens of his own creation. For Arendt (p. 206), through the actions of men like Peters, 'African colonial possessions became the most fertile soil for the flowering of what was later to become the Nazi elite'. In *Covenant*, Scott transposes colonialism to outer space revisiting the engagement with the psychic underpinnings of *Heart of Darkness* he began in *Alien*.

Jacqueline Rose's (1986) remarks on Kristeva's discussion of Céline are pertinent here. For Kristeva, through his writings, Céline (who composed his own *Heart of Darkness*, *Voyage au bout de la nuit* [Journey to the End of the Night] (1932)) exposes a psychic drama of pain and violence that occurs between Mother and child in their early interactions. In *The Monstrous-Feminine*, Creed demonstrates that *Alien* also performs this function. The risk of not exposing this violence is, Rose (1986, p. 155) explains, that it becomes 'projected onto the other, and then played out by culture at large'. For Rose, Céline's writing 'reveals *horror* as a matter of *power* – the power of fascination when we are confronted with the traces of our own psychic violence, the horror when that same violence calls on social institutions for legitimation, and receives it' (p. 155). In contemporary politics, Donald Trump is exploiting such horror, stoking fear of the Other, the 'illegal alien', to justify his border wall. In the past, Hitler took advantage of this horror to support his extermination of the Jews, figuring them as sub-human. Through art, film, and literature, something of this horror can be shown and, perhaps, purged. These cultural forms can therefore embody a political aesthetics crafted to work against paranoid hatred of the Other through exposing the psychic motivations undergirding such hatred and, possibly, purging them. *Alien* gestures towards such a catharsis but *Prometheus* and *Covenant* refuse it. In the prequels, an arrested catharsis is manifest, the films point towards psychic drama but on steadfastly symbolic terms. The semiotic (in Kristeva's sense of the term) as it registers in *Alien* by way of the rhythms of the shadowy mise-en-scènes (the tone of the film) and the noisy soundtrack is minimised in the later prequels.[33] Creed's analysis of *Alien* in *The Monstrous-Feminine* cannot be duplicated in the context of *Prometheus* and *Covenant* because both films seem designed to neuter monstrosity. David masquerades as the archaic mother but his engagement with the abject is neither compelling nor horrifying. Further, and more tellingly, the film deprives the monstrous-feminine of its subversive force, purging the abject of its boundary-troubling potential. Through their frustrated engagement with the feminine, the films betray their hyper-conservative credentials.

Masquerade and the Monstrous-Feminine

Throughout *The Monstrous-Feminine*, Creed draws on the psychoanalytic concept of masquerade or disguise in order to explore the nature of monstrosity. Joan Riviere, was the first to propose that because femininity, particularly excessive displays of femininity, is a construct it can be viewed as a form of masquerade. 'Womanliness therefore could be assumed and worn as a mask' (1929, p. 306). Mary Ann Doane extended Riviere's theory to propose that masquerade is particularly significant in relation to the female spectator:

> The effectivity of masquerade lies precisely in its potential to manufacture a distance from the image, to generate a problematic within which the image is manipulable, producible, and readable by the woman.
>
> (1982, p. 87)

More recently queer theorists have argued that forms of masquerade exist, such as cross dressing, which potentially undermine essentialist notions of gender. We believe that masquerade offers an important theoretical perspective with which to think through the enduring power of the monstrous-feminine in films and works of art, past and present. It is even more relevant to contemporary horror films and artworks in an era in which gender is constantly being questioned. Creed argues that in horror masquerade undermines essentialist notions of gender in that woman's gender identity is never stable; rather it oscillates from one troubling signifier to another. The 'visually horrifying aspects' of the monstrous-feminine 'are offset through the display of woman as a reassuring and pleasurable sign' (Creed 1993, pp. 23–24). In her analysis of the different faces of the monstrous-feminine, she draws attention to the way in which the female protagonists disguise their monstrous identities. Feminine masquerade is generally viewed in two main ways: as the adoption of a feminine appearance signifying a capitulation to patriarchal dictates or as an empowering disguise, perhaps the assumption of masculine dress and codes of behaviour to permit greater freedom. As various theorists have noted, masquerade offers, as proposed by Mikhail Bakhtin, the opportunity for freedom. In the horror film, masquerade is aligned with abjection. Given that the abject emerges through the erosion of boundaries, the horror film plays on this erosion in relation to gender identity.

The monstrous-feminine disguises her abject identity with a display of acceptable femininity, as in *Carrie*, where during the Prom sequence Carrie attempts to cover over her monstrous powers and what she sees as her abject femininity with a display of appealing femininity befitting the newly crowned Prom Queen. Once the masquerade is broken,

Carrie tests her new freedom and lashes out, destroying all before her in an apocalyptic scenario of death and destruction. In *The Exorcist*, Regan dispels all illusions regarding her seemingly sweet feminine nature, performing a display of hyper aggressive 'masculinity', particularly when she speaks in the so-called 'devil's voice'. *Teeth* offers a fascinating display of feminine masquerade in that the heroine's public purity (she leads a chastity group) masks the threat of castration posed by her deadly *vagina dentata* of which she herself is unaware. The horror film also plays with male masquerade as in *Silence of the Lambs* (1991) and *Dressed to Kill* (1980). In *Psycho* (1960), extreme horror is evoked when 'Norman, masquerading as Mother', previously seen through the upstairs window as a frail invalid, bursts into the bathroom in a scenario filled with 'shrill bird-like sounds signalling the presence of the beaked mother' (pp. 146–147).

A male monster such as Norman Bates enacts his masquerade not so much in relation to the abject but more in the context of the uncanny. In *Phallic Panic*, Creed draws on Terry Castle's argument concerning masquerade. 'Castle argues that one of the hallmarks of the uncanny is "masquerade and sexual impersonation"' (Creed 2005, p. 19). For Creed, it is the male monster's feminine aspects which render him both familiar and unfamiliar.

> In particular, the ambivalence underlies the male monster's uncanny alignment with death, the animal and the maternal body-uncanny because the male symbolic order designates these areas as 'other', a being outside the realm of what constitutes proper phallic masculinity.
>
> (Creed 2005, p. viii)

Norman is both himself and his mother, man and woman, castrated and castrating, human and animal. In this way the male monster is aligned with the monstrous-feminine – and the primal uncanny. Both threaten the fragile nature of the symbolic order.

Masquerade, we argue, is central to an understanding of the appeal of the monstrous-feminine. This is particularly true of contemporary films. Whereas in the actual world, as Joan Riviere argues women may adopt a masquerade of ultra-femininity to hide their masculine desires, and win male approval, in the horror film Creed argues masquerade becomes a means of covering over those abject things that the male psyche fears most about woman: her power to incorporate, castrate, and destroy and her alignment with the animal. Masquerade is an important feature of contemporary horror. It is this oscillation between proper and monstrous femininity that *Teeth*, with which we opened this essay, explores. Creed uses theories of masquerade to undermine essentialist notions of castration, notions which have haunted psychoanalysis from its inception. She asks:

> Is woman castrated or does she castrate? Does she use one persona to disguise her hidden and deadly face? What lies behind the veil? (135)

In another contemporary film that explores the power of masquerade, *A Girl Walks Home Alone at Night* (Dir. Ana Lily Amirpour, USA, 2014), directed by Ana Lily Amirpour, the monstrous-feminine is a vigilante vampire who disguises her identity behind a hijab veil as she stalks those she deem to be evil. She adopts a masquerade of piety to allay the fears of her potential victims. Her persona moves into a terrifying state of disguise, an indeterminacy which is irresolvable. As 'woman's nature is represented as deceptive and unknowable' in patriarchal ideology (Creed 1993, p. 136), she must constantly reassure through masquerade and deception. 'She may appear pure and beautiful on the outside but evil may, nevertheless, reside within' – a dominant misogynistic fear (Creed 1993, p. 42). It is when she tears the veil and drops her disguise, Creed argues, that abjection exerts its ambiguous appeal. The monstrous-feminine is compelling yet terrifying. Amirpour's film is also significant to any discussion of the continuing appeal of the monstrous-feminine as more and more women are directing horror films, as well as creating artworks, that explore her significance – as confirmed by many of the essays in this volume.

The Monstrous-Feminine: Past and Present

The chapters that follow either engage directly with ideas articulated in *The Monstrous-Feminine* or with the feminist intellectual ferment out of which they emerged. Many can be seen as adding to recent important scholarship regarding gender and/or motherhood in horror films (Arnold 2013; Grant 2015; Harrington 2016; Schneider 2004). This book is divided into four sections, each with a short introduction that provides an overview of the section as a whole and also of the individual essays it contains. The first section, 'Feminism and Psychoanalysis', offers insight into the socio-historical and political context underpinning *The Monstrous-Feminine*, including the Women's Liberation Movement of the 1960s and 1970s and developments in film studies in the late 1970s and early 1980s. The second section, 'Expanding the Monstrous-Feminine', includes essays that take interpretations Creed develops in *The Monstrous-Feminine* as the starting point for new readings of classic horror films. The third section, 'Reproductive and Post-Reproductive Bodies and the Monstrous-Feminine' explores themes including ageing, dementia, and reproductive bodies as they are depicted in contemporary visual cultures and also considers the role of art, film, and television as modes of resistance to restrictive ideologies. The final section, 'Rethinking the Monstrous-Feminine through a Transnational Frame', examines artworks and films from different cultural and geographic contexts that take up the theme of the monstrous-feminine.

Notes

1 Creed continues her critical engagement with Freud in *Phallic Panic* where she offers a highly insightful reading of the case history of 'The Wolf Man', which he published in 1918 as 'From the History of an Infantile Neurosis'.
2 Our emphasis.
3 A notable exception is Katherine Goodnow. See Goodnow's (2010) *Kristeva in Focus*. Kaja Silverman (1988) also makes extensive and sophisticated use of Kristeva's ideas in *The Acoustic Mirror*, see Chapter 4 in particular. See also Nicholas Chare and Elizabeth Watkins (2013).
4 For a discussion of the importance of the border in contemporary theory and pedagogy, see Audrey Yue (2010, pp. 115–117). Creed (2003) explores the role of boundaries or markers in contemporary media cultures in *Media Matrix*.
5 Emphases in the original. All emphases in the original unless otherwise stated.
6 The choice of Céline as the main exemplar of abjection in literature has not been without controversy because of the writer's notorious antisemitism. For a discussion of this issue, see Chapter 1 'Execrable Speech' in Chare's (2011) *Auschwitz and Afterimages*. See also Kristeva (2010, pp. 160–161).
7 Elsewhere, in an essay co-authored with Jeanette Hoorn, Creed explores how avant-garde art can fulfil this cathartic function (Creed and Hoorn 2016, pp. 90–104).
8 Kristeva (1979, p. 44) signposted such a possibility in her essay 'Ellipsis on Dread and the Specular Seduction' when she suggested that *The Birds* (Dir. Alfred Hitchcock, USA, 1963) and *Psycho* (Dir. Alfred Hitchcock, USA, 1960) now offer catharsis instead of *Oedipus*, *Electra* or *Orestes*.
9 The vagina here, of course, like the phallus, is a symbol and not be confused with the anatomical vagina.
10 Powell's own Deleuzian-inspired readings bring a critical vocabulary to bear on film experience and therefore, arguably, also allegorise it. Visceral responses becoming, for example, emblematic of intensity or of affect.
11 For efforts to link Bracha Ettinger's psychoanalytic ideas to the study of film, see Chare's (2013) essay 'Encountering *Blue Steel*' and Chare's (2015, pp. 157–182) *Sportswomen in Cinema*.
12 For a film analysis inspired by Klein's idea of 'memories in feelings' and by Ruth Riesenberg Malcolm's understanding of transference, see Chare (2017) 'Once More with Feeling: Re-investigating the Smuttynose Island Murders'.
13 For further discussion of asignification, see Simon O' Sullivan's (2006, pp. 70–71) *Art Encounters Deleuze and Guattari*.
14 The lobster has been read by Fèlix Fanés as evoking 'the goddess born from the foam when the genitals of the castrated Uranus fell on the waves' (Venturi 2019, p. 270).
15 Simon Carr, 'Wallis Simpson: The Agony and the Ecstasy', *The Independent*, Monday 1 July 2002.
16 *Alien: Covenant* will henceforth simply be referred to as *Covenant*.

17 The drawings in the film were created by Dane Hallett and Matt Hatton. They were purportedly influenced by Giger's earlier creations for the *Alien* franchise and by the seventeenth-century Dutch artist Rembrandt van Rijn (Ward 2017, p. 138). Rembrandt produced few works that have survived of fauna although there are three versions of a shell, *Het schelpje*, produced in 1650. Rembrandt's shell is depicted side-on. David frequently favours sketching specimens from above. This may be symptomatic of a will to mastery on his part.
18 In the spirit of the monstrous-feminine, we offer femmage rather than homage here. Femmage here meaning an act of honouring. Miriam Schapiro coined this term in the context of the history of art to acknowledge neglected traditions of women's art making (Broude 1982).
19 Early in the film in an archaeological dig on the Isle of Skye, parietal art dated to 35,000 BCE or earlier is discovered. Around 40,000 years ago Neanderthals may have inhabited what is now known as Scotland and this would have to be an example of their visual culture. For much of the Upper Paleolithic period, the region was uninhabitable due to the Last Glacial Maximum. Currently the only known parietal art in the UK, engraved rather than painted, is located at Creswell Crags (Bahn and Pettitt 2009).
20 Lawrence of Arabia's sexuality has been the subject of much historical speculation. He was clearly open-minded about homosexuality, if not gay himself, this at a time when sexual acts between men were illegal in the UK. Sexual acts between two consenting men in private were only legalised in England and Wales in 1967. Christian Destremau (2014, p. 454) has recently argued that Lawrence of Arabia was not a sexual person.
21 Queer here is understood as referring to a mode of being that unsettles heteronormativity. For a discussion of queer as a term, see Yue (2012, p. 4).
22 Here Weyland's possession of the statue may, of course, equally hint at his own sexuality.
23 The phallic symbolism of flutes is commonly remarked. David makes reference to the Montague Rhodes James ghost story 'Oh, Whistle and I'll Come to You, My Lad' when he says to Walter 'Whistle and I'll come'. The story which centres on a mysterious, ancient whistle has been interpreted as articulating fear of homosexuality (Fielding 2000; Richardson 1959).
24 In this, he shares affinities with Weyland, yet Weyland's sadism did not seem to be tinged with erotic pleasure.
25 For a discussion of sadism as it intersects with the gaze, see Chare and Williams (2019, pp. 51–57).
26 Socarides does not countenance the existence of female sadists.
27 Stephen Mulhall (2015, p. 232) suggests that, in *Prometheus,* 'every Engineer we see (alive or dead, in the flesh, fossilized or depicted) looks not only humanoid but male'. For Mulhall, sexual difference is unknown to the Engineers. The varied anatomies of the Engineer corpses in *Alien Covenant*, however, do imply the potential for sexual difference. For a discussion of engineering as a male dominated profession, see Hacker (1990).
28 Vickers is openly dismissive of the paternal. Shaw is shown to mourn her father, an anthropologist killed by Ebola, whereas Vickers' response to the death of her father, Weyland, is indifference.
29 For a discussion of Riefenstahl's fascist politics as they manifest in her films and photography, see Chapter 4 of Chare's (2015) *Sportswomen in Cinema*.
30 Sometimes the alien is still a person in a suit as occurs, at times, in *Covenant*.
31 For a succinct analysis of distancing and Otherness, see Burke (2001, p. 126).

32 As part of his lengthy meditation on histories of genocide and motivations for genocide, Adam Jones (2017, p. 120) discusses how 'solidarity may coalesce around a dominant ethnicity within [a] society, prompting the anathematizing of Other-identified minorities'. This anathematising sometimes contributes to the emergence of genocidal policies and actions.

33 Kristeva (1979, p. 45) discusses colour, 'malleable mass' and sound as semiotic materials in cinema.

References

Ades, D. (1985). 'Web of Images,' in D. Ades and A. Forge (eds.), *Francis Bacon*. London: Tate Gallery and Thames & Hudson pp. 8–23.

Arendt, H. (1968). *The Origins of Totalitarianism*. New York: Harcourt.

Arnold, S. (2013). *Maternal Horror Film: Melodrama and Motherhood*. Houndmills: Palgrave Macmillan.

Bahn, P. and Pettitt, P. (2009). *Britain's Oldest Art: The Ice Age Cave Art of Creswell Crags*. Swindon: English Heritage.

Balanzategui, J. (2018). *The Uncanny Child in Transnational Cinema: Ghosts of Futurity at the Turn of the Twenty-first Century*. Amsterdam: Amsterdam University Press.

Bellour, R. (1979). *L'analyse du film*. Paris: Éditions Albatros.

Broude, N. (1982). 'Miriam Schapiro and "Femmage": Reflections on the Conflict between Decoration and Abstraction in Twentieth-Century Art," in N. Broude and M.D. Garrard (eds.), *Feminism and Art History: Questioning the Litany*. New York: Harper & Row, pp. 314–329.

Brown, S. T. (2018). *Japanese Horror and the Transnational Cinema of Sensation*. Cham: Palgrave Macmillan.

Burke, P. (2001). *Eyewitnessing: The Uses of Images as Historical Evidence*. Ithaca: Cornell University Press.

Butt, G. (2005). *Between You and Me: Queer Disclosures in the New York Art World, 1948–1963*. Durham: Duke University Press.

Céline, Louis-Ferdinand. *Voyage au bout de la nuit*. Paris: Denoël et Steele.

Chare, N. (2011). *Auschwitz and Afterimages: Abjection, Witnessing and Representation*. London: IB Tauris.

Chare, N. (2012). *After Francis Bacon: Synaesthesia and Sex in Paint*. Farnham: Ashgate.

Chare, N. (2013). 'Encountering *Blue Steel*: Changing Tempers in Cinema,' in G. Pollock (ed.), *Visual Politics of Psychoanalysis: Art and the Image in Post-Traumatic Cultures*. London: IB Tauris, pp. 190–207.

Chare, N. (2015). *Sportswomen in Cinema: Film and the Frailty Myth*. London: IB Tauris.

Chare, N. (2017). 'Once More with Feeling: Re-investigating the Smuttynose Island Murders,' in *Intermedialities*, Issue 28–29. Available at http://www.erudit.org/en/journals/im/2016-n28-29-im03201/1041079ar (Accessed 27 February 2019).

Chare, N. and Watkins, L. (2013) 'The Matter of Film: *Decasia* and *Lyrical Nitrate*,' in E. Barrett and B. Bolt (eds.), *Carnal Knowledge: Towards a 'New Materialism' Through the Arts*. London: IB Tauris, pp. 75–88.

Chare, N. and Williams, D. (2019). *The Auschwitz Sonderkommando: Testimonies, Histories, Representations*. Basingstoke: Palgrave Macmillan.
Chaudhuri, S. (2006). *Feminist Film Theorists: Laura Mulvey, Kaja Silvermann, Teresa de Lauretis, Barbara Creed*. London: Routledge.
Chion, M. (1999). *The Voice in Cinema*. Trans. C. Gorbman. New York: Columbia University Press.
Clover, C. (1987). 'Her Body, Himself: Gender in the Slasher Film,' *Representations* 20, pp. 187–228.
Creed, B. (1986). 'Horror and the Monstrous-Feminine: An Imaginary Abjection,' *Screen* 27 (1), pp. 44–70.
Creed, B. (1993). *The Monstrous-Feminine: Film, Feminism, Psychoanalysis*. London: Routledge.
Creed, B. (2003). *Media Matrix: Sexing the New Reality*. Crows Nest: Allen & Unwin.
Creed, B. (2005). *Phallic Panic: Film, Horror and the Primal Uncanny*. Melbourne: Melbourne University Press.
Creed, B. (2017). *Stray: Human-Animal Ethics in the Anthropocene*. Sydney: Power Publications.
Creed, B. and J. Hoorn. (2016). 'Animals, Art, Abjection,' in R. Arya and Nicholas Chare (eds.), *Abjection Visions: Powers of Horror in Art and Visual Culture*. Manchester: Manchester University Press, pp. 90–104.
Deleuze, G. (2006a). 'Four Propositions on Psychoanalysis,' in D. Lapoujade (ed.), *Two Regimes of Madness: Gilles Deleuze, Texts and Interviews 1975–1995*. New York: Semiotext(e), pp. 79–88.
Deleuze, G. (2006b). 'The Interpretation of Utterances,' in D. Lapoujade (ed.), *Two Regimes of Madness: Gilles Deleuze, Texts and Interviews 1975–1995*. New York: Semiotext(e), pp. 89–112.
Deleuze, G. and Guattari, F. (1972). *Capitalisme et schizophrénie: L'anti-Œdipe*. Paris: Minuit.
Deleuze, G. and Guattari, F. (1986). *Kafka: Toward a Minor Literature*, translated from the French by D. Polan. Minneapolis: University of Minnesota Press.
Demos, T.J. (2010). *Dara Birnbaum, Technology/Transformation: Wonder Woman*. London: Afterall.
Destremau, C. (2014). *Lawrence d'Arabie*. Paris: Perrin.
Doane, M.A. (1982) 'Film and the Masquerade: Theorising the Female Spectator,' *Screen* 23 (3–4), pp. 74–87.
Donald, J. (ed.) (1989). *Fantasy and the Cinema*. London: BFI Publishing.
Fielding, P. (2000). 'Reading Rooms: M. R. James and the Library of Modernity,' *MFS: Modern Fiction Studies* 46 (3), pp. 749–771.
Giger, H.R. (1989). *Giger's Alien*. London: Titan Books.
Goodnow, K. (2010). *Kristeva in Focus*. New York: Berghahn.
Grant, B.K. (ed.) (1996). *The Dread of Difference: Gender and the Horror Film*. Austin: University of Texas Press.
Grant, B.K. (ed.) (2015). *The Dread of Difference: Gender and the Horror Film*. 2nd edition. Austin: University of Texas Press.
Grof, S. (2002). 'H. R. Giger and the Soul of the Twentieth Century,' in S. Altmeppen (ed.), *H. R. Giger*. Cologne: Taschen, pp. 13–21.
Hacker, S.L. (1990). *'Doing It the Hard Way:' Investigations of Gender and Technology*. Boston: Unwin Hyman.

Halberstam, J. (1995). *Skin Shows: Gothic Horror and the Technology of Monsters*. Durham: Duke University Press.
Harrington, E. (2016). *Women, Monstrosity and Horror Film: Gynaehorror*. London: Routledge.
Horney, K. (1967). *Feminine Psychology*. New York: W. W. Norton & Co.
Jones, A. (2017). *Genocide: A Comprehensive Introduction*. 3rd edition. London: Routledge.
Klein, M. (1997). 'Envy and Gratitude [1957],' in M. Klein (ed.), *Envy and Gratitude and Other Works, 1946–1963*. London: Vintage, pp. 176–235.
Kristeva, J. (1974). *La Révolution du langage poétique*. Paris: Seuil.
Kristeva, J. (1979). 'Ellipsis on Dread and the Specular Seduction,' *Wide Angle*, 3(2), pp. 42–47.
Kristeva, J. (1982). *Powers of Horror: An Essay on Abjection*, translated from the French by L.S. Roudiez. New York: Columbia University Press.
Kristeva, J. (1995). 'Of Word and Flesh: An Interview with Julia Kristeva by Charles Penwarden,' in S. Morgan and F. Morris (eds.), *Rites of Passage: Art for the End of the Century*. London: Tate Gallery Publications, pp. 21–27.
Kristeva, J. (2010). *Hatred and Forgiveness*, translated from the French by J. Herman. New York: Columbia University Press.
Kuhn, A. (1982). *Women's Pictures: Feminism and Cinema*. London: Routledge & Kegan Paul.
Kuhn, A. (1990). 'Repressions,' in A. Kuhn (ed.), *Alien Zone: Cultural Theory and Contemporary Science Fiction Cinema*. London: Verso, pp. 91–95.
Lacan, J. (1993). *The Psychoses 1955–1956: The Seminar of Jacques Lacan Book III*. Translated from the French by R. Grigg. New York: W.W. Norton & Company.
Lomas, D. (2000). *The Haunted Self: Surrealism, Psychoanalysis, Subjectivity*. New Haven: Yale University Press.
Metz, C. (1975). 'Le signifiant imaginaire,' *Communications*, 23, pp. 3–55.
Mubarki, M.A. (2014). 'The Monstrous 'Other' Feminine: Gender, Desire and the 'Look' in the Hindi Horror Genre,' *Indian Journal of Gender Studies*, 21(3), pp. 379–399.
Mulhall, S. (2015). *On Film*. 3rd edition. New York: Routledge.
Mulvey, L. (1975). 'Visual Pleasure and Narrative Cinema,' *Screen*, 16(3), pp. 6–18.
O'Sullivan, S. (2006). *Art Encounters Deleuze and Guattari: Thought beyond Representation*. Houndmills: Palgrave Macmillan.
Pisters, P. (2003). *The Matrix of Visual Culture: Working with Deleuze in Film Theory*. Stanford: Stanford University Press.
Powell, A. (2005). *Deleuze and Horror Film*. Edinburgh: Edinburgh University Press.
Richardson, M. (1959) 'The Psychoanalysis of Ghost Stories,' *Twentieth Century*, 166, pp. 419–431.
Riviere, J. (1929). 'Womanliness as Masquerade,' *The International Journal of Psychoanalysis*, 10, pp. 303–313.
Rose, J. (1985) 'Introduction – II,' in J. Mitchell and J. Rose (eds.), *Feminine Sexuality: Jacques Lacan and the École Freudienne*. New York: W.W. Norton & Company, pp. 27–57.
Rose, J. (1986). *Sexuality in the Field of Vision*. London: Verso.

Roudinesco, E. and Plon, M. (1997). *Dictionnaire de la psychanalyse*. Paris: Fayard.
Schneider, S.J. (ed.) (2004). *Horror Film and Psychoanalysis: Freud's Worst Nightmare*. Cambridge: Cambridge University Press.
Scott, R. (2017) 'Foreword,' in S. Ward (ed.), *The Art and Making of Alien Covenant*. London: Titan Books, p. 7.
Silverman, K. (1988). *The Acoustic Mirror: The Female Voice in Psychoanalysis and Cinema*. Bloomington: Indiana University Press.
Thomson, D. (2000). *The Alien Quartet*. London: Bloomsbury.
Thurman, J. (2012). 'Twin Peaks,' in A. Bolton and H. Koda (eds.), *Schiaparelli & Prada: Impossible Conversations*. New York: Met Publications, pp. 24–31.
Venturi, R. (2019). 'Into the Abyss: On Salvador Dali's *Dream of Venus*,' in A. Debenedetti and C. Elam (eds.), *Boticelli: Past and Present*. London: UCL Press & Victoria and Albert Museum, pp. 266–289.
Ward, S. (2017). *The Art and Making of Alien Covenant*. London: Titan Books.
Yue, A. (2000). 'Preposterous Hong Kong Horror: *Rouge*'s (Be)Hindsight and *A* (sodomitical) *Chinese Ghost Story*,' in K. Gelder (ed.), *The Horror Reader*. London and New York: Routledge, pp. 364–373.
Yue, A. (2010). *Ann Hui's Song of the Exile*. Aberdeen: Hong Kong University Press.
Yue, A. (2012). 'Queer Singapore: A Critical Introduction,' in A. Yue and J. Zubillaga-Pow (eds.), *Queer Singapore: Illiberal Citizenship and Mediated Cultures*. Aberdeen: Hong Kong University Press, pp. 1–25.

Part I

Introduction

Feminism and Psychoanalysis

Nicholas Chare, Jeanette Hoorn, and Audrey Yue

In *Recording Reality, Desiring the Real*, Elizabeth Cowie (2011, p. 159) observes that '[t]o remember is to bring back to the present something of the past, but it is also to engage the pastness of the event and its meanings and emotions'. The three essays in this section display both these aspects of remembrance, reviving something of the excitement and originality of intellectual enquiry that characterised the historical and political moment from which *The Monstrous-Feminine* emerged while also acknowledging today's changed times and linked but specific challenges. The three essays, by some of the pioneers of feminist film theory, Elizabeth Cowie, Annette Kuhn, and Laura Mulvey, each look back appreciatively to critical approaches to the study of culture fostered and honed during second-wave feminism. As is clear from all the essays, second-wave feminism as it was taken up within film-making and film studies provided an invaluable means of identifying and reflecting on structures of sexual difference, power, and representation.

The section begins with an interview with Laura Mulvey, 'Symmetry and Incident', in which she reflects on themes including her style of writing, her film-making, and the importance of *The Monstrous-Feminine* to her own thinking. The interview's title is taken from the title of an essay by one of Mulvey's ancestors, Alice Meynell. Meynell's (1897, p. 82) essay is a meditation on European and Japanese aesthetics, a thoughtful exploration of difference, one that is judgemental yet also knowing of its limitations: '[Japanese] beauty is remote from our sympathy and admiration; and it is quite possible that we might miss it in pictorial presentation'. Meynell ultimately celebrates Greek 'symmetry' over Japanese 'incident', yet it is possible to find inspiration in her willingness to acknowledge another culture's perspective. She is attentive to how ways of seeing are varied, embodying cultural specificities. Mulvey perceives no direct legacy between her writing and Meynell's but rather an affinity in terms of both women favouring the essay format to express their ideas. For Mulvey, the essay provides an important space for women to articulate their thoughts from within a patriarchal culture. Judy Maloof (2000, p. 247) has noted in the context of Latin American women writers, that '[c]ertain characteristics of the essay as a form – its flexibility, exploratory nature and subjective tone – have made it particularly attractive to women'. For Mulvey, similarly, the less rigid conventions of the essay render it a powerful medium of intellectual expression.

Mulvey (2007) herself briefly discusses Japanese art as part of an essay exploring works by the Canadian artist Jeff Wall. The essay centres upon Wall's 1993 artwork *A Sudden Gust of Wind (After Hokusai)* which was inspired by Katshusika Hokusai's woodcut *Travellers caught in a Sudden Breeze at Ejiri* (c1832). In both these works, a sudden incident is rendered by way of a process of composition that is its antithesis: gradual, carefully deliberated, and studious. As part of her discussion of Hokusai, Mulvey (2007, p. 36) draws attention to the influence of modernity upon the artist, not solely in terms of his subject matter but also in relation to the process of production of his artworks. Technological changes in the nineteenth century transformed Japanese artists such as Hokusai into purveyors of mass-marketable commodities. Wall's work is also made possible by technological change, the advent of digital imaging processes that enable him to collage images and create a composition which, as Mulvey puts it, 'fuses the old and the new through a conjuring up of a collective memory of the photographic aesthetic, not by a means of indexical inscription, but by its representation' (p. 33). For Mulvey, Wall's works also speaks to her of the impact of technological change on cinema. She observes that the arrival of the digital era led to a 'blurring of boundaries between a collective, historic experience of film as movement and its new, improbable mutation into stillness' (p. 33). Mulvey (2006) analyses the ways in which digital technology has transformed the reception of film in *Death 24x a Second*. The transformation, however, as she makes clear in the interview, has also registered in her film-making. One of her remixes, one of her films that use footage from earlier films in novel ways, influenced her thinking on new modes of spectatorship in *Death 24x a Second*. A short film, here, forming a crucial mode of analysis in its own right rather than merely something to be subject to analysis.

Mulvey moves on from a discussion of film-making to offer an extended consideration of the importance of Creed's work for her own thinking. The essay 'Horror and the Monstrous-Feminine' (Creed 1986) introduced Mulvey to Kristeva's thinking on abjection and was a touchstone for her renewed interest in psychoanalytically informed readings of images of women in art and film. Mulvey describes how she developed a fresh understanding of the female body in which Woman functions in the patriarchal imagination not solely as spectacle but also as a figure 'divided between exterior and interior'. This new understanding features prominently in Part 2, 'Dialectics of Division', of *Fetishism and Curiosity* (Mulvey 1996). It is there that Mulvey offers her inspirational reading of Pandora as a prototype for the 'exquisite female android' and the '*femme fatale*', both iconographies that 'depend on an inside/outside topography' (p. 55). Pandora's story installs her 'as a mythic origin of the surface/secret and interior/exterior topography' (p. 55). As she explain in the interview, Creed's notion of the monstrous-feminine led Mulvey to reflect on the split in the depiction of some women 'between an alluring, cosmetic surface and an abject, concealed but threatening, interior'. In *Fetishism and Curiosity*, this split is explored most notably in Mulvey's reading of the art of Cindy Sherman where she suggests that 'Creed's argument that abjection is central to the recurring image of the "monstrous feminine" in horror movies is also applicable to the monstrous in Sherman' (p. 74). Mulvey concludes the interview with a consideration of *Phallic Panic* (Creed 2005) and its exploration of deviant masculinity.

In *Fetishism and Curiosity*, Mulvey also discusses the importance of Joan Riviere's conception of 'womanliness as masquerade' for the study of cinema. She notes of 'films which acknowledge, self-consciously, an awareness of femininity as masquerade [that they] create "a distanciation effect" so that different facets of performance (the social, the spectacular and the narrative) are made visible' (p. 30). The next essay in this section, Annette Kuhn's 'A Dream of Bare Arms', takes Riviere's essay 'Womanliness as masquerade' as its starting point. 'Womanliness as masquerade' was first published in 1929 yet would become the subject of important feminist debates in the 1970s and 1980s. As Kuhn explains,

> with the rise of second-wave feminism, the idea of femininity as a masquerade or performance was enthusiastically taken up within an emergent strand of feminist film criticism interested in mining psychoanalytic thinking on sexual difference for insights on the relationship between women, femininity, films and cinema.

In 'A Dream of Bare Arms', Kuhn revisits Riviere's essay from a fresh perspective, beginning with a consideration of the figure of Riviere herself and her own potential acts of masquerade. Through exquisite close readings, Kuhn attends to descriptions of Riviere by men and women who knew her in a way comparable to that of an analyst listening to their patient. She is careful to register the potential psychic significance of particular emphases and details, on the lookout for screen memories, for apparently insignificant content that conceals unconscious phantasies. Processes of screening are explored through writings, paintings, and photography. Kuhn moves on from writings referring to Riviere to analyses of Édouard Manet's painting *Bar at the Folies-Bergère* (1882) and the photographic collaborations and literary outputs of Hannah Cullwick and Arthur Joseph Munby. In Manet's *Bar*, Kuhn discusses the significance of the barmaid's uncovered arms, initially depicted folded then overpainted in their current position leaning against the bar's marble counter. The arms would have been registered as sexual by a bourgeois spectator in nineteenth-century Paris, serving as a metonym for nakedness, but this sexual charge passes unremarked today (Pollock 1996). Comparably, in the eighteenth century, as Carolyn Steedman (2007, p. 45) remarks, '[t]he hand mattered in ways that have now disappeared from our own erotic registers' and the display of a well-toned arm and a heaving bosom during labours such as spinning may well have held allure. In nineteenth- and early twentieth-century bourgeois culture, women were expected to wear gloves. The exposed forearms and tell-tale hands of the barmaid in Manet's *Bar* therefore betray her class, this despite the bourgeois veneer she perfects by way of her dress, jewellery, and coiffure. Manet has painted a gold bangle on the woman's right forearm, the auriferous ornament rhyming with the foil of the champagne bottles, encouraging a sense of equivalence between the woman and the other wares on display yet also, crucially, drawing the eye of any customer (and, by extension, any spectator) to the fleshy substantiality of the arm, its circumference and colour.

The barmaid's bangle serves a function akin to that of the leather strap around Hannah Cullwick's right wrist which is visibly prominent in many of the photographs that Cullwick and Munby staged together. These were mainly produced in the studios of cheap trade photographers (Dawkins 1987, p. 171). Cullwick, Munby's servant, entered into a clandestine relationship with the bureaucrat and would subsequently marry him although the formalising of their union also appears to have led to their quasi-permanent separation. As Kuhn explains, Munby had a penchant for seeing working women 'in their dirt'. To this end, he collected photographs of pit girls and servants. The photographs of Cullwick, which form part of this collection, are varied in theme, sometimes showing her dressed as a lady and sometimes as a servant (these contrasting images, Kuhn notes, were often juxtaposed). In those of her as a servant, the 'dirty pictures', she is shown at work polishing, scrubbing, sweeping. It is in these images, arms bare, that the wrist band is visible, a black strap conspicuous against white flesh, enticing the eye. In these pictures, like Manet's *Bar*, arms are an index of class and a source of erotic interest. Hands too are often a key focus. Lynda Nead (2018, p. 653) finds a close-up of Cullwick's hands, 'cut off from the rest of her body and displayed like specimens, with callouses and dirt caught by the recording process' to be 'one of the most extraordinary images of Victorian class and gender'.

In a sophisticated reading, Kuhn describes all the photographs by Cullwick and Munby as forms of performance rather than mere documentation. The couple seemingly explored dominance and submission through their photographs and writings, their collaborations signalling a complex power dynamic in which they clearly switched roles. At least two of the photographs of Cullwick in the role of servant are crafted to showcase her biceps, the size of which (measured at 13 and a half inches) was plainly of note (Mavor 1995, p. 73). In the first she stands slightly at an angle rather than head-on, her right hand loosely gripping what may be a mop or broom. With her left hand she is rolling up the sleeve of her blouse, revealing her right bicep which was hitherto veiled by the fabric. The photograph represents something akin to a strip-tease yet without the need for disrobing. In the second, she is seated, 'her right fist pushing out the muscles of her left arm' (Dawkins 1987, p. 183). Munby also delighted in being lifted up by Cullwick, in her shows of strength (Atkinson 2003). His desires seem, in part, akin to those of the contemporary muscle worshipper although, as Pierre Samuel's (2000) examines through the works of literary figures such as Louis-Ferdinand Céline and Émile Zola, bourgeois male erotic fascination with working-class female muscularity has a long history.

The photographs by Cullwick and Munby often seem to turn on class as masquerade, the pairing of Cullwick 'passing' as a lady with Cullwick performing as a scullery maid, the index of transformation, clearly key to the couple's fantasy role-playing. Class, Kuhn suggests, is also key to Riviere's conception of masquerade. Turning to a dream featuring bare arms recounted by one of Riviere's patients, Kuhn subtly teases out how, through her interpretation, the analyst seeks to screen her own her dirty thoughts. As Patrick Boucheron (2013, p. 38, our translation) has noted, 'words sometimes cover over as surely as cloths or overpainting that which we do not wish to see'. Although Kuhn's focus is not the abject, there are clear points of connection with the monstrous-feminine in terms of discourses of the clean and proper, the pure and virtuous, as against the unclean, the improper and the repellent. Masquerade, as we discuss in our Introduction to this volume, is also crucial to Creed's thinking although her conception of it differs from Riviere's. For Riviere, women may adopt exaggerated forms of behaviour culturally coded as feminine as a means to offset qualities deigned masculine and garner male approval whereas for Creed, masquerade forms a means by which to veil abject qualities feared by the male psyche.

In the final essay in this section, 'Feminism, Film, and Theory Now', Elizabeth Cowie centres a series of reflections on film, feminism, femininity, and subjectivity around the question of horror. Cowie combines ideas from philosophy and psychoanalysis, demonstrating the productive potential of dialoguing across these fields of knowledge. The essay offers in microcosm something of Cowie's own development as a thinker with the use of psychoanalysis in works such as *Representing the Woman* (1997) now increasingly supplemented by ideas from philosophers including Gilles Deleuze, Jacques Rancière, and Bernard Stiegler, among others. Cowie's engagement with Stiegler is motivated by a need to address the impact of technological change upon the fantasy-life of the self. For Stiegler, as Marcel Swiboda summarises succinctly, technology is not something that defines the human after the fact but 'a defining quality through which the human thinks and *becomes*' (Swiboda 2012, p. 116). Understanding contemporary subjectivity therefore necessitates attending to technology's role in its fashioning. Like Mulvey, Cowie's thinking has increasingly sought to address the complexities of the contemporary viewing subject through exploring the effects of technological innovations upon that subject, including their reception of film.

For Cowie, feminism 'is a politics of sexual difference'. This politics revolves around issues of sayability and visibility, around what can be said and seen in a given socio-historical context. It is therefore, in significant part, an aesthetic project. For this reason, Rancière has become an increasingly important interlocutor. For Mulvey (2018, p. 87), Cowie's turn to Rancière with his 'demand that the invisible should be made visible and the unsayable [...] be spoken' is one that evokes 'aspects of 1970s feminist political aesthetics that demanded an end to women's silences, the invisibility of their everyday lives and their exclusion from the Symbolic order'. Rancière provides a crucial vocabulary for apprehending and describing the 'unincluded' (Cowie 2015, p. 49). It is necessary here to refer to the 'unincluded' rather than the excluded, as exclusion already presumes recognition and rejection. It therefore already implies a kind of visibility even if that visibility is registered through turning away or ignoring. In this sense, the 'unincluded' is never the abject. The abject is indisputable, it shows itself, it can be known, perceived, but is expelled and repressed. Here there is therefore a measure of difference with Creed's project and the monstrous-feminine although Cowie derives inspiration from Creed's capacity to explore the politics of sexual difference and its representation as it manifests in horror films.

Drawing on Stanley Cavell's thinking, horror, for Cowie, is a phenomenon that registers the precariousness of human identity. In this sense, there is crossover with the monstrous-feminine as an embodiment of the horrific in that encounters with the monstrous-feminine necessitate a skirting of the dissolution of those boundaries that guarantee the self. A comparable confrontation with identity's precariousness is involved. For Cowie, horror as experience is profoundly affective and also empathic (rather than sympathetic). To be horrified in an encounter with film or art or another medium of imaging is to identify with another's anxiety, to share their feelings. This other is not known, not possessed, but felt. Representation as a practice of coding requires knowledge of its subject. The affective dimension to horror is therefore beyond representation, existing alongside the represented but not subsumed by it. Cowie employs the language of trauma to describe this unknown felt. The traumatic is often conceived as the unsymbolisable. For Cowie, therefore, the 'unique role of the horror film [...] is not its symbolizations as such, but its enjoining the spectator to symbolize'.

Cowie builds on her 2003 essay on the horror film *Eyes without a Face* (Dir. George Franju, France, 1960) in which she analyses anxiety to consider a different register of horror that of 'ravage'. Ravage, as Cowie explains, is a term Lacan associates with feminine jouissance, with feminine pleasure, and which he links to the death drive. Through compelling analyses of the figure of the monstrous woman in *In the Realm of the Senses* (Dir. Nagisa Oshima, Japan, 1976) and *Trouble Every Day* (Dir. Claire Denis, France, 2001), she mulls over whether or not they can be considered feminist horror films. This feminist dimension emerges by way of the affective engagement each film encourages. It is an engagement which elicits an encounter with sexual difference in the viewer, an encounter which moves beyond what is currently knowable or sayable regarding sexual difference. Drawing on Jacques Lacan's idea of the sinthome [the symptom, Man the Saint, artificial man] to argue that 'what we name as our sexual difference is itself a sinthome', Cowie postulates sexual difference as a 'not', as a phenomenon not bound by the Symbolic but existing outside of it. Through encounters with sexual difference, a gap is opened within the factual known of everyday life, a gap that demands 'a thinking otherwise and anew' (Cowie 2015, p. 49). In this sense, Cowie, like Creed, foregrounds how horror films often perform important psychic work for the viewer, work which has potentially vital political implications. Cowie's essay, along with those of Kuhn and Mulvey, signals the ongoing importance of thinking about and through feminist theory in relation to the visual.

References

Atkinson, D. (2003) *Love and Dirt: The Marriage of Arthur Munby and Hannah Cullwick*. Houndmills: Palgrave Macmillan.

Boucheron, P. (2013) *Conjurer la peur: Essai sur la force politique des images*. Paris: Éditions du Seuil.

Cowie, E. (1997) *Representing the Woman: Cinema and Psychoanalysis*. Minneapolis: University of Minnesota Press.

Cowie, E. (2003) 'The Lived Nightmare: Trauma, Anxiety, and the Ethical Aesthetics of Horror,' in S. Schneider & D. Shaw (Eds.), *Dark Thoughts: Philosophic Reflections on Cinematic Horror*. Lanham: Scarecrow Press, pp. 25–46.

Cowie, E. (2011) *Recording Reality, Desiring the Real*. Minneapolis: University of Minnesota Press.

Cowie, E. (2015) 'The Difference in Figuring Women Now,' *Moving Image Review and Art Journal* 4(1&2), pp. 46–60.

Creed, B. (1986) 'Horror and the Monstrous-Feminine: An Imaginary Abjection,' *Screen* 27(1), pp. 44–70.

Creed, B. (2005) *Phallic Panic: Film, Horror and the Primal Uncanny*. Melbourne: Melbourne University Press.

Dawkins, H. (1987) 'The Diaries and Photographs of Hannah Cullwick,' *Art History* 10(2), pp. 154–187.

Malouf, J. (2000) 'Recovering and Discovering another Perspective: Recent Books on Latin American Women Writers,' *Latin American Research Review* 35(1), pp. 243–255.
Mavor, C. (1995) *Pleasures Taken: Performances of Sexuality and Loss in Victorian Photographs*. Durham: Duke University Press.
Meynell, A. (1897) 'Symmetry and Incident,' in A. Meynell (Ed.), *The Colour of Life and Other Essays of Things Seen and Heard*. London: John Lane, pp. 73–87.
Mulvey, L. (1996) *Fetishism and Curiosity*. Bloomington: Indiana University Press.
Mulvey, L. (2006) *Death 24x a Second: Stillness and the Moving Image*. London: Reaktion.
Mulvey, L. (2007) '*A Sudden Gust of Wind (After Hokusai)*: from After to Before the Photograph,' *Oxford Art Journal* 30(1), pp. 27–37.
Mulvey, L. (2018) 'Afterword: Some Reflections on the Engagement of Feminism with Film from the 1970s to the Present Day,' *Moving Image Review and Art Journal* 7(1), pp. 83–90.
Nead, L. (2018) 'The Extraordinary Archive of Arthur J. Munby: Photographing Class and Gender in the Nineteenth Century,' *Victorian Studies* 60(4), pp. 651–653.
Pollock, G. (1996) 'The "View from Elsewhere": Extracts from a Semi-public Correspondence about the Visibility of Desire,' in B.R. Collins (Ed.), *12 Views of Manet's Bar*. Princeton: Princeton University Press, pp. 278–314.
Samuel, P. (2000) 'Amazons in Fiction: A Bibliography,' in J. Freuh, L. Fierstein & J. Stein (Eds.), *Picturing the Modern Amazon*. New York: Rizzoli International Publications, pp. 168–174.
Steedman, C. (2007) *Master and Servant: Love and Labour in the English Industrial Age*. Cambridge: Cambridge University Press.
Swiboda, M. (2012) 'Life and Thought in the Rushes: Mnemotechnics and Orthographic Temporal Objects in the Philosophy of Bernard Stiegler,' *New Formations* 77, pp. 111–126.

2 Symmetry and Incident

Laura Mulvey in Conversation with Nicholas Chare

Laura Mulvey

Nicholas Chare: I first studied your work in depth for a course at the University of Leeds, entitled 'Reading Laura Mulvey,' that was run by Griselda Pollock.[1] I'd like to begin by asking you what it is like writing as Laura Mulvey? In *Visual and Other Pleasures*, you discuss the role of language in feminist film analysis, drawing attention to the need to find an adequate and appropriate conceptual vocabulary as a means to articulate the influence of patriarchy upon film form. In the Introduction to that volume, you describe how structuralism and semiotics permitted a previously invisible world in images to be 'materialised with the language that could name its objects, like the appearance of invisible ink in front of a flame' (Mulvey 1989, p. xiii). You clearly reflect carefully on how words relate to images. Do you think your approach to writing, including your style of writing, has changed over the years in parallel with changing emphases and approaches to images in your research? You've also called yourself an essayist, therefore expressing a preference for shorter pieces of writing. What do you perceive to be the benefits of the essay form for yourself as a film scholar?

Laura Mulvey: Various events in 2015 marking the fortieth anniversary of the 1975 publication of 'Visual Pleasure and Narrative Cinema' brought me back yet again to some of these questions about writing and style. In the Introduction to *Visual and Other Pleasures* (Mulvey 1989) that you refer to, I reminisced about the particular difficulties that I had with writing during my time at school and university. As I was a precocious, intellectual child/young woman who benefited from a family with a strong tradition of intellectual women as well as a very privileged education, this was specifically a difficulty with, even perhaps, in retrospect, a resistance to writing and self-expression. When I joined the Women's Liberation Movement in the early 1970s, I found new ways of thinking that were enormously exciting; and feminist ideas, as drawn for instance from psychoanalytic theory, did have the illuminating effect you mention above. It was in this polemical and feminist context that I saw some point in trying to put ideas into words, as though, at last, I had found something to say. This exhilarating new experience might have influenced the imagistic kind of style I think you're referring to and that I invested a lot of thought and imagination into at the time. Since then, now I come to think about it, 'writing as Laura Mulvey' has changed. I've tried to simplify my style and tend to edit out any too obvious flourishes, which is part of a search for an economical form of expression that's part, in turn, of a commitment to writing about ideas and theory directly and 'unacademically'. I'm not at all sure if this has always been successful but it's a continuing aspiration.

You are right that I have fallen instinctively into an essay form. I have always seemed to work better with ideas than, for instance, careful historical research. In some ways, this has been a disappointment to me. I studied history, my first intellectual passion, at university but my lack of success with it might well be symptomatic of my mentality, which seems to be more suited to a style in which a personal point of view co-exists with a commitment to ideas. Furthermore, I didn't do a PhD. I didn't have an academic position until 1979, that is, 16 years after I left Oxford. I was fortunate that new film studies programmes depended on amateurs, rather than proper academics, to get established in their very early years! My great-grandmother, my mother's maternal grandmother, Alice Meynell, was an essayist who wrote about art and literature but also everyday life from a woman's point of view and very often about women.[2] Reading her essays recently I have felt some affinity with her approach to writing, but rather than any direct legacy, I think that her presence persisted in my family through the intellectual women who brought me up and strongly influenced me, as I mentioned earlier. To say that the essay as a form lacks intellectual ambition might seem disparaging, but it is, in fact, a strength and perhaps has enabled some women writers to find a way of writing within an overwhelmingly patriarchal culture. I should mention here, in the context of this interview, that I have the greatest admiration for Barbara Creed as an outstanding example of the 'extended essayist'; she builds on a thorough and complex initial idea, which is then argued through specific examples into a carefully researched, fascinating book length exposition.

NC: Another similarity between yourself and Barbara is your shared interest in film-making. You have always made films as well as thinking critically about them. In part, the films enabled you, in your own words, to express what your writings could not, 'reaching out beyond the limits of the written word' (Mulvey 1989, p.ix), providing another mode of activism and of investigation. In the 1970s and 1980s, you co-wrote and co-directed a number of very important works of avant-garde cinema with Peter Wollen and you continue to produce films in the present including your 'remixes' (as you have called them) of *Gentlemen Prefer Blondes* (Dir. Howard Hawks, USA, 1953) and *Imitation of Life* (Dir. Douglas Sirk, USA, 1959). Your work in the 1970s and

1980s, as avant-garde, seem very much to be working from the without of mainstream cinema, whereas your more recent projects start within Hollywood productions. How do you conceptualise your career as a film-maker? What are the continuities and/or differences between your earlier and more recent film-making?

LM: I haven't always made films. In fact, my film-making has always been dependent on an outside initiative or context. For instance, Peter and I were able to make films during the 1970s in the context of a flourishing British independent film movement, which had come into being due to a combination of circumstances. Speaking for myself (rather than Peter), these circumstances opened up possibilities: there was a collective energy and commitment to political film (in all its varied forms) in the UK at the time, funding was available (briefly) for the kind of 'theory' films that interested Peter and me. As images of women were a site of feminist struggle and as psychoanalysis had raised the question of language (through the Lacanian concept of the Oedipus Complex), we took advantage of this extraordinary and unusual opportunity to think about, for instance, word and image, representation and myth, through the flexibility and ingenuity of film form. Working with and collaborating with Peter was, of course, a special circumstance of its own and the dialogue between our ideas and interests, in the context of the politics of the time, was exciting and definitely enabling. But everything changed after the election of Margaret Thatcher in 1979... the earlier possibilities for theoretical avant-garde films closed down. Our late films show an attempt to adapt to changing circumstances. But it was a disorientating time. Although for a short time Channel 4 offered a haven for independent film-makers of the 1970s, I personally found it hard to make the move. The shift to television demanded a level of dedication and professionalisation that I just didn't have... Perhaps this relates back to my preference for the dilettantism of the essay that I mentioned above.

Much later, I made two films with my friend Mark Lewis that mix the documentary and the essay forms. *Disgraced Monuments* (Dirs. Mark Lewis & Laura Mulvey, UK, 1994) also came about due to chance circumstances: Mark asked me to collaborate on his project for a film about the removal of the old Soviet monuments. We were fascinated by their visual power (whether you liked them or not) and, more conceptually, their personification of the problem of continuity and discontinuity within history, the literal falling of the (even if debased) communist idea. I got back some of my old enthusiasm for transforming ideas into film images in *Disgraced Monuments*. In this case, it was interesting to think about the spaces of historical time, how the Soviet monuments both marked and occluded earlier histories. Mark, much more recently (in 2013), helped me make *23 August 2008* (Dirs. Mark Lewis & Laura Mulvey, UK, 2013), in which Faysal Abdullah, in single shot monologue, talks about Iraq, exile, and the life and death of his brother Kamel. This is a project I have always wanted to follow up and expand...and still hope to, if possible.

My remixes do, as you point out, go back to the Hollywood of the studio system and movie cinephilia; they are a direct product of my experiments in the early to mid-1990s with new kinds of spectatorship, that is, watching favourite and very familiar old movies on electronic or digital formats. These experiments led to and formed the basis of my 2006 book *Death 24 x a Second: Stillness and the Moving Image*. I made the 30 seconds of Marilyn (in *Gentlemen Prefer Blondes)* stretched into a three-minute remix before writing the book where I refer to it briefly as an example of both pensive and possessive spectatorship. I found that this mode of spectatorship fragmented the narrative homogeneity of a movie, and it was possible to detach a sequence from its place in the original film and turn it into an object in its own right. The remix of the four opening shots in *Imitation of Life* came later, out of the analysis that makes up a chapter of *Death 24*. I hadn't really looked back at these favourite Hollywood films for some time. More and more, I became conscious of the whiteness of Hollywood, that its apartheid nature was confirmed, with few exceptions, by the subservient images of African Americans that dominated this cinema. I had tried to conceptualise Marilyn as a racially marked image in an essay, 'Close-ups and Commodities,' published in *Fetishism and Curiosity* (Mulvey 1996). I came to see this fetishistic, highly constructed vulnerable façade to be signalling racial disavowal as well as the male castration anxiety that was more familiar from my background. But I haven't pursued this further, anyway as yet... *Imitation of Life* is a rare Hollywood film in that it actually engages with day to day racism, beyond the emotional implications of the story, in a violent and vivid series of 'tableaux'. In my last work with the film, I re-edited it to show only Sarah Jane's story. It comes out in an exact pattern of sequences that works as a contained and conceptual realisation of American racism in the 1950s.

NC: Picking up on your reference to *Fetishism and Curiosity*, Barbara Creed is an important interlocutor for you in that book, with her writings about abjection and the monstrous-feminine cited several times. In what ways did you find Barbara's work enabling for you as a feminist in the 1990s?

LM: The essay 'Horror and the Monstrous-Feminine', the basis for Barbara's future book, published in *Screen* in 1986, introduced me to Julia Kristeva's *Powers of Horror* (1982) and the concept of abjection. When we were working on *Riddles of the Sphinx* (Dirs. Laura Mulvey & Peter Wollen, UK, 1977), Peter and I had been influenced by Kristeva's work on the semiotic and the *chora*, which was important for our thinking about language outside the Symbolic order. Retrospectively, Barbara's discussion of the archaic mother would also have been relevant to *Riddles of the Sphinx*, especially the concept of a pre-phallic, pre-Oedipal maternal. And she does, indeed mention the figure of the Sphinx in her essay. But as I only encountered her ideas later, here I would like to focus specifically on the concept of abjection and its influence on the development of my work in the late 1980s and early 1990s.

To reiterate: I only encountered the concept of abjection through Barbara's essay. I was deeply impressed by the way she developed Freudian psychoanalysis through Kristeva to formulate her own specifically feminist film analysis of this particular representation of the female body and, furthermore, its cinematic narrativisation. Her essay drew my attention, retrospectively, to a theoretical lack in the arguments that I had begun to develop in my article on Allen Jones (Mulvey 1973) as well as 'Visual Pleasure and Narrative Cinema' (Mulvey 1975).

A background aside: in the early 1970s, I read Mario Praz's *The Romantic Agony* (1933), which, with its detailed analysis of a phobic misogyny at the heart of late nineteenth-century culture, vividly documented the disgust with which the male unconscious contemplated the female body. Although I don't mention Praz in either of those early essays, his cultural criticism supplemented Freudian theory, particularly the effects of male castration anxiety, which he, Freud, would also have encountered around the same, late nineteenth century, time. The cultural phenomena that Praz analysed pre-figure the idea of the female body as abject: castration anxiety fuses with the disgust aroused by the maternal body and fits, for instance, with Barbara's analysis of the Medusa image and her reading of Freud's reading of the myth. I think she included in the book *The Monstrous Feminine* an extraordinary and typical Symbolist image of snakes writhing out of a beautiful woman's vulva – with castration anxiety explicit without resorting, that is, to the displacement intrinsic to the Medusa.

Retrospectively (again), I realise that I had been, in those two 1970s essays, in search of a theoretical concept, such as abjection, that would have taken my ideas beyond an initial engagement with fetishism and woman as spectacle. But my interests then veered away towards Hollywood melodrama, the avant-garde, and finally an attempt to face the political, social, and economic tragedies of Thatcherism. During the late 1970s and early 1980s, furthermore, I had started to make films with Peter Wollen and had become involved with the radical independent film movement in the UK, as I mentioned above. But by the mid to late 1980s, the political and economic climate had changed, rendering independent film-making much more difficult and avant-gardist aspirations foundered ... That's another story. But it might have been that enforced abandonment of film-making that precipitated my return to my early interests, that is, to images of women in film, art, etcetera, and to feminist engagement with psychoanalytic theory. Barbara's essay was probably the crucial influence on this phase of my thinking.

As you point out in your question, the impact on 'The Monstrous Feminine' emerges quite suddenly in Part 2 of my 1996 collection of essays *Fetishism and Curiosity*, later subtitled *Cinema and the Mind's Eye* (2nd edition 2013). The essays in Part 2 (on Pandora's Box, on Cindy Sherman and on late 1980s Godard) all revolve around a new kind understanding of the female body, not simply as spectacle, but figured by the patriarchal imagination as divided between interior and exterior – as I explain further below. The crucial influence of Barbara's work emerges immediately in the Preface: I point out that, as I shifted away from my longstanding concern with male spectatorship and the female body as spectacle to 'the "rebus" of the fetishized female body', it was Barbara's work that 'helped me find a figure for the space into which the fetish collapses' (Mulvey 1996, p. xii; 2013, p. xxiv). That is, male castration anxiety, once complicated by the place of the maternal body in the male unconscious, demanded the further theorisation that Barbara offered via Kristeva. As my ideas developed under these influences, my earlier work on woman as spectacle moved towards a 'topographical' image of the female body. While, for instance, the image of the Medusa seemed to arise as a horrific phantasmagoria, abjection seemed to occupy an inside, an interior space concealed by the surface glamour of the phantasmatic female body.

This preoccupation with 'an imaginary spatial relationship and a phantasmatic topography' (Mulvey 1996, p. xii; 2013, p. xxiv) first appears in the chapter on Pandora's Box (first published in 1992), where I specifically use Barbara's articulation of the abject as emanating from varying images of the maternal body, as she puts it 'the horrifying image of woman as archaic mother, phallic woman and castrated body represented in a single figure' (quoted in *Fetishism and Curiosity* (Mulvey 1996, p. 64; 2013, p. 83)).[3] While Barbara's analyses of the horror movie led her to explicit representations of the 'monstrous feminine', her ideas influenced me rather towards this split between an alluring, cosmetic surface and an abject, concealed but threatening, interior, which I developed through my analogy between Pandora and her box. In my chapter on Cindy Sherman, I refer back to Pandora, once again citing Barbara, to discuss Sherman's photographs as a collapse of the body's boundaries, revealing the internalisation of abjection within a woman's own psyche: 'The images of decaying food and vomit raises the spectre of the anorexic girl, who tragically acts out the fashion fetish of the female body as an eviscerated, cosmetic and artificial construction, designed to ward off the "otherness" hidden inside her' (Mulvey 1996, p. 72; 2013, p. 93).

I was interested in two aspects of the relation between Pandora and her box: first of all, there was the spatial analogy, that I mentioned above, but the association between Pandora and curiosity led to a woman's look that, in the first instance, was turned towards the enigma that her body represented for the patriarchal unconscious. If the box, as I argue in the essay, is a metaphor for the female genitalia, Pandora can look inside it without fear or disgust. Her look into the space of the male-designated abject enables its mutation into a symptom, and the 'phantasmatic topography' can be reconfigured into a riddle. Ultimately this offered an image of feminist curiosity, addressing and articulating the vast mass of displacements behind representations of the feminine across patriarchal culture, and psychoanalytic theory could provide a code, of a kind, to initiate the process. Although Barbara took the horror film as the object to be deciphered, whereas I continued to focus on a variation of woman as erotic spectacle, we shared a political commitment to 'feminist curiosity'. I would like to quote the last lines of 'Horror and the Monstrous-Feminine' essay:

> We can see its [the horror film's] ideological project as an attempt to shore up the symbolic order by constructing the feminine as an imaginary 'other' which must be repressed and controlled in order to secure and protect the social order. Thus, the horror film stages and re-stages a constant repudiation of the maternal figure.
>
> But the feminine is not per se a monstrous sign; rather, it is constructed as such within a patriarchal discourse which reveals a great deal about male desires and fears but tells us nothing about feminine desire in relation to the horrific. When Norman Bates remarked to Marion Crane in *Psycho* that: 'Mother is not herself today', he was dead right. Mother wasn't herself. She was someone else. Her son – Norman.
>
> (Creed 1986, p. 70)

To my mind, these lines sum up precisely the kind of sleight of hand that feminist theory and criticism must always perform. And however wary feminism should be of Freud, psychoanalytic theory has offered feminism, to quote your quotation above: 'a language that could name its objects, [materialising] like the appearance of invisible ink in front of a flame'.

The idea of a 'phantasmatic topography,' that is the idea of woman's exterior and interior split between a perfect and alluring mask concealing an abject interior, has stayed with me and contributed to my thought about two other topographical configurations that do not at first glance relate to the image of woman. By the time I wrote the Introduction to *Fetishism and Curiosity*, I had absorbed the concept of abject and was, as it were, 'recycling' its implications, perhaps stretching at the limits of the theory. But I would like to note the way that Barbara's original influence carried on in these rather different contexts. The idea of 'an inside/outside' opposition, an alluring surface that conceals something, 'unsightly' allowed me to make an analogy between Marxist and Freudian fetishisms. I summed up the relation between the two fetishisms in the Introduction to the second edition of *Fetishism and Curiosity*:

> Fetishisms disguise, on the one hand, (Marx) the workers' labour as productive of value under capitalism and, on the other, (Freud) the anxiety provoked by the maternal body perceived as castrated. These, too real, material bodies disappear into the spectacular forms of commodity fetishism and fetishised femininity…'.
>
> (Mulvey 2013, p. vii)

It was not until I wrote this second Introduction, in 2013, that I paid any attention to that most repressed mechanism of the cinema, the projector, that then suggested a third topographical pattern. The worker's labour power, hidden by the commodity fetish, suggested an analogy with the labour of the projector and projectionist, hidden, or, in psychoanalytic terms, repressed in a box at the back of the cinema. Here the image of woman returned. I began to think about the screen and most of all, the 'to-be-looked-at' female star, as the site of cinema's own, material and specific fetishism, disavowing the labour power of the projector that lay behind its very existence. So the fetishism invested in the female star and of the apparatus creates the circuit of 'visual pleasure'. In another aside: I noticed that this sense of a circuit was lacking in 'Visual Pleasure and Narrative Cinema', where my understanding of the cinematic apparatus was restricted, simply and only, to the camera. In a form of repression of my own, I ignored the process of projection. Retrospectively, of course, how the still images of the film strip are transformed into the fascinating, moving, illusion on the screen seems much more vital for an analysis of spectatorship than the registration of the original film by the camera. In films such as *Deux ou trois choses que je sais d'elle* (Dir. Jean-Luc Godard, France, 1967), Godard came close to bringing all three fetishisms into visibility. As he 'defetishized' the cinematic apparatus, he also linked a cosmetically constructed female sexuality to a female, domestic consumption of commodities, weaving the 'phantasmatic topography' across Marx, Freud, and the cinema itself.

I would like to add a few final words about the great originality and importance of Barbara's 2005 book *Phallic Panic: Film, Horror and the Primal Uncanny*. The book takes feminist psychoanalytic theory and criticism to a further stage, examining the flaws and weaknesses of the Symbolic order as personified by deviant masculinity (beyond those personified by the feminine, by now a more established discourse). In both *The Monstrous-Feminine* and *Phallic Panic*, I have been impressed by Barbara's ability to use the Lacanian orders, especially the symbolic (she uses the lower case), an essential concept for feminist political, cultural critique, of the system on which patriarchy is constructed and sustained. Freud's 1919 essay 'The Uncanny' is her major point of psychoanalytic reference. I also used 'The Uncanny' in *Death 24 x a Second: Stillness and the Moving Image* (Mulvey 2006) and I also discuss E.T.A Hoffmann's story 'The Sandman' and although I have a rather different reading of the automaton Olympia, we both use Freud's association of uncanniness with the maternal body. From the perspective of criticism, I was struck not only by her emphasis on 'feeling' but also by her careful attention to its textual construction, to its filmic materiality, the specificity of the cinema's embodiment of monstrosity, and those feelings of fear and the frightening that define the horror genre. And she goes on to analyse a primal uncanny and male monstrosity that the horror film brings to the surface and into the light of day.

Barbara's key idea is that the primal uncanny emerges when aligned with the three principle figures of symbolic taboo: 'The male monster is made monstrous when he enters the domain of woman, death and nature' (Creed 2005, p. 17). But in her discussion of Jack the Ripper, she suggests that there is also something essentially and necessarily masculine to this thing that 'strikes at the heart of the symbolic order' at the masculinity that 'embodies phallic power and asserts masculine qualities of power, rationality, ascendency and control' (p. 201). That is, the monster threatens the 'ruin of representation', standing for 'the point where meaning collapses' (p. xviii). She sums up: 'If inscription in language – in the symbolic – is almost always phallocentric and designed to shore up the power and authority of the symbolic, then the monster's nonmeaning, which includes enjoyment, is designed to unsettle the symbolic order and as such is ideological' (p. xviii). Finally, in the closing paragraphs of the Introduction, Barbara wonders whether the monster is designed to act as a safety valve for the Symbolic order or whether in the last resort 'the male monster signifies a desire for the collapse of patriarchal civilisation' (p. xix). As well as the variety of monstrous forms that Barbara discusses throughout the book (all of whom are threatening to women), to my mind she also conjures up the pre-Oedipal father from whose rage and irrationality civilisation has always been supposed to offer a safe-guard.

I was deeply impressed by *Phallic Panic* when I first read it. But reading it again it seems to have a new relevance. As I read the Introduction a particular figure rose in my mind, one who is flamboyantly unconstrained by any patriarchal inhibition, who has brought nonmeaning into the public sphere, who, in a return of the Symbolic repressed, fuses lies with incoherent speech, who can only actually conceive of objects (a wall) unable to handle the abstract (administrative rules and regulations)… that is, (you've doubtless guessed) the present President of the US. It's very likely that he does want to bring about the collapse of patriarchal civilisation. Probably only an alliance between women and non-patriarchally invested men can construct, with difficulty, an alternative symbolic and a transformed public sphere.

Notes

1 [NC] I am grateful to Michelle Gewurtz and Silvestra Mariniello for their help and advice in preparing the questions that formed the basis for this conversation.
2 [NC] The title of this conversation, 'Symmetry and Incident', is also the title of one of Alice Meynell's (1897) essays from the collection *The Colour of Life and Other Essays*. For further discussion of Meynell's essay, see the introduction to Part 1 of the present volume.
3 [NC] The essay 'Pandora: Topographies of the Mask and Curiosity' (Mulvey 1992) was published in the volume *Sexuality & Space*.

References

Creed, B. (1986) 'Horror and the Monstrous-Feminine: An Imaginary Abjection,' *Screen* 27(1), pp. 44–70.

Creed, B. (2005) *Phallic Panic: Film, Horror and the Primal Uncanny*. Melbourne: Melbourne University Press.

Kristeva, J. (1982) *Powers of Horror: An Essay on Abjection*. Translated from the French by L.S. Roudiez. New York: Columbia University Press.

Meynell, A. (1897) 'Symmetry and Incident', in A. Meynell (ed.), *The Colour of Life and Other Essays of Things Seen and Heard*. London: John Lane, pp. 73–87.

Mulvey, L. (1973) 'You Don't Know What Is Happening, Do You, Mr Jones?' *Spare Rib* 8, pp. 13–16.

Mulvey, L. (1975) 'Visual Pleasure and Narrative Cinema', *Screen* 16(1), pp. 6–18.

Mulvey, L. (1989) *Visual and Other Pleasures*. Basingstoke: The Macmillan Press.

Mulvey, L. (1992) 'Pandora: Topographies of the Mask and Curiosity,' in B. Colomina (ed.), *Sexuality & Space*. New York: Princeton Architectural Press, pp. 53–72.

Mulvey, L. (1996) *Fetishism and Curiosity*. Bloomington and Indianapolis: Indiana University Press.

Mulvey, L. (2006) *Death 24X a Second: Stillness and the Moving Image*. London: Reaktion.

Mulvey, L. (2013) *Fetishism and Curiosity: Cinema and the Mind's Eye*. 2nd ed. Basingstoke: Palgrave Macmillan.

Praz, M. (1933) *The Romantic Agony*. Translated from the Italian by A. Davidson. London: Oxford University Press.

3 A Dream of Bare Arms

'Womanliness', Dirt, and a Quest for Knowledge

Annette Kuhn

When Joan Riviere's paper 'Womanliness as a masquerade' was published in 1929, it was intended as a salvo in the interwar debate within the pyschoanalytic movement about the nature of femininity and its mental aetiology and organisation. Freud's more widely known contributions to this debate are his 1931 paper 'Female Sexuality' (Freud 1977a) and his 1933 lecture 'Femininity' (Freud 1973). Other key interventions were made by Karen Horney (1926) and Helene Deutsch (1930).[1]

The argument in 'Womanliness as a masquerade' is based upon material arising in the analysis of one of Riviere's patients, a professional woman who, despite considerable ability and success as a writer and speaker, craved reassurance from men by seeking sexual and professional compliments from them after any public engagement: this she would do by flirting and generally presenting herself as ultra-feminine. Riviere's conclusion was that for this patient, womanliness could be assumed and worn like a mask, 'both to hide the possession of masculinity and to avert the reprisals expected if she was found to possess it' (Riviere 1986, p. 38). Decades later, following Lacan's 'retrieval' of her notion of the masquerade in his seminar series from 1958 to 1959, Riviere's paper was reprinted in a 1966 anthology on psychoanalysis and female sexuality.[2] Subsequently, with the rise of second-wave feminism, the idea of femininity as a masquerade or performance was enthusiastically taken up within an emergent strand of feminist film criticism interested in mining psychoanalytic thinking on sexual difference for insights on the relationship between women, femininity, films, and cinema.[3] So it was that Riviere's clinical interpretation of 'womanliness' and the concept of the masquerade were taken up in Anglophone cultural theory, notably in feminist and psychoanalytic thinking around sexual difference, gender performativity, female spectatorship in cinema, and the role of fantasy in the constitution of sexual and gender identity.[4] Interestingly, though, it is rarely, if ever, referenced in these contexts today.

This chapter will make a return visit to Riviere's paper, approaching it from a fresh angle, to reflect on the enigma of Riviere herself, and to scrutinise some of the detail of the case history she sets out in 'Womanliness as a masquerade'. Who was Joan Riviere? In his 1986 essay, 'Joan Riviere and the masquerade', Stephen Heath notes that she was born Joan Verrall, but does not indicate how she came by a different name. In fact, Riviere was born in 1882 into an established Sussex county family and acquired her slightly exotic surname when she married a barrister, Evelyn Riviere, at the age of 23. Heath sifts through the literature on the psychoanalytic circles of the early decades of the twentieth century, in search of clues in the correspondence between the 'great men' of the movement about Riviere, who became a founding member of the British Psychoanalytical Society and a lay analyst. He comes up with some intriguing fragments, among them that Freud's biographer and epigone, Ernest Jones, wrote to Freud in 1921 about her: she had been in analysis with Jones since 1916. Jones recommended Riviere to Freud as a potential analysand, describing her as colossally narcissistic and masculine-identified. He regarded her analysis as a 'failure' (Heath 1986, p. 45).

Heath also mentions a brief reference in Jones's book *Sigmund Freud: Life and Work* to the sort of woman that Freud was attracted to: Freud, says Jones, liked to surround himself with 'intellectual', 'masculine' women (among them his sister-in-law, Minna Bernays, and indeed Joan Riviere herself) (Jones 1984, p. 474). Jones is at pains to emphasise, however, that this was not an erotic attraction. Finally, Heath quotes a striking, almost cinematic, image in a 1958 memoir by Katherine West, in which Riviere is remembered as a 'tall, Edwardian beauty with a picture hat and scarlet parasol – walking up and down the seashell path in lively conversation with a gentleman' (Heath 1986, p. 47).

Joan Riviere, then, certainly according to some of the men in her life, was narcissistic, intellectual, and masculine-identified: in their eyes, these qualities made her both admirable and troublesome. One wants to know more; and in their study of Freud's women, Lisa Appignanesi and John Forrester (1993) flesh out Heath's tantalising sketch. Ernest Jones had referred Riviere to Freud for further analysis after he had himself 'failed' with her, due (in Freud's view at least) to his, Jones's, mishandling of the transference. Freud rebukes Jones for his 'technical error' in befriending his patient before her analysis was brought to a close (Jones had recruited her as a lay analyst, allowed her to use his country cottage, and in several other ways breached the boundary between an analyst-client relationship and friendship) (Appignanesi and Forrester 1993, p. 355).[5] Freud took Riviere on as his analysand, and she was in analysis with him for a year or so in the early 1920s. It is clear that he had considerable respect for her intellect, and persuaded Jones to offer her the important post of translations editor on the *International Journal of Psychoanalysis*. Riviere had in fact already translated some of Freud's works into English, and was later to be Melanie Klein's principal translator. In later years, she would cross swords with Freud over her espousal of the Kleinian view on the development of the superego in infancy. Ernest

Jones, for his part, spoke of the 'elegant and acerbic' Riviere's 'disdainful way of treating other people, *like dirt beneath her feet*' (Quoted in ibid. p. 354; emphasis added). Despite her high-handed manner – she was, it seems, a perfectionist who did not suffer fools gladly – her role within the psychoanalytic movement was in many respects a classically feminine one: as a translator, she was in effect a channel or conduit for the words and ideas of others. There is clearly an element of handmaidenliness, and even of servitude, in such a role; though the issue is obviously far from clear-cut in Riviere's case.

Besides all this, it appears that Riviere was a sharp dresser. Heath relates that she liked cosmetics, too (rather unusual, perhaps, in a woman of her class and generation), and had once worked as a dressmaker (couturier would probably be a more appropriate term, since after being 'finished' in Germany she served an apprenticeship to a court dressmaker); not something one would normally expect to find on the CV of a psychoanalyst, even a lay one. Riviere is altogether fascinating, and remains something of a puzzle.

The vivid memory-image of Joan with her hat and parasol in 'lively conversation' with a gentleman places her at a moment in history that evokes less the post Jazz-age moment of the masquerade paper than the pre-First World War moment of another of Freud's women, the hysteric 'Dora', whom Freud had analysed in 1901 – indeed Joan and Dora would have been similar in age. The picture of Joan and her gentleman companion, fixed forever in an era conventionally remembered as one of innocence and leisured cultivation (for a certain class, at least), recalls nothing so much as Freud's Dora's lakeside strolls with her dodgy 'suitor' Herr K (Freud 1977b, pp. 55–56). The hat and the parasol – remembered as scarlet (not merely red), with all the overtones of that colour-name – suggest, aside from an evident elegance and style, a certain occlusion. Does Joan have something to hide? Are we perhaps not seeing everything there is to see about Joan? Could she be a 'scarlet woman'? A picture hat (a woman's elaborate hat with a wide brim) *and* a parasol seem too much: either one would be enough on its own, surely? There are too many clothes in this picture, and perhaps a certain flashiness as well. If Joan is exhibiting elegance through her attire, its excessiveness suggests that there is also something else afoot, that the clothes could be a cover-up as well as a display – in several senses. We might recall that in the course of one of his repeated puzzlings over the 'enigma' of femininity, Freud (1973, p. 146) quotes some lines from a poem by Heine:

> Heads in hieroglyphic bonnets
> Heads in turbans and black birettas,
> Heads in wigs and thousand other
> Wretched, sweating heads of humans.[6]

The remembered scarlet 'bonnet' sported by Joan is itself something of a hieroglyph – the memory-image is a code, condensing a riddle whose solution, in the classic manner, lies concealed within itself.

The picture hat and the parasol also bring to mind other devices of female costume that conceal or occlude or otherwise get in the way of the gaze – while at the same time alluding to something that cannot be seen: the veil, the hijab, even the fetishist's furs and feathers. Riviere's *picture* hat – aptly, even symptomatically, named – is exactly a *screen*, in several senses of the word. In the Victorian drawing room, a screen hides something, interrupts the gaze; in cinema, on the other hand, the screen is a site for exhibition, for display; in psychoanalysis (as indeed in cinema), a screen is a *tabula rasa* onto which fantasies are projected. Concealment, display, fantasy – all of these are condensed in Joan's hieroglyphic bonnet-fetish.

***

Édouard Manet's painting 'A Bar at the Folies Bergère' was made in the early 1880s.[7] It portrays a woman, a barmaid, standing behind a bar counter, engaging the spectator's gaze. Her hands are braced on the counter as she appears to lean slightly forward. Behind her is a mirror in which her back view is reflected, along with the theatre audience and – at top left of the picture – the shins and feet of the acrobat who is performing. The woman presents herself to the gaze, we may assume, of a male spectator, a customer at the bar, and steadily returns that gaze. But there is more to it than is visible on the picture's surface. The art historian Griselda Pollock (1995) notes that an X-ray of the canvas reveals an earlier version of Manet's painting, in which the barmaid stands with folded arms.[8] Pollock's interpretation of the change in the way the woman's arms are painted turns on the meanings – in social-historical context – of certain gestures of arms and hands in women; of sleeves and gloves; and of their presence or absence.

> In the paradoxical conventions of bourgeois society, women could bare their chests and upper arms in ballgowns, but their lower arms and hands had to be gloved.... Hands thus acquired a symbolic significance in the sexual geography of the female body totally unfamiliar to us today. To go about ungloved was akin to leaving your body naked. Such exposure was a classed sign which functioned metonymically for both nakedness and vulgarity.
>
> (Pollock 1995, pp. 26–27)

The barmaid's fully visible gloveless hands signal the erotic charge, for the *fin-de-siècle* man of the world, of the lower-class or *declassée* woman's bare hands and forearms. Semiotically speaking, the exposed forearms and the frank outward gaze are mutually reinforcing. This woman is no lady – unlike Joan Riviere, whose hands, we may safely assume, would have been discreetly gloved as she strolled along the sea-shell path with her gentlemen interlocutor. But Joan's gloves, like her hat and parasol, and like the extra layer of paint on 'A Bar at the Folies Bergère', are screens in every sense of the word: they hide, they display, they inscribe fantasy; they do all of those things at the same time.

Once you become aware of it, the trope of the bare arms seems to surface everywhere. Certainly from the standpoint of nineteenth-century bourgeois masculinity, it figures recurrently in imaginings of transgression – transgression above all of the limits of respectability and of divisions between social classes, as well as, relatedly, in fantasies of forbidden sexuality. From the standpoint of the feminine, on the other hand, and on either side of the dividing line between the working and the middle classes, the bare arms trope stands for the absolute necessity of recognising one's proper place as a woman of a particular class.

The fantasy, the dream, of bare arms condenses many layers of meaning, then; some of them unconscious. I want now to look at an intriguing nineteenth-century case in which the meanings of bare arms, and their associated psychical energies, underlie and structure certain kinds of activities and enthusiasms. For the time being, we can leave Joan Riviere to her conversations with the men in her life; but she will be back.

***

> For she is still a working wench
> And sits with hands still bare,
> O' Sundays, on the poor folk's bench:
> But he is with her there.

This verse was written by Arthur Munby (1828–1910), a quintessential Victorian gentleman: respectable civil servant, barrister, teacher, amateur artist. In common with many others of his caste, Munby was also a man with a hobby. His was one that preoccupied him to the point of obsession: throughout his life, he was powerfully drawn to working women. Munby's copious journals record innumerable encounters with such women – colliery women, fishwives, farm workers, dairymaids and acrobats, as well as servant women – whom he names, describes in detail, interviews, and sometimes befriends (Hudson 1974). Munby commissioned photographs of dozens of his 'subjects', and executed sketches of many more. He was particularly fascinated by the trouser-wearing pit girls of Wigan, and visited his contacts there repeatedly over a number of years. He especially liked to see them, and have them photographed, 'in their dirt'. Munby's quest was only in part, if indeed at all, a documentary one, *à la* Henry Mayhew. Like Mayhew's, Munby's encounters largely took place in public, and were – by definition, in Victorian class terms – with strangers. Like Baudelaire's *flâneur*, though perhaps more purposeful in his pursuit of a particular desire, Munby haunted city streets and places of public entertainment and resort.

Here he describes an encounter which took place in May 1860:

> [A]bout eleven I went to see a masquerade of a very singular character at the Victoria Theatre. The ball took place on stage, the house itself being densely crowded with spectators of the lowest class, many of them young women – orange girls, coster girls, servants and the like. The masqueraders, whose costumes when they wore any were absurd enough; were of a somewhat better class. I was in a private stage box (price sixpence) and to me entered two uninteresting young women, rather tawdrily dressed, one of whom, though not at all immodest, paid me the most unnecessary & undesired attentions. They were hat trimmers, working for Christy the hatter; earning some 15/ a week: all the lining and braid of hats are made up by women, it appears. They said that most of the young women masquerading were envelopefolders [sic] and bootbinders, earning from 15/[sic] to £1 a week: these have the reputation, said the hat trimmers of being 'fast' and fond of dancing....
>
> (Hudson 1974, pp. 60–61)

Munby's reports are somewhat ethnographic in character (indeed the tone of this passage is highly reminiscent of reports by the amateur Mass-Observers of the 1930s and 1940s), and there is no suggestion that he is engaged in any sexual quest. The reference to 'undesired attention' is characteristic: Munby insists on a certain distance between himself and his subjects. This, however, is by no means to deny the possibility of a sexual – or more accurately, perhaps, a libidinal – energy behind Munby's researches. On the contrary: his activities suggest classic sublimation, of the sort that would be described by Freud some decades later:

> [T]he libido evades the fate of repression by being sublimated from the very beginning into curiosity and by becoming attached to the powerful instinct for research as a reinforcement. Here, too, the research becomes to some extent compulsive and a substitute for sexual activity.
>
> (Freud 1985 [1910], p. 180)

To the extent that the specific objects of such a powerful drive for research are distinctive or particular, though, they may productively be treated as symptomatic. In Munby's case at least, other aspects of his life suggest that this is appropriate; for his 'researches' overlapped with, and fed into, his emotional life in a quite extraordinary manner.

From his mid twenties, Munby enjoyed a secret liaison with his maidservant, Hannah Cullwick. The couple eventually married and, by their own accounts (Hannah also kept a diary), enjoyed a contented life together.[9] Throughout their relationship, even after they were married, Hannah insisted on remaining Munby's servant (she called him 'Massa'), and it seems that – unlike, say, the upwardly mobile partners of a number of her husband's acquaintances among the pre-Raphaelites – she refused to try and turn herself into a 'lady', and intended this refusal as a gesture of independence. Indeed this appears to be the secret of the longevity of Hannah's and Arthur's deeply mutually loving (if perhaps in the Freudian sense deeply perverse) relationship.

Munby's verse, which is of course dedicated to Hannah herself, eulogises her 'hands still bare'. These same bare hands (and forearms) feature prominently in many of the photographs the couple collaborated over the years in producing. They include portraits of Hannah in her work clothes and at work, 'in her dirt' (Figures 3.1–3.3). Elsewhere, Hannah appears in a range of other guises – as a 'lady', in men's clothing, as a chimney sweep, a peasant.

It has been rightly suggested that these photographs, of which Hannah should certainly be regarded as co-creator, 'rupture the politics of visibility and representation of the bourgeois household...at a time when household dirt, servants and their work were to be invisible' (Dawkins 1986, p. 1).[10] It is perhaps also worth pointing out, however, that the

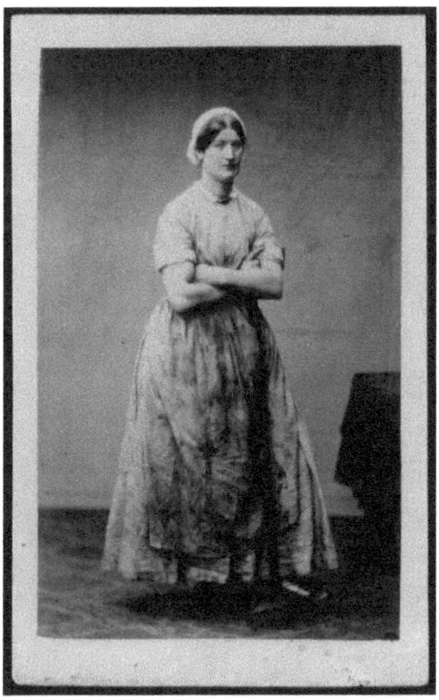

Figure 3.1 Hannah Cullwick in work clothes, 1864.

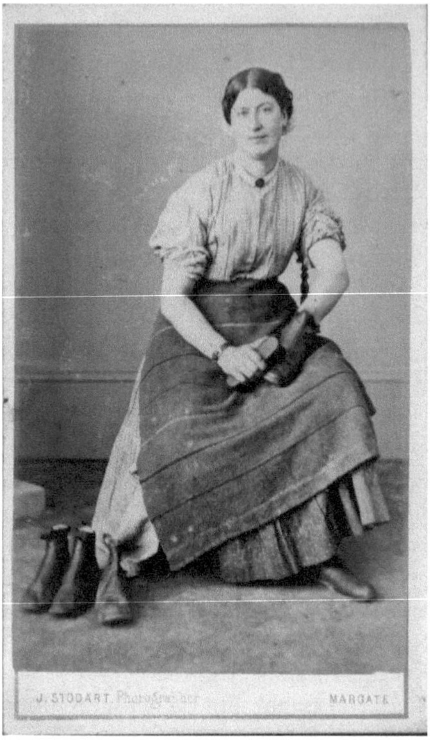

Figure 3.2 Hannah Cullwick seated, cleaning boots, 1864.

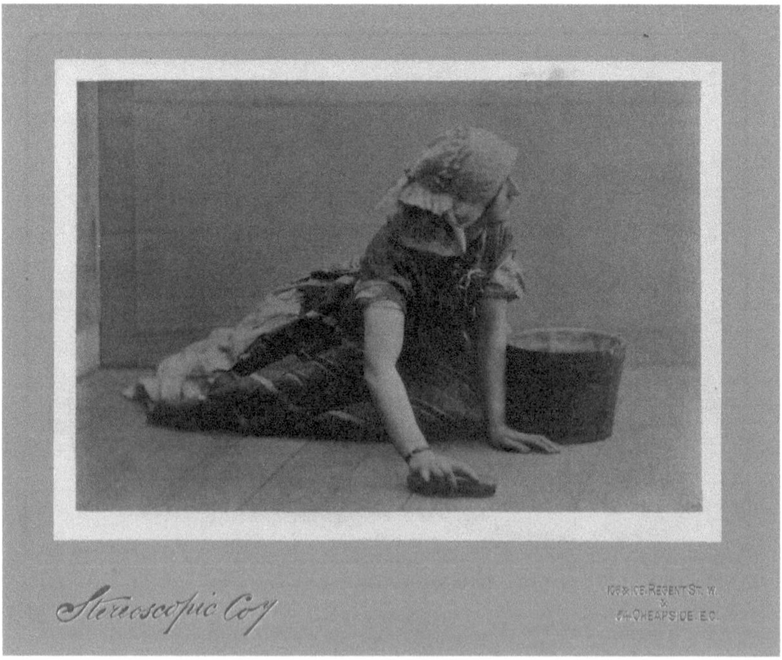

Figure 3.3 Hannah Cullwick scrubbing the floor, no date.

photographs are conventional in the sense that some are reminiscent of a type of popular imagery prevalent at the time in mass-produced sentimentalised vignettes, in various media, of peasant and lower-class persons and lives. Perhaps more significantly, Munby's photographs, and especially his collaborations with Cullwick, embody elements of performance in their staging of a range of different activities and identities. These are certainly not documentary images, in the twentieth- and twenty-first-century sense of the word: indeed the category of documentary had yet, in Munby's time, to be invented.

A fetishisation of the bare hands of working women is apparent also in Munby's writings; as, for instance, in an account of a visit to a large gathering of 'the English working classes' at Crystal Palace:

> ...I passed a tallish woman, evidently a servant, who was noticeable for the size of her gloveless hands. She seemed to be alone in the crowd, and (with a view to her hands) I asked her if she meant to dance? No, she couldn't dance at all – only liked to look on: for which I was not sorry. So after a little chat we walked away, and I (still with a view to my hobby) proposed to rest n the bank near, under the trees. She gave me her hand to help her up – and, oh ye ballroom partners, what a breadth of massive flesh it was to grasp! She sat down by me, ready to talk, after the blunt fashion of such maidens, but not forward...She was a maid of all work at Chelsea, it seemed....I looked at her hands, and spoke my opinion of them. 'How can you like them?' she says, like Margaret in the garden; 'they are so large and red, I'm ashamed of them'. 'They are just the hands for a servant,' say I: 'they show you are hardworking, and you ought to be proud of them. You wouldn't wish them to be like a lady's?' 'Yes I should!' said she, bitterly: 'and I should like to be a lady, and I wish my hands were like yours!' [....] Her right hand lay, a large red lump, upon her light-coloured frock: it was very broad and square & thick – as large and strong & coarse as the hand of a sixfoot [sic] bricklayer...the skin was rough to the touch, and hard & leathery in the palm: there was nothing feminine about it in form or texture....
>
> (Hudson 1974, pp. 71–72)

This passage, in common with others like it, suggests that it is precisely the hands – gloveless and work-worn – which alert Munby to his quarry, and which then become the object of his questing gaze. Like the passage quoted earlier, this one also evidences Munby's sensitivity to details of female attire. His photographic collaborations with Hannah Cullwick suggest that they were both alert to the potential of clothing to effect mutations of identity: significantly in this regard, in Munby's albums, photographs of Hannah in her work clothes were often juxtaposed with portraits of her as a lady. At the same time, hands and arms may speak a truth which costume can dissemble. In her own diary, Hannah describes an incident of class 'passing' on a friend's part:

> Well she said how Mrs Shepherd borrow'd an opera cloak for her – she's got one for herself & a black velvet skirt, what she wears to go into the theatres. And Ellen wore her black silk frock, white gloves, & her hair was done up with a bow of ribbon somehow, & they left their bonnets in the cloakroom. Then Ellen said they was shown up an elegant staircase with flowers each side of it, & to a row of chairs, so fine, & when they sat down it was like a down pillow they sank down so. She said to herself, 'Can it be myself that's here?' And she felt so comfortable that she wanted the acting to have no end, & yet uncomfortable too, for she was afraid to turn or speak for fear of the rest seeing she was a servant [....] Ellen seem'd to rather like being a lady – if her hands wasn't so red she said, & if she'd plenty o' money.
> (Stanley 1984, p. 156)

Hannah herself 'passed' from time to time; often describing the great sense of relief she felt on dropping her masquerade and going back to being a servant ('...I actually jumped for joy & felt as if I was let out o' prison. The feeling is dreadful – that being stuck in a drawing room and having a fussy fine lady talking to you....' (Stanley 1984, p. 74)). It is the tension between the masquerade of the clothes on the one hand and the 'truth' of the hands and arms on the other that organises the pleasures and the productivities of Munby's researches and of his relations with Hannah Cullwick.

***

We may now return to Joan Riviere, for whom the masquerade is, on the face of it, about gender identity rather than class. But on closer inspection it transpires that class does indeed lurk beneath the story she tells in 'Womanliness as a masquerade'. It is insistently present in a dream – significantly, a dream of bare arms – produced by Riviere's professional woman patient, who is the dream's protagonist. It is recounted by Riviere:

> She was in terror alone in the house; then a negro came in and found her washing clothes, with her sleeves rolled up and arms exposed. She resisted him, with the secret intention of attracting him sexually, and he began to admire her arms and caress them and her breasts.
> (Riviere 1986, p. 37)

In this intensely erotic scenario, the dreamer declasses herself – not just by performing menial domestic work, but also, and especially, by exposing her arms, which then figure centrally in the ensuing sexual encounter. At the same time, the dreamer takes up at least two enunciative positions at once: she is both *observer of* the scene, and *observed within* it. In a scenario which recalls a peepshow, the dreamer/narrator is at one and the same time maidservant and voyeur. This dream mirrors, and perhaps even sheds light on the workings of, the fantasies that power the Munby-Cullwick collaborations. But there is something more here as well.

The dream's content and emotional colour call to mind some of the anxieties Riviere reports in her client, notably the woman's fear of the otherness of certain forms of masculinity *for a woman*. According to Riviere, she 'had great anxiety in dealings with men such as porters, waiters, cabmen, tradesmen' (Riviere 1986, p. 39). From a middle-class lady's standpoint, the bare arms of the dream stand for disgrace, for 'falling' in class terms and/or sexually. But the sibling of fear ('she was in terror alone in the house') is, of course, desire, which is perhaps where the 'negro' of the dream comes in. Riviere rather too hastily explains away his appearance by noting that the patient had spent her youth in the southern states of the US. While this makes sense at the first level of dream interpretation, Riviere chooses not to acknowledge the condensation and displacement which characterise the dream-work. There is surely more to the 'negro' image than a reference to the dreamer's background. In recruiting a black man to the erotic scenario of this dream of bare arms, its enunciation calls on positionalities of race and ethnicity as well as of class and gender in a scenario that mixes up, confirms, and at the same time, upends, culturally conventional positions of dominance and servitude. Who, to appropriate Munby and Cullwick's fantasy scenarios, is the 'Massa' in this dream of bare arms?

***

Taken together, the 'negro' and the bare forearms of the dreamer/maidservant are clearly fetishes that point towards a fear of, and a simultaneous desire for, relegation to the social and sexual margins, to the place where dirt proliferates and must be swept out of sight. Eroticisation of dirt seems an appropriate enough fantasy for an analysand to offer up to a woman analyst who treated those she considered her inferiors 'like dirt beneath her feet'. It perhaps ultimately provides a key to Munby's and Cullwick's secret liaison and shared interests, the illicitness of which was grounded in, and produced, a nexus of energy in which fantasies centring on dirty work and the mutability of class, gender, and even racial, identity are bound together in displaced form in an obsessive quest for knowledge – a quest to see, to know, and to record all.

Acknowledgement

Photographs from the Munby Papers are reproduced by kind permission of the Master and Fellows of Trinity College, Cambridge.

Notes

1 Joan Riviere (1929), 'Womanliness as a masquerade.' Page references throughout the present chapter are taken from the version reprinted in Victor Burgin et al. (eds.) (1986), *Formations of Fantasy*. See also Freud (1977a), 'Female sexuality'; Freud (1973), 'Femininity'; Horney (1926), 'The flight from womanhood'; Deutsch (1930), 'The significance of masochism in the mental life of women'.
2 Lacan (1977), 'The signification of the phallus'; Hendrik M. Ruitenbeek (ed.) (1966), *Psychoanalysis and Female Sexuality*.
3 An early example is Claire Johnston (1975), 'Femininity and the masquerade'.
4 For example, Mary Ann Doane's (1982) influential 'Film and the masquerade: theorising the female spectator', brought Riviere's article to the centre of feminist debate on cinema. Judith Butler (1990, pp. 50–54) set out a critique of Riviere's notion of masquerade in *Gender Trouble*. In Burgin et al. (eds) (1986), *Formations of Fantasy*, Riviere's article was reprinted and commented upon in relation to the instrumentality of fantasy in shaping mental life and cultural experience.
5 See also Athol Hughes (1991).
6 'Häupter in Hieroglyphenmützen/ Häupter in Turban und schwarzem Barett/ Perückenhäupter und tausend andre/Arme, schwitzende Menschenhäupter'.
7 The painting is in the collection of the Courtauld Gallery in London: see https://courtauld.ac.uk/gallery/collection/impressionism-post-impressionism/edouard-manet-a-bar-at-the-folies-bergere [accessed 29 July 2018].
8 The X-ray can be viewed online at https://courtauld.ac.uk/gallery/collection/impressionism-post-impressionism/edouard-manet-a-bar-at-the-folies-bergere [accessed 25 July 2018].
9 See, for example, Davidoff (1979) and Atkinson (2003).
10 Dawkins (1986), *Purloined Portraits*. Available online at https://e-artexte.ca/id/eprint/173/1/PurloinedPortraits.pdf [accessed 26 July 2018].

References

Appignanesi, L. and J. Forrester (1993) *Freud's Women*. London: Virago.
Atkinson, D. (2003) *Love and Dirt: The Marriage of Arthur Munby and Hannah Cullwick*. London: MacMillan.
Burgin, V., J. Donald and C. Kaplan (eds.) (1986) *Formations of Fantasy*. London: Methuen.
Butler, J. (1990) *Gender Trouble: Feminism and the Subversion of Identity*. New York: Routledge.
Davidoff, L. (1979) 'Class and gender in Victorian England: the diaries of Arthur J. Munby and Hannah Cullwick', *Feminist Studies* 5 (1), pp. 86–141.
Dawkins, H. (1986) *Purloined Portraits*. Halifax: The Art Gallery, Mount Saint Vincent University.
Deutsch, H. (1930) 'The significance of masochism in the mental life of women,' *International Journal of Psychoanalysis* 11, pp. 48–60.
Doane, M.A. (1982) 'Film and the masquerade: theorising the female spectator', *Screen* 23 (3–4), pp. 74–87.
Freud, S. (1973) 'Femininity', in J. Strachey and A. Richards (eds.), *Pelican Freud Library*, vol. 2. Harmondsworth: Penguin, pp. 145–169.
Freud, S. (1977a) 'Female sexuality', in A. Richards (ed.), *Pelican Freud Library*, vol. 7. Harmondsworth: Penguin, pp. 367–392.

Freud, S. (1977b) 'Fragment of an analysis of a case of hysteria', in A. Richards (ed.), *Pelican Freud Library,* vol. 8. Harmondsworth: Penguin.

Freud, S. (1985) 'Leonardo da Vinci and a memory of his childhood', in A. Richards (ed.), *Pelican Freud Library*, vol. 14. Harmondsworth: Penguin, pp. 151–231.

Heath, S. (1986) 'Joan Riviere and the masquerade', in V. Burgin, J. Donald and C. Kaplan (eds.), *Formations of Fantasy*, London: Methuen, pp. 45–61.

Horney, K. (1926) 'The flight from womanhood', *International Journal of Psychoanalysis* 7, pp. 324–339.

Hudson, D. (1974) *Munby: Man of Two Worlds*. London: Abacus.

Hughes, A. (1991) 'Joan Riviere: her life and work', in A. Hughes (ed.), *The Inner World and Joan Riviere: Collected Papers 1920–1958*. London: Karnac Books, pp. 1–43.

Johnston, C. (1975) 'Femininity and the masquerade: *Anne of the Indies*', in C. Johnston and P. Willemen (eds.), *Jacques Tourneur.* Edinburgh: Edinburgh Film Festival, pp. 36–44.

Jones, E. (1984) *The Life and Work of Sigmund Freud.* Harmondsworth: Penguin.

Lacan, J. (1977) 'The signification of the phallus', in *Ecrits: A Selection.* London: Tavistock Publications, pp. 281–291.

Pollock, G. (1995) 'The "view from elsewhere": extracts from a semi-public correspondence about the politics of feminist spectatorship', in P. Florence and D. Reynolds (eds.), *Feminist Subjects, Multi-media: Cultural Methodologies.* Manchester: Manchester University Press, pp. 2–38.

Riviere, J. (1929) 'Womanliness as a masquerade', *International Journal of Psychoanalysis* 10, pp. 303–313.

Riviere, J. (1986) 'Womanliness as a masquerade', in V. Burgin, J. Donald and C. Kaplan (eds.), *Formations of Fantasy.* London: Methuen, pp. 35–44.

Ruitenbeek, H.M. (ed.) (1966) *Psychoanalysis and Female Sexuality.* New Haven, CT: College and Universities Press.

Stanley, L. (ed.) (1984) *The Diaries of Hannah Cullwick, Victorian Maidservant.* New Brunswick, NJ: Rutgers University Press.

4 Feminism, Film, and Theory Now

Elizabeth Cowie

In these notes I explore current questions of feminism and femininity as well as subjectivity and film, drawing on my work over a number of years and in recently published essays. These notes are themed around the question of horror – the horrible – in an engagement with the groundbreaking study of the horror film by Barbara Creed. They address the seen and the heard – the gaze and the voice – in film and new media.

What has remained for me a central issue for film and feminist theory is the concept of the subject who is addressed. In the work of Michel Foucault and Gilles Deleuze the subject is posited as an effect of practices, while Actor–network theory describes and analyses not the cognising subject but the networks of relations arising between agents, human and non-human that produce a performativity of subjectivity as agency. The subject is an effect and not agent of these networks and discourses, indeed she is herself a 'network' of affect arising through her rhizomatic interaction with the world. Yet the subject is at the same time someone who laughs, or cries, and who desires. It is this subject and her desires that psychoanalysis attends to and which I continue to draw upon in thinking about moving images and sounds and photography. In our era of multiplying technological media forms of address and interaction the question then arises: what does the addressee want – desire – to hear, to see, to know or to not know? What does the addressor want – desire – of the other as a response to their address via Facebook, Twitter, Instagram, Tumbl, etcetera? And how is difference engaged, for the subject of address is always a subject in difference and subject to the difficulties of difference, of sexuality and gender, of class and wealth, of race and colour. Social media connects people, just as the letter in the post or the telephone has in the past, but now as a kind of 'conference call', in a performance of the self in the theatre of the accumulated photos, mementoes, and anecdotes of everyday life uploaded onto Facebook, or Instagram, which had always also been part of our postings to friends and family via mail – and even now continues in the round-up of ones activities over the year sent at Christmas. What is engaged is a being seen and known by the other – our friends and acquaintances – and what is different is the temporality of social media. A tap on a keyboard or phone instantly communicates to friends and groups online.

Bernard Stiegler has proposed that the relation of the human subject and the technical is co-originary, and that each tool or artefact is a form of memory of the consciousness that produced it, and thus can be re-examined. In his concept of the 'mnemo-technical system', he addresses the way in which in each epoch there is also a technology by which memory is exteriorised and is central to the way we adopt and adapt to new technology that introduces new knowledge and new ways of life. He argues that 'The concept of desire is the key to understanding the relation between economics and psychoanalysis, that is, between social and psychic investment, or between productive and libidinal economies' (2011, p. 150). In question here is not specific objects of desire, but 'desire' as a psychological category, and our embodied engagement with technology, for which scale, temporality and our embodied relation are central, hence for Stiegler, cinema is a key 'mnemotechnical system'. For it combines a technology as memory-machine while engaging the spectator as herself a 'memory machine', in 'the coincidence between the film's flow and that of the film spectator's consciousness, linked by phonographic flux, initiating the mechanics of a complete adoption of the film's time with that of the spectator's consciousness – which, since it is itself a flux, is captured and 'channelled' by the flow of images. This movement, infused with every spectator's desire for stories, liberates the movements of consciousness typical of cinematic *emotion* (Stiegler 2011, p. 12; italics in original).[1]

Christian Metz (1985, p. 81), writing on the differences between the photograph and cinema, addresses these in terms of the kinds of ways we engage with each form, as a socialised unit of reading, that is, the mode of reception or reading of works – in sculpture the scale, material, and siting of works, in music the performance heard and setting, and 'the photograph, a silent rectangle of paper ... much smaller than the cinematic lexis'. Scale of image, the presence of sounds, speech and music, of duration – and thus temporality, as well as mode of engagement – holding a photo, or visiting a cinema, all distinguish photography from film and video. For new media and the internet, what comes into play is interactivity, and our tactile relation to the mobile phone, computer, lap top or iPad or tablet, access – like a book, or photograph – anywhere and anytime. These new forms of social interaction, with new limitations on that interaction, open new ways to fantasy, to narratives of the self and others that are addressed to a fantasmatic audience of interlocutors. They also engage us in new ways of remembering, as Stiegler notes, and which Sigfried Kracauer (1947) had explored in relation to photography that in the 1910s and 1920s was seen by many to be a threat to memory, and remembering.[2]

Following Laura Mulvey's (1975) groundbreaking essay, 'Visual Pleasure and Narrative Pleasure', the gaze has been a central focus of analyses of film, media, and new technology. While most certainly there are power relations involved in who holds the gaze, and whose look is dominant in the cinematic narrative, these cannot be simply reversed in gender terms because of wider social assumptions that still obtain regarding the power of the male look. What I have been concerned to address is not simply the look as such but the look of the represented or imagined other, the look back. Andrea Mubi Brighenti (2010, p. 185) suggests that through 'the uncanny fact that in some way, through the technological setup, the object stares back.... It is a feeling of Unheimlichkeit, which questions the changing boundaries of the human itself within complex socio-technical assemblages'.[3] For Slavoj Žižek (1994, p. 194), 'Specters belong to the Real, they are the price we pay for the gap that separates reality from the Real'.[4] It is a gap arising as well in relation to the voice such that, he suggests, it too is spectral:

> An unbridgeable gap separates forever a human body from "its" voice. The voice displays a spectral autonomy, it never quite belongs to the body we see, so that even when we see a living person talking, there is always a minimum of ventriloquism at work: it is as if the speaker's own voice hollows him out and in a sense speaks "by itself", through him.
>
> (Žižek 2001, p. 58)

Dolar (2006, p. 70), drawing on Žižek, goes on to argue that,

> Ventriloquism pertains to voice as such, to its inherently acousmatic character: the voice comes from inside the body, the belly, the stomach – from something incompatible with and irreducible to the activity of the mouth. The fact that we see the aperture does not demystify the voice: on the contrary, it enhances the enigma.[5]

Dolar explores the voice not only as a vehicle of meaning or as a source of aesthetic admiration, but also as an object cause of desire, in the sense that Jacques Lacan gives this, drawing on Freud, of the little object other, *objet petit a,* that, Dolar suggests, can be seen as the lever of thought for the subject who speaks. For to speak is first of all to desire to be heard by an other, to engage an encounter with an other. The voice itself, however, *is what does not contribute to making sense.* It is the material element recalcitrant to meaning, and if we speak in order to say something, then the voice is precisely that which cannot be said' (Dolar 2006, p. 15; italics in original). And, *it is precisely the voice that holds bodies and language together* (ibid., p. 60; italics in original).

Derrida (1973, p. 85), too, posits a gap that language institutes,

> this pure difference, which constitutes the self-presence of the living present, introduces into self-presence from the beginning all the impurity putatively excluded from it. The living present springs forth out of its nonidentity with itself and from the possibility of a retentional trace. It is always already a trace.

This is a subject divided, as the one who speaks, but who also hears her own words as if another's. Žižek (1996, p. 90) emphasises that 'gaze and voice are *objects*, that is, they do not belong on the side of the looking/seeing subject but on the side of what the subject sees or hears'. Moreover, Alice Lagaay (2008, p. 59) notes, 'it is not a particular person's gaze, and not a particular sounding voice, that these objects refer to. Instead, gaze and voice have a quasi-fundamental status in Lacan's theory insofar as they refer to the fundamental relation from outside (the other) to inside (the self), which in constituting the subject at the same time defines it as lack'.[6]

What then of sexual difference? Difference is heard in the first words introducing the new-born baby, 'it's a boy' or 'it's a girl', instituting difference as performance for another that realises, or not, that first invocation of sexual difference. It was Sigmund Freud who placed sexuality as a central term in understanding the human mind, and it was also Freud who displaced it as a unified phenomenon, instead proposing a polymorphous sexuality, and arguing that it is the drive and desire, and not instinct, that is central to sexuality, while sexuality is but one aspect of human desire. Lacan, in his rethinking of Freud, further emphasises that we are formed psychically through our relations to others and the desire of the other. With his concept of the *objet petit a* as cause of desire Lacan posits the human subject as a subject of lack, not of the object lost but of the lostness of the object, such that every replacement object nevertheless signifies that 'lostness'.[7] Lacan (2006, p. 147) famously insisted that *Il n'y a pas de rapport sexuel* 'there is no sexual relationship'; instead there is the possibility of love.[8]

In Lacan's (2016, p. 68) late Seminar XXIII, *The Sinthome,* the consequences for the subject that the sexual relation does not exist are explored in relation to the psychoanalytic concept of the symptom. Lacan uses the term sinthome to mark a difference in the psychical formation of the symptom in that the sinthome, unlike the symptom, involves a creative process that upholds the consistency of reality for a subject, 'knotting' the Real, the Imaginary and the Symbolic through an identification with one's symptom. The symptom, as Žižek (1991, p. 207) notes, is a particular pathological signifying formation in the unconscious which enjoys, resisting interpretation, 'a stain which cannot be included into the circuit of discourse, of social bond/network', that is the Symbolic, 'but which is at the same time a positive condition of it'. Identifying with one's sinthome is a way of managing one's symptom, of managing that which intrudes upon, and defines one. Lacan develops this concept subject through an exploration of the writings of James Joyce and he not only develops his conceptualisation of the Real but also addresses how art – the artifices of art – might be engaged through the symptom in relation to Joyce's writing, while at the same time Lacan complicates the role of the phallus and The-Name-of-the-Father. As a result, Lacanian analyst Geneviève Morel

(2005, p. xvi) suggests that Lacan's theory of the symptom 'allows us to think the relations between the sexes and the generations without necessarily referring to the Name-of-the-Father nor to the phallus, as transcendent norms of a symbolic order'. While Paul Verhaeghe and Frédéric Declercq (2002, p. 76) refer to the sinthome as, 'a particular process that is situated entirely in the line of femininity'.[9] For what Lacan introduces through this term is the subject's individuation without the phallic signifier. I see this, however, not as a 'feminine way' (op. cit., p. 59), but rather as other or as indifferent to the sexual difference that is posited by the Symbolic order, namely as Lacan (1993, p. 171) asserts: 'The subject's sexual position.... is tied to the symbolic apparatus'. For Lacan there is no feminine outside language because, as Jacqueline Rose (1982, p. 55) notes, first 'the unconscious severs the subject from any unmediated relation to the body as such ... and secondly because the "feminine" is constituted in a division in language'. Yet difference is present, as Lacan argues in *Seminar XXIV,* 'the Other with a capital O that is at stake in the unconscious. I do not see how one could give a sense to the unconscious, except by situating it in this Other, the bearer of signifiers'. This Other, which is also the m/Other, introduces the Real of lack in that it desires. The naming and names of sexual difference both institutes and attempts to assuage this lack, and it is the symptom that, for the subject, attests to the failure of such naming – of woman, or man, and the object choices of the other sex, or the same sex. For Lacan, the concept of the sinthome as knotting the Real, Symbolic and the Imaginary is a naming of one's Real, one's lacking, that is, it seems, indifferent to sexual difference. I speculate that what we name as our sexual difference is itself a sinthome. In one sense both Freud and Lacan have queered sexuality, in making it 'strange', and in terms of contemporary queer politics.

It is the namings of sexual difference and their imagining that Barbara Creed (1993) addresses in her groundbreaking study, *The Monstrous-Feminine.* She argues that the horror film, 'is populated by female monsters, many of which seem to have evolved from images that haunted dreams, myths and artistic practices of our forebears' for, as she notes, 'All human societies have a conception of the monstrous-feminine, of what it is about woman that is shocking, terrifying, horrific, abject' (Creed 1993, p. 1) She uses the term 'monstrous-feminine' because

> the term "female monster" implies a simple reversal of "male monster". The reasons why the monstrous feminine horrifies her audience are quite different from the reasons why the male monster horrifies his audience. A new term is needed to specify these differences. As with all other stereotypes of the feminine, from virgin to whore, she is defined in terms of her sexuality. The phrase "monstrous feminine" emphasises the importance of gender in the construction of her monstrosity. (Creed 1993, p. 3)

In the subtitle of her book – 'Film, Feminism, Psychoanalysis' – Creed poses psychoanalysis as the theoretical space in which to explore the question of the monstrous-feminine in film, at the same time as she introduces the question of the politics of sexual difference and its representation. She suggests,

> It may be that the horror genre is more directly responsive to questions of sexual difference, more willing to explore male and female anxieties about the "other", than film texts which belong to mainstream genres such as the detective, suspense thriller, comedy and romance films.
>
> (Creed 1993, p. 152)

For me the feminist claim of the 1970s that 'the personal is political' addressed what it is to experience being a woman and its anxieties, that is, the shaping of our experience through norms of representation – images of women – in society as a product of 'patriarchal ideology'. Laura Mulvey (1973) analysed the gaze of patriarchy that forms and deforms the feminine for masculine pleasure and control, noting later in 1978 that 'Patriarchal ideology is made up of assumptions, "truths" about the meaning of sexual difference, women's place in society, the mystery of femininity and so on ... However, ideology – whether bourgeois or patriarchal – is not a blanket-like or eternal totality and it is crucial for feminists to be aware of contradictions within it' (Mulvey [1978] 1989, p. 121; Cowie 2015c).

It is the work of Michel Foucault – which was a central focus of the journal *m/f* that I was co-founder and co-editor of 1976–1986 – that offered a new understanding of our discursive construction and the politics of representation as not simply that of a patriarchy controlling our images but more complexly as the discursive ordering that figures daughter, sister, girl, woman, mother, wife, femme fatale, whore, harridan, crone, and which names how we should be. Here it is not a question of equality, or of an injustice that could be righted, but of how we learn, or not, to be 'a woman', 'feminine', or a 'mother' in relation to an other in a field of possibilities in which our biology is only one element. The politics of feminism relates not to a unified subject, a singular identity of woman, nor is it simply plural; it is a distributed subjectivity in process. We are 'hailed' (Althusser 1971), for example, as a daughter or we enact 'hailing' as a mother: 'be tidy/good/pretty'. Judith Butler, in her concept of gender performance, draws on Foucault's work in her rejection of gender as an essential difference. Further, she uses Friedrich Nietzsche's (1969, p. 45) claim in *On the Genealogy of Morals* that 'there is no "being" [or "I"] behind doing, effecting, becoming; "the doer" is merely a fiction added to the deed – the deed is everything', when she argues: 'There is no gender identity behind the expressions of gender; that identity is performatively constituted by the very "expressions" that are said to be its results' (Butler 1990, p. 25).[10] What is not addressed by Butler is the way our performance is for another, and how our sense of ourselves that we call our 'identity' is experienced performatively through our relation to others, and how others bring to us ways of knowing ourselves through interactions that are figured through a desire to be for the other, to be the other's desire. The question is then, how to be in the world as a body that is 'female'? That is, how to perform for the gaze of others by which we know and tell others 'who I am' as a person who is a 'woman', which may be as lesbian or heterosexual, or transgender. Yet we are formed as much by our resistance as by our acquiescence to the constructions our affective relations give rise to.

This is equally the case in relation to our political subjectivisation which is also, Jacques Rancière (1992, p. 62) argues, 'a logic of the other', because 'it is never the simple assertion of an identity; it is always, at the same time, the denial of an identity given by an other'. Rancière calls this a heterology, namely, a lack of correspondence between apparently similar bodily parts due to differences in fundamental makeup or origin. He argues that subjectivisation is also 'a demonstration, and a demonstration always supposes an other' (p. 62). Even if that other refuses the demonstration, what is established is a 'polemical commonplace' for addressing the 'wrong' of difference. Rancière asserts that, 'the logic of subjectivisation always entails an impossible identification' (p. 62).

Feminism is a politics of sexual difference and, drawing on the work of Rancière, I want to characterise the politics of feminism as one which is not simply a struggle for power or rights or equality but, rather, an engagement with the political whereby, as Rancière (2004, p. 13) proposes, 'politics revolves around what is seen and what can be said about it, around who has the ability to see and the talent to speak, around the properties of spaces and the possibilities of time'. It 'consists in refiguring space, that is, in what is to be done, to be seen and to be named in it. It is the instituting of a dispute over the distribution of the sensible' (Rancière 2010a, p. 37). Feminism is such a dispute about the norms of sexual division and difference, of who can speak, and who can act within the social. It is also an ethos in relation to living, that is, in a dwelling, in a being and a doing as a woman. Rancière posits man, or woman, or citizen as 'political subjects' not 'definite collectivities':

> They are surplus names, names that set out a question or a dispute (*litige)* about who is included in their count. Correspondingly, *freedom* and *equality* are not predicates belonging to definite subjects. Political predicates are open predicates: they open up a dispute about what they exactly entail and whom they concern in which cases.
>
> (Rancière 2004, p. 303)

For Rancière (2004, p. 309), what is central is not ethics but politics:

> Ethics is indeed on our agendas. Some people see it as a return to some founding spirit of the community, sustaining positive laws and political agency. I take a fairly different view of this new reign of ethics. It means to me the erasure of all legal distinctions and the closure of all political intervals of dissensus. Both are erased in the infinite conflict of Good and Evil.

The current focus on equality of pay and opportunity in Hollywood and in film and television production more widely, as well as the issues of sexual harassment and the Me Too movement is the constitution of a dispute in Rancière's sense. It is a challenge to the lack of women behind the camera, as directors, writers, directors of photography, sound, as well as the lack of women in film, not only as central characters but even as extras in scenes.[11] The inclusion of women does not just even things up with men, however, but more importantly it opens up opportunities for film-makers and audiences that can also be challenges to think ourselves within these stories as agents in the world and in our relationships to others.

Feminism is also an aesthetic project in relation to the understanding of, and intervening in, the representation of woman and her imagining, her difference, and practices of art are political not because they promote political awareness or provoke political actions but insofar as, Rancière (2010a, p. 149) writes, 'they contribute to the constitution of a form of common sense that is "polemical", to a new landscape of the visible, the sayable and the doable'. Feminist politics, therefore, involves not only disputing existing canons of film or literature, and challenging norms of representation, but also in posing the difficulties of difference and desire for women (and men) as social beings and exposing the contradictions of 'femininity', of motherhood and gender, in the production and circulation of images of women.

Rancière (2004, p. 38) argues that, 'The real must be fictionalised to be thought', and the '"fictions" of art and politics are heterotopias' (p. 41) that introduce dissensus, 'the "heteron" or the "other": the other as the effect of a reconfiguration of the distribution of places, identities, and capacities' (2010b, p. 21).[12] Rancière here draws on Lacan's conceptualisation of the Real as the unrepresentable that haunts the subject. Dissensus for Rancière (2010a, p. 38) names the process of a fissuring of the sensible order made possible not by a perception of a new 'fact' but by the perception of an incompleteness, 'a gap in the sensible itself'.[13] The political effect of films arises not through the words or actions of their participants, or as a knowledge that seeks to persuade. Rather, as Rancière (2009, p. 72) argues, it arises through 'a multiplicity of folds and gaps in the fabric of common experience that change the cartography of the perceptible, the thinkable and the feasible'. The folds entwine elements that are incommensurable, disturbing the commonsense of the knowable – the 'distributed sensible' of sexual difference – that bears on how one looks and how one is engaged by an art work, thus producing a gap in knowledgeability. This is the 'good' of my affectual experience, and it is feminist in engaging the viewer in her or his difference. It is a politics, a dissensus.

We experience film, and art, cognitively as affect as well as the thought, and here I turn to the question that Sigfried Kracauer (1960, p. 285) posed in *Theory of Film,* 'which is the most central of all: what is the good of our experience of film?' The 'good' is how film engages us in our dwelling, being and doing, namely to social and thus the political. Kracauer (p. 308) goes on to argue that,

> much as the images of material moments are meaningful in their own right, we actually do not confine ourselves to absorbing them but feel stimulated to weave what they are telling us into contexts that bear on the whole of our existence.

Kracauer (p. 305) also notes that,

> In acquainting us with the world we live in, the cinema exhibits phenomena whose appearance in the witness stand is of particular consequence. It brings us face to face with the things we dread. And it often challenges us to confront the real-life events it shows with the ideas we commonly entertain about them.

Philosopher Stanley Cavell (1979, p. 419) writes that,

> Horror is the title I am giving to the perception of the precariousness of human identity, to the perception that it may be lost or invaded, that we may be, or may become, something other than we are, or take ourselves for; that our origins as human beings need accounting for, and are unaccountable.

Here is the underbelly of affect, those states we term fear or terror, horror and anxiety that are engaged through performance art, photography, and film. How are these feelings reconciled or repudiated? Can images be too disturbing? What is the relation of Cavell's horror to anxiety, trauma, and mourning, and to the other represented?

Kracauer's question, 'what is of the good of our experience?' poses not only a question about our evaluation of what we have experienced as art – image, sound, film, or video – but also the experience itself and the temporal and emotional relation between affect that gives rise to thought as an understanding that is also an interpretation, and affect as a 'felt' that arises with thought, but which we might think of as ostensibly independent of thought. Affects are our experiences of the world, how we are touched by the world, viscerally as hot or cold, or fainting at the sight of blood, but also as we are touched by the coldness of a stare or the warmth of a gaze that we receive. Affect is the mind caught by the scene, both sound and image, experienced in the body. For sympathy often leads us to turn away from the abjection of the other in a horror which is disavowed. Affect is not singular, it is a process in time whereby feelings are continuous with one another, interpenetrate one another, and may even be opposed to one another. It is not a question of ethical 'thought', but of 'being', in an experiencing that becomes an action of felt being, for example in an identification – 'that could be me' – giving rise to empathy for another or of anxiety at the very thought – 'that could be me'. Or the felt being experienced as anger – against those others who drive badly, or do not pick up litter, or take our jobs or who in other myriad ways may prevent me enjoying/being. It is this complexity that Henri Bergson (2002, p. 73) describes when he notes: 'We instinctively tend to solidify our impressions in order to express them in language, hence we confuse the feeling itself, which is in a perpetual state of becoming, with its permanent external object, and especially with the word which expresses this object'. We actualise our responses, as 'this', and then as another 'this'.[14]

Vikki Bell (2008) writing about Andrew Jarecki's documentary film, *Capturing the Friedmans* (Dir. Andrew Jarecki, USA, 2003) draws on Gilles Deleuze and Félix Guattari (1994, p. 175) who write that artists are 'presenters of affects, the inventors and creators of affects. They not only create them in their work, they give them to us and make us become with them, they draw us into the compound'. The work of art is 'a being of sensation and nothing else' (p. 164). Bell (2008, p. 100) concludes: 'what is unsettling about this particular film is that, as viewers, we are also captured in the cinema assemblage in terms of its percepts and affects.... And if it makes one feel uncomfortable, the burden of that sensation is also a movement and in itself an ethics; having looked at this picture/film, who – or more properly the question, for all the reasons I have argued here, is how – do we become?'

The debates and different concepts of 'affect' are themselves a symptom of the complex issues – and politics – surrounding the concept of affect in cognitive theory, in philosophy and ethics, but with which psychoanalysis is much more comfortable. The felt which is not immediately subsumed to knowledge is the sublime of the eighteenth-century writers and later romantics – a wonder, an awe, a terror, a sudden upwelling of tears, or laughter, and thus of the unconscious. It is the felt of the 'real', Lacan's term for the felt that is unrepresentable, unsymbolisable. This is not the 'unrepresentable' in art of Theodor Adorno, which Rancière (2010a, p. 195) argues conflates impossibility and interdiction.

Instead Rancière posits the unrepresentability of trauma, drawing on Lacan's discussion of Sophicle's play Antigone, which replaces Oedipus in Freud's thinking as a new form of secret,

> one that is irreducible to any salvational knowledge. There is neither beginning nor end to the trauma encapsulated in Antigone. The tragedy bespeaks the discontent of a civilization in which the laws of social order are undermined by the very things that support them.

Which are the powers of affiliation. Rancière (2010a, p. 187) argues that for Lacan, Antigone 'is not the heroine of human rights created by modern democratic piety. Instead she is the terrorist, the witness of the secret terror that underlies the social order. Terror is precisely the name that trauma takes in political matters'. If, in the play by Sophocles, Antigone is monstrous then perhaps the monstrous woman of the horror film, too, is a terrorist.

What role might the art work play in relation to the traumatic remembered? What I suggest is that the anxiety – horror – of the art work as traumatic does not involve a remembering of a past trauma as a kind of recovery of an experience. It is the experience and as such may produce a remembering, as *Nachträglichkeit*, or, as psychoanalyst Jean Laplanche (1999, p. 165) terms it, 'afterwardsness',[15] which haunts the subject but which can become translated, symbolisable, enabling us to move beyond imaginary captivation. This symbolisation, however, bears the trace of the Real thereby rendering it into the reality of its sounds and images. The art work, too, enables the apprehension of the Real in dreadful anxiety without losing oneself as a subject, through a form of sublimation in which one confronts, but is not overwhelmed by, the limits of one's existence.[16] This is not a matter of rational explanation, yet the processes of thought here are not without reason, that is, of cause and effect, such that, moreover, they produce purposive action and understanding on the part of the subject. The art work confronts us, therefore, in a way which opens us psychically – like the joke! – as Freud (1905/1960: p. 161, 165) argues, to a repressed wish better understood through Lacan's concept of the Real, which is not sublimated in or through the art object, or the images and sounds, but rests in us. Not 'as if' but 'as me'.

But what of fear, and fear of the horrible? For Lacan, the anxiety that exceeds reasonable fear 'is not a symbolic phenomenon, but is situated at the border of the imaginary and the real' (Shepherdson 2013, p. lx). Trauma is a symptom of the Real, it is not a simply past event, it is 'the experience you are awaiting' (Hernandez 1998, p. 139),[17] namely, an annihilation. It is not the infraction – the wound – as such but the possible *future* wound that will destroy, just as *this* wound might have; it is the unrepresentable of anxiety, whereby the subject herself or himself is placed as lack, as *objet petit a*, in relation to the desire of the Other that the subject desires.[18] Lacan (Harari 2001, p. 108) refers to Georg Wilhelm Friedrich Hegel's classic dialectic between the master and the slave, developed in the *Phenomenology of Spirit*, in which desire is for recognition – the desire of desire, to 'be' for the Other. Yet, in this, I become the object of the Other's desire in a recognition that thereby denies me the subjectivity I desire in desiring the Other's desire. Lacan identifies a fundamental asymmetry here, as the result of which a reciprocity of recognition is impossible. Instead, he argues, what I seek in desiring the Other's desire is to find myself in the other, in which I thereby also seek the Other's loss. The reverse is thus that what the Other seeks, desires, in desiring me is to find itself in me, 'for which it solicits my loss' (Harari 2001, p. 108). In desiring the desire of the Other, I confront the Other's desire, which Lacan (1979, p. 263) characterises as 'I love you but, because inexplicably I love in you something more than you – the *objet petit a* – I mutilate you'.

Georges Franju writes of his film, *Eyes without a Face* [*Les Yeux sans visage*] (Dir. Georges Franju, France, 1960), 'It's an anguish film. It's a quieter mood than horror, something more subjacent, more internal, more penetrating. It's horror in homeopathic doses' (Quoted in Durgnat 1967, p. 83). Franju's comments on *Eyes Without a Face* suggest an approach to horror that, perhaps not coincidentally, closely relates to Lacan's view of anxiety:

> In my experience, it is necessary to canalise it [anxiety] and, if I may say so, to take it in small doses, so that one is not overcome by it. This is similar to bringing the subject into contact with the real'. Homeopathy – established on the principle of 'Let likes cure likes' – seeks to heal through the similar, prescribing a remedy that will *cause* the symptom in a healthy person, and thus in the ill body stimulate it to restore itself to health. Yet for psychoanalysis this cannot be a form of inoculation against or resistance to anxiety, or the real, as if it were a pathogen, which could be removed. The experiencing of "small doses" must, rather, bring about some accommodation with the real of anxiety, circumscribing anxiety so that it no longer floods the subject or defines every encounter with others in everyday reality as always being in the service of the *jouissance* of the Other.
> (Lacan 1979, p. 41)

Indeed, this film was my own encounter with the horrific that I wanted to look away from. But while the horrible evokes visceral revulsion it is not simply the body torn, but rather it arises from an identification, of my own body torn, for certain stories and images don't go away when you stop looking. The horror film's monstrous figures of abjection and scenes of terrifying destruction and chaos, by engaging us in a compulsive return to look, to watch, to know what we dread, snare us in the uncanny, and in the pleasure/unpleasure of repetition.[19] That is, they snare us in the repeated re-encounter of the *jouissance* of the Other, which I serve insofar as I find my enjoyment, my *jouissance*, in the desire of the Other, and resist by attempting to master the Other – to abject her.[20] Rather, what is necessary is a re-figuring of my relation to the desiring Other through symbolisation and not as *jouissance*. The unique role of the horror film here is not its symbolisations as such, but its enjoining the spectator to symbolise. Public performances of horror address us as both traumatic and as symbolising, translated. Both its compulsive attraction and its ethical dimension lie in this double role of horror. That we can find the fictitious terrors of the horror film traumatic testifies not to the success of its illusionism – its 'realism' – nor to the humanist truths of its fabrications, but to the appearance of the uncanny Real that is never either reality or fiction.

Where my discussion in my essay 'The Lived Nightmare: Trauma, Anxiety, and the Ethical Aesthetics of Horror' (Cowie 2003) focussed on anxiety, I now want to draw upon the idea of 'ravage' in Lacan and the monstrous feminine. In his seminar on *The Sinthome*, Lacan (2016, p. 107) speaks of being 'stupefied' on seeing Nagisa Oshima's *In the Realm of the Senses* [*Ai no korīda*] (Dir. Nagisa Oshima, Japan/France, 1976), because 'it was feminine eroticism', and that 'In it feminine eroticism ... seems to be carried to its extremes'. Lacan suggests that 'this extreme is the fantasy, no more or less, of killing the man. But even that does not suffice. Having killed him, she goes further still. Afterwards – why after?'.[21]

The film is based on a real event in Tokyo reported by newspapers in 1936 – recounted by Oshima's voice-over at the end of the film – of a woman named Sado found after wandering through Tokyo for several days with a man's penis inside her. Lacan (2016, p. 107) comments that 'We all know it's a fantasy', but a fantasy of what is less clear to him, for he suggests that there 'is a shade of what I just now called doubt. This is where one can clearly see that castration is not the fantasy'. He does not explore this further but says that, 'As for what the woman fantasises, if this is really what the film presents us with, it is something that, either way, impedes the encounter' (p. 108).

Philosopher Jean-Luc Nancy (2008, p. 2), writing on *Trouble Every Day* (Dir. Claire Denis, France/Germany/Japan, 2001), is equally visceral in writing about the film's fatal carnality, arguing that,

> We must understand that the bite of the kiss here, devours the sexes (their organs), not by castration, but by an absorption which opens on to a kind of horrific sublimation: not that of sex in which a body takes pleasure, but that of an entire body in which sex bursts out and is spattered with the body's blood, with its life/death and with that which explodes it: that which exposes it in splashes, drops, streams

> and stains, clots and ribbons that will never again be restored to a form. We might say that the film's entire story is the allegory, and its entire image the literality of this: the unbearable tearing apart of orgasm.

Both these films centre a fatal – indeed monstrous – woman, each of whom realise Lacan's (1979, p. 263) aphorism: 'I love you but, because inexplicably I love in you something more than you – the *objet petit a* – I mutilate you'. While Lacan is 'stupified', and foregrounds the issue of feminine desire, Nancy declares 'This film is shattering', just as 'Ecstasy shatters the image of itself (the image of self and the proper image of ecstasy)', the film shuts 'out the gaze by opening it onto a wound, a bite mark'. While Nancy does not address the obsession of the film's murderess, Coré, or that of Dr Shane Brown, in terms of their difference, Douglas Morrey (2008, p. 18), in his essay 'Open Wounds: Body and Image in Jean-Luc Nancy and Claire Denis' does when he asserts 'If Coré's kill shows sex as killing, Shane's murder of the hotel chambermaid, Christelle, presents killing as sex'. Morrey (p. 16) comments that, 'A body never penetrates or opens up another, wrote Nancy (2006, p. 27) in *Corpus, except in murder.* But in his text on Denis's *Trouble Every Day,* this comes across as the truth of desire'. And it is a truth that is, nevertheless, marked by sexual difference.

Shane had been obsessed by Coré some years before his return to Paris with his newly married wife, and he now seeks Coré out. She has been imprisoned by her husband (a former colleague) to prevent her murdering further men, and when he finds her she is in the sexual act with a young male intruder she is gorging, and as she turns to him, he strangles her as she moves to bite him. The house is then enveloped in flames. Unable or unwilling to realise sexual relations with his wife earlier – we see him frantically masturbating in the hotel bathroom after failing to consummate lovemaking with his wife – the vampiric desire suggested in the kiss she receives from him on their plane to Paris is realised when, after killing Coré, he first seduces then rapes a maid before biting her to death, starting with her sexual organs.

What might it mean to view each film as a feminist horror film? Certainly each is a 'splatter' movie, with grisly scenes of blood and organs spilt, and each presents awful sexual violence, while centring a woman and addressing us with her story, her desire, and the puzzle of her identity, thereby raising issues of feminist politics. For each film complicates how we can make her the object of our gaze, of our desire to know her, to fix her identity, or to be or to have her. It is thereby engaging us affectually through the ways that we encounter her desire in the film, as well as that of the men for whom she is an object of desire. And each film is feminist in engaging the viewer in her or his difference in the sense I suggested earlier, whereby the folds of cinematic expression entwine elements that are incommensurable, disturbing the common sense of the knowable – the 'distributed sensible' of sexual difference – that bears on how one looks and how one is engaged by an art work, thus producing a gap in knowledgeability.

In *In the Realm of the Senses*, which relates a true incident, Kichi's submission to Sada's demands, and her ecstasy when she playfully, but finally mortally, gently strangles him with a cord, disturbs, and delights. *Trouble Every Day*, however, poses sexual ecstasy as death in the context of a risible plot – noted by many reviewers as incomprehensible – that centres on a brain disorder arising from the research Shane (who is employed by a pharmaceutical firm) and Coré's husband had been working on together in South America that a former colleague Shane meets in Paris accuses Shane of stealing. But such a possible rational explanation is left shadowy in contrast to the ecstasy of vampirism. Sada and Coré each ravage their lovers, destroying as they enjoy him sexually in a ravishment, and this is their 'monstrousness'. In both English and French, the two terms overlap in their meanings. The adjective ravishing comes from the verb ravish, which is from the Latin word *rapere*, meaning to seize, as a verb, either to seize and take away by violence, to be raped; or to overcome with emotion (such as joy or delight), ravished by the scenic beauty. Ravage also derives from *rapere*, taking the first meaning, to be plundered, laid waste. And it is ravage that is the term Lacan uses in relation to a feminine jouissance that is not erotic – phallic pleasure, and not subject to the Name-of-the-Father, instead ravage has to do with the death drive.[22] It is this ravishing ravage that I suggest is also in play for each woman in these two films. And it is ravage that engages us in the horror of the horror film.

Central to Barbara Creed's discussion of horror is Julia Kristeva's theory of abjection, which, Creed (1993, p. 14) writes, 'provides us with an important theoretical framework for analysing, in the horror film, the representation of the monstrous-feminine, in relation woman's reproductive and mothering functions. However, abjection by its very nature is ambiguous; it both repels and attracts'. The abject, as explored by Kristeva (1982) in her book, *Powers of Horror*, in its literary and metaphorical appearances, has been a compelling concept and account for discussions of the horror film, articulating the fascination as well as the horror of the abject. The abject, or abjection, refers to two distinct phenomena for Kristeva. The first is the act of abjection in which the subject separates itself from the object and thereby designates it as abject, the 'horrible', thus also instituting a distinction of inside/outside but where what is put outside is abjured, evicted, and effaced. Yet in this process of abjecting, the abject retains a dreadful fascination. The second is the state of abjection, of being the lost, abjected, reviled object.

Where abjection is the experience of borders disrupted, unsettled, made disturbingly permeable, ravage is the perpetrator of abjection.

While Kristeva emphasises the body as surfaces and drives, Lacan's concept of the Real addresses the emergence of the child as a subject in language in his triad of Real, Imaginary and Symbolic. The Real is the unrepresentable, the felt but unnamed of the body that is experienced psychically. It is our terror of the Real, the taint of which always remains attached to the *objet a*, not the projections of the abject, that is central for understanding the unpleasures and pleasures of horror. For both Lacan and Kristeva, the maternal is linked to the experiencing of ravage and/as abjection for men and women. Lacan (1973, p. 21) refers to, 'the ravage that in a woman is her relation to her mother' where it is the child who is abject, who is 'laid waste' by the mother. Kristeva (1982, p. 5) writes of this as the abjection of the self,

> If it be true that the abject simultaneously beseeches and pulverizes the subject, one can understand that it is experienced at the peak of its strength when that subject, weary of fruitless attempts to identify with something on the outside, finds the impossible within; when it finds that the impossible constitutes its very *being*, that it *is* nothing other than abject (italics in original).

For Lacan (1998, p. 271), it is not the mother's body, but her desire that is central to the experience of ravage,

> the subject's primary dependency in reference to the Other's desire .... Here is what is being inscribed in the structure through the subject's history: the fortunes and misadventures of the constitution of this desire as subjected to the law of the Other's desire.

Lacan rephrases the question of the primary relation to the mother as one where, for the subject,

> what matters is to finally acknowledge – with reference to what is an x of desire in the mother, that which made it possible to become or not become the one who responds to it, to become or not become the desired being.

Hence the question that Lacan places in the foreground of the psychoanalytic experience: what does the (m)Other want from me?

It is not only the mother that effects ravage for the woman (and indeed for the man) however, for Lacan (2016, p. 84) writes of the sexual relation, 'If a woman is a sinthome for any man, it's quite clear that another name needs to be found for what's involved in man for a woman, since the sinthome is characterised precisely by non-equivalence. One can say that for a woman, man is anything you please, specifically an affliction that is worse than a sinthome. A ravage, even'. The sinthome knots the

Real, imaginary and symbolic registers, while ravage exposes the subject to the Real, to horror, to the death drive.

In each film desire, and sexual ecstasy, is also deathly for the other of the woman's desire. Sada and Coré each realise Lacan's (1979, p. 263) verdict on desire, that in desiring the other they nevertheless want something more than the other – the *objet petit a* – and thus mutilate, indeed destroy, the other of their desire. It is the spectator's journey with Sada and Coré that engages her with the symptom, the ravage, articulated by each character's story and imaged by each film. Oshima prefaces *In the Realm of the Senses* with a shot from the end of the film of Sada lying down, gazing out off screen to a space that is, in effect, that of the spectator, and repeated as the film's final shot, but now we see, traced in red – the blood of Kichi's severed genitals – the words 'Sada, Kichi together the two of us only', while Oshima's voice-over relates the aftermath, as reported in the news, of Sada found wandering in Tokyo with his penis. Coré, too, narrates her symptom in her victim's blood – through her paintings on the wall of her room. Each film engages us in a cinematically narrated ecstasy that is also deathly, posing the question of desire and the fatal implications of desire and difference enacted through the symptom.

Stephen Heath (1981, p. 160) argues what is at stake *In the Realm of the Senses* is, 'throughout, that is, evidently (but with great difficulty) the whole problem of representation and sexual difference in cinema'. This is no less true for *Trouble Every Day*, where Shane's devouring of the maid is off-screen, unlike the graphic image of Coré's ecstasy, and instead Denis' camera simply gives us the woman's transformation from ecstasy to agony. At the end of the film, Shane is washing away his victim's blood in the shower, when his wife appears and asks: are you happy? He replies that yes, he's happy, and that he's now ready to go home, as the camera shows her noticing watery blood on the shower. While Coré dies, immolated in flames, Shane returns home with the 'happiness' that he's found from their visit to Paris, that is, a pleasure, the nature of which remains ambiguous.

Each film incites and excites, requiring the spectator to manage the folds of audio-visual representation entwining elements that are incommensurable, that disturb the commonsense of the knowable – the 'distributed sensible' of sexual difference – that bears on how one looks and how one is engaged by an art work, producing a gap in knowledgeability that is the Real, namely the possibilities and impossibilities of what we call sexual difference in relation to the deathly ecstasies of passion.

My thanks to Nicholas Chare for all his help with this article, and to the editors of the journals and books in which my articles that I quote from were published. In each case their comments and support have been invaluable.

Notes

1 On Stiegler and film, see Roberts (2006) and Stiegler (1998).
2 On this, see Kracauer (1947). Also, Leslie (2010).
3 I explored this further in 'The World Viewed: Documentary Observing and the Culture of Surveillance' (Cowie 2015a).
4 Jacques Derrida observes in the film *Ghost Dance* (Dir. Ken McMullen, UK/West Germany, 1983) that 'A specter is ... a trace that marks the present with its absence in advance. The spectral logic is de facto a deconstructive logic ... Film plus psychoanalysis equals a science of ghosts ... a trace that marks the present with its absence in advance'.
5 I discussed the question of voice in documentary in 'The ventriloquism of documentary first-person speech and the self-portrait film' (Cowie 2015b).
6 The letter *a* refers on the one hand to the a of *l'autre* (other); on the other hand, as the first letter of the alphabet, it stands for both the beginning of a symbolic system and the algebraic place-holder, meaningless in itself, but essentially open to take on significance in a particular context.
7 I explored desire and the Real in chapter 4, 'Documenting the Real', in *Recording Reality, desiring the real* (Cowie 2011, pp. 118–134).
8 The phrase is used in following Seminars, especially in *Encore* in relation to the sexual relation not being 'able to write the sexual relationship' (Lacan 1999, p. 35).
9 The sinthome is thus, for Lacan, a new way to understand the end of analysis. The conclusion of the treatment is 'the identification with the Real of the symptom, the choice of jouissance, and the creation of a neo-subject' I am drawing here on my essay on sexual difference, desire and the symptom/sinthome (Cowie 2019).
10 In *Bodies that Matter*, Butler (1993, p. 6) argues that, 'if gender is constructed, it is not necessarily constructed by an 'I' or a 'we' who stands before that construction in any spatial or temporal sense of 'before'. Indeed, it is unclear that there can be an 'I' or a 'we' who had not been submitted, subjected to gender, where gendering is, among other things, the differentiating relations by which speaking subjects come into being ... the 'I' neither precedes nor follows the process of this gendering, but emerges only within the matrix of gender relations themselves'. Butler draws from J. L. Austin's work on performative speech, the non-necessity of an 'inward' performance to accompany the 'outer' performative. It is a move to go against the simple binary: Do I make or cause myself and my identity, or am I made or caused by factors – social or biological – outside of my control? Instead, the 'interiority' of subjectivity is displaced to be an effect of the performativity that is undertaken without any 'inward act', that is, in doing this I do not think or reflect that I am doing something that 'makes' me; I just do it, but in doing it I become 'made'. The problem of the origin of subjectivity continues to haunt, notwithstanding Judith Butler's later work that incorporates an account of melancholia, of a lost object, and thus of identification, for she fails to address the identifying that arises with the wish to be what the other wants, to be for the other. See on this Butler's (1997) *The Psychic Life of Power*, especially chapters 3 and 4.
11 For more on this, see Geena Davis Institute on Gender in Media, online:http://seejane.org/research-informs-empowers/. Accessed 19 November 2015.
12 Rancière's concept here of heterotopia is quite different from that articulated by Foucault (1986, p. 24) in his essay 'Of Other Spaces', in which he argues that 'whereas utopias are unreal spaces whose alternative worlds contest by remaking reality, heterotopias are real spaces, locatable sites, that enact

contestation in which the real sites, all the other real sites that can be found within the culture, are simultaneously represented, contested, and inverted. Places of this kind are outside of all places, even though it may be possible to indicate their location in reality. Because these places are absolutely different from all the sites that they reflect and speak about, I shall call them, by way of contrast to utopias, heterotopias'.

13 The gap in the sensible that is dissensus, like Lacan's concept of the Real, arises not before but after symbolisation. Here, we might also think of Deleuze's (1989, p. 214) account of the 'irrational' cut, or interval, of film that is also the opening of a gap, and a thinking of what is not yet, and not yet thought – and a movement between before and after in the now.

14 This is central for Deleuze's distinction between the affection image of the movement cinema and the affect of time cinema. My discussion here draws on my arguments in 'The difference in figuring women now' (Cowie 2015c).

15 I explore more fully Laplanche's idea of afterwardsness in 'The Lived Nightmare: Trauma, Anxiety, and the Ethical Aesthetics of Horror' (Cowie 2003, p. 33), and draw on this essay in the following discussion of horror and film.

16 This idea is explored in Philippe Van Haute's (1998, pp. 115–116) 'Death and Sublimation in Lacan's Reading of Antigone'.

17 Hernandez is referring here to the work of Alvin Frank (1969) in 'The Unrememberable and the Unforgettable: Passive Primal Repression'.

18 The subject is thus what Julia Kristeva terms *abject*. As explored in her book *Powers of Horror* (Kristeva 1982), in its literary and metaphorical appearances, the abject has been a compelling concept and account for discussions of the horror film, articulating the fascination as well as the horror of the abject. The abject, or abjection, refers to two distinct phenomena. The first is the act of abjection in which the subject separates itself from the object and thereby designates it as abject, the 'horrible', thus also instituting a distinction of inside/outside but where what is put outside is abjured, evicted, and effaced. Yet in this process of abjecting, the abject retains a dreadful fascination. The second is the state of abjection, of being the lost, abjected, reviled object. Lacan's concept of the *objet a* makes clear its role as cause or support of desire, avoiding (Kleinian) implications of the object abjected as bad. It is our terrors of the Real, the taint of which always remains attached to the *objet,* not the projections of the abject, which are central for understanding the unpleasures and pleasures of horror.

19 The terror and dread of the specular and its fascinating seduction in cinema are vividly articulated in Kristeva's (1979) essay, 'Ellipsis on Dread and the Specular Seduction'. The specular seduction brings identity, meaning, and symbolisation, so that 'The glance by which I identify an object, a face, my own, another's, delivers my identity which reassures me: for it delivers me from frayages, nameless dread, noises preceding the name ... name ... Intellectual speculation derives from this identifying, labelling glance' (ibid, p. 42). The specular is the point of origin not only of signs, and of narcissistic identifications, but also for 'the phantasmatic terror one speaking identity holds for another'. Once that terror, which is the incursion of the other, 'erupts into the seer, that seen stops being simply reassuring, trompe-l'oeil, or invitation to speculation, and becomes the fascinating specular. Cinema seizes us precisely in that place' (ibid, p. 45). The specular for Kristeva here marks that which is beyond identification, unverbalised, unrepresented, namely, the Real. It represents the unrepresented because it 'includes an excess of visual traces' (ibid, p. 42), useless for signification, but insistently there and naming the before of symbolisation.

20 Seduced to speculate, Kristeva (1979, p. 45) labels terror as 'to do with the dependency on the mother', while seduction lies with 'an appeal addressed to the father'. While she invites a dangerous homogenisation in the categories 'man' and 'woman' here, she goes on to say, in an important qualification, 'But if they enter the game, they will both be led to cross both zones and attempt both identifications – maternal, paternal. Test of sexual difference – of homosexuality, that brush with psychosis—they never stop letting it be intimated, even when they don't let it be seen: Eisenstein, Hitchcock.

21 I have used here the unauthorised translation by Cormac Gallagher from unedited French manuscripts, http://www.lacaninireland.com/web/wp-content/uploads/2010/06/Book-23-Joyce-and-the-Sinthome-Part-2.pdf, p55 uploaded 13/12/2018. In the Jacques Alain-Miller authorised translation by A.R. Price, Lacan was 'taken aback' (2016, p. 107).

22 Patrick Monribot (2013, p. 15) writes that, for Lacan, 'love has to do with speech, whereas ravage has to do with the death drive', and he characterises what Lacan speaks of as 'feminine jouissance' as feminine ravage. Thus, for Lacan, 'the end of analysis "feminises" the speaking-being: the treatment pushes the analysand to name his or her link to the real of feminine jouissance'. See also the work of Bracha Lichtenberg Ettinger who, while drawing closely on Lacan's work, has introduced the concept of the 'matrix', as the encounter with the mother and mother-tongue, drawing as well on Lacan's concept of the sinthome. 'A border-Other I becoming-together between presence and absence' is developed in The *Matrixial Borderspace* (2008, p. 163).

References

Althusser, L. (1971) 'Ideology and Ideological State Apparatus (Notes Towards an Investigation),' in L. Althusser (ed.), *Lenin and Philosophy and Other Essays*. Translated from the French by B. Brewster. London: New Left Books, pp. 121–176.

Bell, V. (2008) 'The Burden of Sensation and the Ethics of Form: Watching *Capturing the Friedmans*,' *Theory, Culture and Society* 25 (3), pp. 89–101.

Bergson, H. (2002) 'The Idea of Duration,' in K. Ansell Pearson & J. Mullarkey (eds.), *Henri Bergson: Key Writings*. London: Continuum, pp. 49–80.

Brighenti, A.M. (2010) 'Artveillance: At the Crossroads of Art and Surveillance', *Surveillance & Society* 7 (2), pp. 175–186.

Butler, J. (1990) *Gender Trouble: Feminism and the Subversion of Identity*. London: Routledge.

Butler, J. (1993) *Bodies That Matter: On the Discursive Limits of "Sex"*. New York: Routledge.

Butler, J. (1997) *The Psychic Life of Power: Theories In Subjection*. Stanford: Stanford University Press.

Cavell, S. (1979) *The Claim of Reason: Wittgenstein, Skepticism, Morality and Tragedy*. Oxford: Clarendon Press.

Cowie, E. (2003). 'The Lived Nightmare: Trauma, Anxiety and the Ethical Aesthetics of Horror,' in S.J. Schneider & D. Shaw (eds.), *Dark Thoughts: Philosophic Reflections on Cinematic Horror*. Lanham: Scarecrow Press, pp. 25–46.

Cowie, E. (2011) *Recording Reality, Desiring the Real*. Minneapolis: Minnesota University Press.

Cowie, E. (2015a) 'The World Viewed: Documentary Observing and the Culture of Surveillance,' in A. Juhasz & A. Lebow (eds.), *A Companion to Contemporary Documentary*. London: Routledge, pp. 580–610.
Cowie, E. (2015b) 'The Ventriloquism of Documentary First-person Speech and the Self-portrait Film,' in A. Piotrowska (ed.), *Embodied Encounters: New Approaches to Psychoanalysis and Cinema*. London: Routledge, pp. 36–50.
Cowie, E. (2015c) 'The Difference in Figuring Women Now,' *The Moving Image Review and Art Journal* (*MIRAJ*) 4(1–2), pp. 46–61.
Cowie, E. (2019) 'The Certainties of Difference and Their Difficulty: Desire and the Symptom', in A. Piotrowska and B. Tyrer (eds.) *Femininity and Psychoanalysis: Cinema, Culture, Theory*, London: Routledge, pp. 8–36.
Creed, B. (1993). *The Monstrous-Feminine: Film, Feminism, Psychoanalysis*. London: Routledge.
Deleuze, G. (1989) *Cinema 2: The Time-Image*. Translated from the French by H. Tomlinson & R. Galeta. Minneapolis: University of Minnesota Press.
Deleuze, G. & F. Guattari. (1994) *What is Philosophy?* Translated by H. Tomlinson & G. Burchell. New York: Columbia University Press.
Derrida, J. (1973) *Speech and Phenomena and Other Essays on Husserl's Theory of Signs*. Translated from the French by D.B. Allison & N. Garver. Evanston: Northwestern University Press.
Dolar, M. (2006) *A Voice and Nothing More*. Cambridge, MA: MIT Press.
Durgnat, R. (1967) *Franju*. London: Studio Vista.
Foucault, M. (1986) 'Of Other Spaces,' Translated from the French by Jay Miskowiec. *Diacritics* 16 (1), pp. 22–27.
Frank, A. (1969) 'The Unrememberable and the Unforgettable: Passive Primal Repression,' *The Psychoanalytic Study of the Child* 24, pp. 48–77.
Freud, S. (1905/1960) *Jokes and Their Relation to the Unconcious: The Standard Edition of the Complete Works of Sigmund Freud*. London: Hogarth Press.
Harari, R. (2001) *Lacan's Seminar on Anxiety: An Introduction*. Translated from the Spanish by J.C. Lamb-Ruiz. New York: The Other Press.
Haute, P.V. (1998) 'Death and Sublimation in Lacan's Reading of *Antigone*,' in S. Harasym (ed.), *Lévinas and Lacan: The Missed Encounter*. Albany: State University of New York Press, pp. 102–120.
Heath, S. (1981) *Questions of Cinema*. London: Macmillan.
Hernandez, M. (1998) 'Winnicott's "Fear of Breakdown": On and Beyond Trauma,' *Diactritics* 28 (4), pp. 134–143.
Kracauer, S. (1947). *From Caligari to Hitler: A Psychological History of the German Film*. London: Dennis Dobson.
Kracauer, S. (1960) *Theory of Film: The Redemption of Physical Reality*. New York: Oxford University Press.
Kristeva, J. (1979) 'Ellipsis on Dread and the Specular Seduction,' Translated by D. Burdick. *Wide Angle* 3 (3), pp. 42–47.
Kristeva, J. (1982) *Powers of Horrors: An Essay on Abjection*. Translated from the French by L.S. Roudiez. New York: Columbia University Press.
Lagaay, A. (2008) 'Between Sound and Silence: Voice in the History of Psychoanalysis,' *Episteme* 1 (1), pp. 53–62.
Lacan, J. (1973) *L'étourdit*. Paris: Seuil.

Lacan, J. (1979) *The Four Fundamentals of Psychoanalysis*. Translated from the French by A. Sheridan. Harmondsworth: Penguin.
Lacan, J. (1993) *The Psychoses, 1955–1956: The Seminar of Jacques Lacan Book III*. Translated from the French by R. Grigg. New York: W.W. Norton and Company.
Lacan, J. (1998) *Le Seminaire, Livre V, Les formations de l'inconscient*. Paris: Seuil.
Lacan, J. (1999) *On Feminine Sexuality, The Limits of Love and Knowledge (Encore): The Seminar of Jacques Lacan Book XX*. Translated from the French by B. Fink. New York: W.W. Norton & Company.
Lacan, J. (2006) *Le séminaire. Livre XVIII. D'un discours qui ne serait pas du semblant*. Paris: Seuil.
Lacan, J. (2016) *The Sinthome: The Seminar of Jacques Lacan XXIII*. Translated from the French by A.R. Price. Cambridge: Polity.
Laplanche, J. (1999) *Essays on Otherness*, London: Routledge.
Leslie, E. (2010). 'Siegfried Kracauer and Walter Benjamin: Memory from Weimar to Hitler,' in S. Radstone & B. Schwartz (eds.), *Memory: Histories, Theories, Debates*. Fordham: Fordham University Press, pp. 123–135.
Metz, C. (1985) 'Photography and Fetish,' *October* 34, pp. 81–90.
Monribot, P. (2013) '"There Is No Sexual Relation" What Does It Mean? Clinical Consequences of Lacan's Formulae of Sexuation,' This Paper Was Presented on the 28 September 2013 in Dublin as Part of the ICLO-NLS Annual Seminar. Downloaded 3/3/2019: www.iclo-nls.org/wp-content/uploads/Pdf/HB10%20Monribot%20Eng%20FINAL.pdf
Morel. G. (2005) 'Sex, Gender and Identity: From Symptom to Sinthome,' *Cités* 21, pp. 61–78.
Morrey, D. (2008) 'Open Wounds: Body and Image in Jean-Luc Nancy and Claire Denis,' *Film-Philosophy* 12 (1), pp. 10–31.
Mulvey, L. (1973) 'You Don't Know What Is Happening, Do You, Mr Jones?,' *Spare Rib* 8, pp. 13–16.
Mulvey, L. (1975) 'Visual Pleasure and Narrative Cinema.' *Screen* 16 (1), pp. 6–18.
Mulvey, L. (1989) [1978] 'Film, Feminism and the Avant-Garde,' in L. Mulvey (ed.), *Visual and Other Pleasures*. Basingstoke: Macmillan, pp. 111–126.
Nancy, J-L. (2006) *Corpus*. Translated from the French by R.A. Rand. Fordham: Fordham University Press.
Nancy, J-L. (2008) 'Icon of Fury: Claire Denis,' *Trouble Every Day*' *Film-Philosophy* 12 (1), pp. 1–9.
Nietzsche, F. (1969) *On the Genealogy of Morals*. Translated by W. Kaufmann. New York: Vintage.
Rancière, J. (1992) 'Politics, Identification and Subjectivization,' *October* 61, pp. 58–64.
Rancière, J. (2004) 'Who Is the Subject of the Rights of Man?' *South Atlantic Quarterly* 103 (2/3), pp. 297–310.
Rancière, J. (2009) *The Emancipated Spectator*. London: Verso.
Rancière, J. (2010a) *Dissensus: On Politics and Aesthetics*. Translated from the French by S. Corcoran. London: Continuum.
Rancière, J. (2010b) 'The Aesthetic Heterotopia.' *Philosophy Today* 54, pp. 15–25.

Roberts, B. (2006) 'Cinema as Mnemotech: Bernard Stiegler and the Industrialisation of Memory,' *Angelaki* 11 (1), pp. 55–63.

Rose, J. (1982). 'Introduction II,' in J. Lacan (ed.), *Feminine Sexuality*. Translated from the French by J. Rose, New York: W.W. Norton & Company, pp. 27–58.

Shepherdson, C. (2013) 'Foreword,' in R. Harari (ed.), *Lacan's Seminar on Anxiety*. New York: Other Press, pp. ix–lxxix.

Stiegler, B. (1998) *Technics and Time, 3: Cinematic Time and the Question of Malaise*. Translated from the French by Stephen Barker. Stanford: Stanford University Press.

Stiegler, B. (2011) 'Pharmacology of Desire: Drive-based Capitalism and Libidinal Dis-economy,' *New Formations* 72, pp. 150–161.

Van Haute, P. (1998) 'Death and Sublimation in Lacan's Reading of *Antigone*,' in S. Harasym (ed.), *Levinas and Lacan: The Missed Encounter*. New York: SUNY, pp. 102–120.

Verhaeghe, P. & Declercq, F. (2002) 'Lacan's Analytical Goal: "Le Sinthome" or the Feminine Way,' in L. Thurston (ed.), *Re-Inventing the Symptom: Essays on the Final Lacan*. New York: Other Press, pp. 59–83.

Žižek, S. (1991) 'The Truth Arises from Misrecognition,' in E. Ragland-Sullivan & M. Bracher (eds.), *Lacan and the Subject of Language*. London: Routledge, pp. 188–212.

Žižek, S. (1994) *The Metastases of Enjoyment: Six Essays on Women and Causality*. London: Verso.

Žižek, S. (1996) '"I Hear You with My Eyes": or, the Invisible Master,' in R. Salecl & S. Žižek (eds.), *Gaze and Voice as Love Objects*. Durham: Duke University Press, pp. 90–128.

Žižek, S. (2001) *On Belief*. London: Routledge.

Part II

Introduction

Expanding the Monstrous-Feminine

Nicholas Chare, Jeanette Hoorn, and Audrey Yue

Many of the analyses of films offered in *The Monstrous-Feminine* have become classics shaping subsequent readings of those same films or, at the very least, acting as their foils. The three essays in this section either reflect on or build upon some of these benchmark analyses. The section begins with a lively and thought-provoking interview with Creed herself, '*The Monstrous-Feminine*, Then and Now' in which she reflects on a variety of themes. The interview starts by looking back on the genesis of the 'monstrous-feminine', tracing the influence of Elizabeth Cowie's, Laura Mulvey's, and Julia Kristeva's work upon her groundbreaking 1986 *Screen* article 'Horror and the Monstrous-Feminine' and the 1993 book, *The Monstrous-Feminine*, that developed out of that. Creed then tracks how she has gone on to develop ideas latent in *The Monstrous-Feminine* in later work.

Creed's current interest in representations of non-human animals, for example, already registers within many of the analyses offered by the book. *Cat People* (Dir. Jacques Tourneur, USA, 1942), for instance, is read as offering a portrayal of 'woman as non-human animal' (Creed 1993, p. 1). The film *The Brood* (Dir. David Cronenberg, USA, 1979) also figures the central character Nola as 'like an animal' at one point (47). *Carrie* (Dir. Brian de Palma, USA, 1976), which is analysed by Patricia Pisters in her essay in this section, depicts Carrie as pig-like (p. 80). Were-creatures such as the werewolf are entities 'whose bodies signify a collapse of the boundaries between the human and the animal' (p. 10). Citing Freud, Creed also links the primal scene with the child observing sexual intercourse between animals (p. 17). Non-human animals and humans becoming non-human animals, boundary breakdowns between human and animal, in varied manifestations the animal is a recurring presence, if not a major theme, in *The Monstrous-Feminine*. Creed explains that her third book, *Phallic Panic* (2005), fleshes out this theme, examining how the monstrous masculine is allied with the feminine and the animal. In more recent works the animal has increased in importance, with *Darwin's Screens* (Creed 2009) exploring the role of fictional or 'screen animals' in cinema. For Creed (2009, p. 178), through its use of 'screen animals' cinema can potentially challenge 'the bases on which the differences between human and animal have historically and philosophically been founded'. This belief in cinema's capacity to effect social change also features in Creed's later discussion of her own film-making.

Creed moves on to reflect about the role of sound in horror films, foregrounding sound as a 'crucial dimension' of the abject. The abject as it relates to sound has not attracted considerable scholarly interest although Creed draws attention to notable exceptions in the essays of Deborah Dixon (2011) and Elizabeth Fairweather (2014). Additionally, Greg Hainge (2013, pp. 67–68) has examined noises that might be thought of as abject in relation to nausea in *Noise Matters*. Abject sounds are qualitatively different to sounds which register as disgusting. In an undated letter, the eighteenth-century naturalist Gilbert White (1987, p. 226) observed of sounds that '[w]e are more apt to be captivated or disgusted with the associations which they promote, than with the notes themselves'. This prefigures Andras Angyal's (1941, p. 402) observation that '[s]ensory qualities as such are never disgusting', but they may contribute to the disgusting qualities attributed to an object by way of their being 'specifically associated with disgusting material'. Abject sounds, however, do not operate by association. They rather function as a force of meaninglessness within the Symbolic, a troubling semiotic (in Kristeva's sense of the term) upsurge.

The shifting nature of the horror film as a genre is then explored. Creed discusses changes in the way the monstrous-feminine is articulated in some recent horror films. She attributes these changes, in part, to the growing number of women directors working in the genre. The increasing number of women directors making use of formal and thematic elements from the horror genre is a phenomenon also discussed by Patricia Pisters in her essay in this section. For Creed, the horror film provides an important space within which women can push boundaries relating to gender, desire, and female agency. In this sense, horror as a genre has a potentially vital contribution to play in feminist film-making both now and in the future. In this regard, her position resonates strongly with that articulated by Elizabeth Cowie in her essay for this volume. Creed concludes by discussing her preparations for a new edition of *The Monstrous-Feminine* in which she will examine ways in which the concept resonates with many of the pressing concerns of our time relating to human and animal rights. The new edition will place greater emphasis on the 'radical potential' of the abject, exploring its revolutionary promise in greater depth.

The next essay, Mark Nicholls' 'Abjection beyond Tears', builds on Creed's reading of *The Exorcist* (Dir. William Friedkin, USA, 1973) in *The Monstrous-Feminine*, providing an inspired reading of the actor's craft as it is embodied in Ellen Burstyn's interpretation of her role as Chris MacNeil, the mother of a daughter, Regan (Linda Blair), possessed by demons. Nicholls foregrounds the complexity of Burstyn's role, with Chris functioning as an interface between good and evil and also confronting symbolic (in Kristeva's sense of the term) collapse through her daughter's abject appearance and behaviour. This behaviour involves emitting abject substances and inflicting violence. In *The Monstrous-Feminine*, Creed (1993, p. 40) explores the acoustic dimension to this behaviour, discussing Regan's 'snarling, grunting voice'. She returns to this theme in her interview for this section, identifying vocalisations of this kind as abject sounds. For Nicholls, Regan's possession causes Chris to become literally and emotionally soiled. Through her portrayal of Chris, Burstyn must attest to this process of sullying. Nicholls focusses on the experiences and techniques she drew upon to create the role. Her fashioning of the emotional reality of the situation, an extraordinary case of demonic possession, can be seen as central to the film's success.

In analyses of film, the roles of actors are often viewed as peripheral, the skills necessary to their craft frequently overlooked and undervalued. The common emphasis placed on narrative analysis and cinematography is often to the detriment of acting. Nicholls' subtle and sophisticated essay, however, speaks powerfully to the importance of attending to how roles are created and interpreted. In *The Exorcist*, Nicholls demonstrates how personal experiences play into Burstyn's performance, the breakdown of her marriage to Neil Nephew informing her portrayal of her relations with her estranged husband in the film. In this sense, the emotional tenor in some scenes can be understood as autobiographical. The feelings are from life but find expression through fiction. The extent to which they can be called 'staged' is questionable. The emotional veracity of Burstyn's performance is undeniable. This contrasts with Linda Blair's interpretation of Regan. As Nicholls discusses, there is considerable argument over how 'knowing' her portrayal is, over whether she is a consummate professional imitating behaviours of which she is ignorant or a faux-naïf (in which case her dissimulation, her playing at obliviousness to the devilishness of her behaviour, also merits credit). Nicholls' attentiveness to Regan's 'sexual gestures' in this context is invaluable. Gesture is often sidelined in film analysis yet as Carol Mayo Jenkins (2015) has eloquently attested it forms a crucial component of any actor's artistry. Regan's gestures, such as stabbing herself in the crotch with a crucifix, embody her moral corruption and may also embody Blair's awareness of that corruption. This gesture, as Nicholls implies, is sexual. Teenage knowledge of sexuality is therefore being employed to signify Regan's fallen status (with potentially negative ramifications, through guilt by association, for Blair). Using *The Monstrous-Feminine* as a point of reference, Aviva Briefel (2005) has traced the conservative politics often underpinning such acts of self-mutilation in horror films, including in *The Exorcist*.

Nicholls also notes moments where Burstyn improvises within the film, adlibbing, deviating from the script. This is, again, a key dimension to acting yet one which can frequently only be recognised and appreciated through archival work of the kind practised in 'Abjection beyond Tears'. In the context of theatre, Denis Podalydès (Stiegler 2018, p. 230) has observed that 'an actor's capacity to go beyond the template provided by the stage directions is [...] crucial'. He explains that it is through improvisation that performance rises above the automatic. Nicholls provides the cinematic example of Burstyn as Chris on the telephone to her estranged husband. In this scene, through improvisation, breaking with the script and drawing on her lived experience, Burstyn gives her character an emotional roundness which acting by rote would be unable to achieve. Burstyn also encouraged Blair to improvise. Improvisation, as a mode of interpretation, encourages the emergence of the extraordinary (Stiegler 2018, p. 239). Through analysing elements of Burstyn's performance and her personal reflections on the process, as well as those of her colleagues, Nicholls offers a creative practice account which demonstrates the subtlety and intelligence of her approach towards the creation of Chris as abject mother. Her reactions to the image of female monstrosity embodied by Blair as Regan, her ability to register the process of degradation this confrontation with monstrosity prompts in Chris, demonstrate that Burstyn is an actor of the highest order.

In the final essay in this section, 'Carrie's Sisters', Patricia Pisters explores the significance of the appropriation of horror aesthetics by female directors, arguing that their work demonstrates the ongoing relevance of the monstrous-feminine for film analysis. She begins by revisiting Creed's celebrated analysis of *Carrie* and also examining Kimberly Pierce's 2013 remake. Pisters then goes on to consider *In the Cut* (Dir. Jane Campion, USA, 2003) and *Evolution* (Dir. Lucile Hadžihalilović, France, 2015) Her conception of the monstrous-feminine, however, is one that seeks to move beyond the Freudian, Lacanian, and Kristevan framework employed in *The Monstrous-Feminine* offering alternative perspectives that look beyond the abject as anxiety-inducing and repulsive. In a beautifully crafted analysis, Pisters links her case studies by way of a common thread, the appearance of blood red, which is visible across her corpus.

Pisters (2003, p. 49) has previously discussed blood as a theme in *Carrie* in *The Matrix of Visual Culture*, explaining how traditional fears of witchcraft are 'explicitly related to all kinds of blood (menstrual blood, pig's blood, birth blood, the blood of sin, the blood of death)'. In a psychoanalytic reading, she explains, bodily material such as blood comes to stand for 'what is outside the subject but nevertheless also constitutes the subject' (p. 49). In patriarchal ideology of the kind embodied in the 1976 version of *Carrie*, for instance, blood comes to figure Woman as unruly body, as uncontrollable and monstrous by nature, the antithesis of rational Man. For Pisters, however, this negative portrayal contrasts markedly with the 2013 remake. In *Carrie* as directed by Pierce, monstrosity is viewed from a woman's perspective and there is considerable emphasis on female agency. Qualitative differences between the two films have important implications for issues of female empowerment.

Empowerment and agency, Pisters shows, are also noteworthy themes in *In the Cut*. The sophisticated chromatics of *In the Cut* have already attracted considerable and considered attention (Bolton 2011; Watkins 2007, 2013). Pisters' approach is markedly different, however, in its focus on gendered violence as it is explored by way of the film's use of colour. Through a compelling close reading of its chromatics, Pisters traces how the film explores the significance of the colour red by way of both the fantasy life of the central character, Frannie Avery, and her real-world experiences (which are tinged by that fantasy life). Pisters' reading, her tracing of the colour red across varied forms as something in excess of them, possesses parallels with Jean-Louis Schefer's attention to red as an enigmatic quality in paintings that cannot be captured by way of an iconographic approach. For Schefer, red forms part of a picture's economy of intensities. He repeatedly links red with blood, exploring the religious connotations of the colour in Renaissance art, its sacred and profane qualities (Schefer 1995, 2007; Bann 2010; Rifkin 2005). His analysis of Paolo Uccello's *Profanation of the Host* (1467) in *L'Hostie profanée* includes a section that traces how the emergence of the vampire as a monstrous figure paralleled and was shaped by mediaeval debates regarding the Eucharist, debates which can be seen to inform elements of Bram Stoker's epistolary novel *Dracula*. In this sense, blood as a staple of the horror genre has an often disavowed link to the sacred.

Pisters looks beyond historical aspects to consider the affective qualities held by the colour red in contemporary horror aesthetics and how these link with violence and sexuality. For her, these affective qualities can be read as registering a monstrous-feminine but one incompatible with the disgusting affects associated with the abject. In this sense, she can be seen to identify a turn away from the religious underpinnings of much modern horror, underpinnings central to *The Exorcist* and also strongly present in *Carrie* through Carrie's religious mother who identifies red with fallen womanhood, with profanation and sin (Greven 2011, p. 4). In *In the Cut* and also *Evolution*, red no longer operates in a religious register. Pisters' final case study, *Evolution*, which also builds out from inspiring close readings of the film's use of the colour red, examines the theme of motherhood. For Pisters, *Evolution* again borrows elements from horror aesthetics but transforms them, expanding the affective potential of these elements. To appreciate this enhanced affect, Pisters suggests, it is necessary to think 'horror' anew. Her call echoes that of Cowie in her essay in the previous section as does the overall emphasis on the importance of attending to affect. For Pisters, the films by women directors that she analyses are united by a desire to provide a female perspective on the monstrous-feminine and to offer visions of female agency that are of considerable contemporary importance. Each of the essays in their different way therefore revisit familiar case studies yet explores the monstrous-feminine in those studies across new terrain, sound in Creed, actors in Nicholls and colour in Pisters.

References

Angyal, A. (1941) 'Disgust and Related Aversions,' *The Journal of Abnormal and Social Psychology* 36(3), pp. 393–412.

Bann, S. (2010) 'A New Orientalism?' *History and Theory* 49, pp. 130–138.

Bolton, L. (2011) *Film and Female Consciousness: Irigaray, Cinema and Thinking Women*. Houndmills: Palgrave Macmillan.

Briefel, A. (2005) 'Monster Pains: Masochism, Menstruation, and Identification in the Horror Film,' *Film Quarterly* 58(3), pp. 16–27.

Creed, B. (1993) *The Monstrous-Feminine: Film, Feminism, Psychoanalysis*. London: Routledge.

Creed, B. (2005) *Phallic Panic: Film, Horror and the Primal Uncanny*. Melbourne: Melbourne University Publishing.

Creed, B. (2009) *Darwin's Screens: Evolutionary Aesthetics, Time and Sexual Display in Cinema*. Melbourne: Melbourne University Publishing.

Dixon, D. (2011) 'Scream: The Sound of the Monstrous,' *Cultural Geographies* 18(1), pp. 435–455.

Fairweather, E. (2014) 'Jerry Goldsmith and the Sonification of the "Monstrous-Feminine" in his Science Fiction Scores,' *Divergence Press* 2 [online]. Available at http://divergencepress.net/articles/2016/11/3/jerry-goldsmith-and-the-sonification-of-the-monstrous-feminine-in-his-science-fiction-scores (Accessed: 8th March 2019)

Greven, D. (2011) *Representations of Femininity in American Genre Cinema*. New York: Palgrave Macmillan.

Hainge, G. (2013) *Noise Matters: Towards an Ontology of Noise*. New York: Bloomsbury.

Jenkins, C.M. (2015) 'A Mark on the Canvas,' *Journal for Cultural Research* 19(1), pp. 110–113.

Pisters, P. (2003) *The Matrix of Visual Culture: Working with Deleuze in Film Theory*. Stanford: Stanford University Press.

Rifkin, A. (2005) 'From Structure to Enigma and Back, Perhaps,' *Journal of Visual Culture* 4(3), pp. 365–381.

Schefer, J-L. (1995) *Question de style*. Paris: L'Harmattan.

Schefer, J-L (2007) *L'Hostie profane: Histoire d'une fiction théologique*. Paris: Éditions P.O.L.

Stiegler, B. (2018) 'Out Automated Lives: An Interview with Denis Podalydès,' *Liminalities: A Journal of Performance Studies* 14(1), pp. 229–247.

Watkins, L. (2007) 'The (Dis)Articulation of Colour: Cinematography, Femininity and Desire in Jane Campion's *In the Cut*,' in W. Everett (ed.), *Questions of Colour in Cinema from Paintbrush to Pixel*. Oxford: Peter Lang, pp. 202–213.

Watkins, L. (2013) 'Disharmonious Designs: Colour Contrast and Curiosity in Jane Campion's "In the Cut,"' *NECSUS* 2(1), pp. 197–212.

White, G. (1987) [1788] *The Natural History of Selborne*. London: Penguin.

5 *The Monstrous-Feminine*, Then and Now

Barbara Creed in Conversation with Nicholas Chare

Barbara Creed

Nicholas Chare: I'd like to begin by asking you about the genesis of your idea of the monstrous-feminine, the subject of your groundbreaking article (Creed 1986) in *Screen* and your subsequent book (Creed 1993). Did the idea emerge gradually or was there a moment of epiphany?

Barbara Creed: A complex question – many factors were involved. I loved horror movies. And I had always been interested in psychoanalytic theory. I recall that I gave my first public lecture on the monstrous-feminine in 1985. I was invited by Sneja Gunew to present a keynote at the Australia-Europe Cultural Crossroads Conference run by the Victorian Ministry of Arts. The title was 'The Monstrous-Feminine in Film: Julia Kristeva's *Powers of Horror*'. Why Kristeva? I had recently attended a public lecture in Sydney by Liz Grosz in which she presented Julia Kristeva's theory of the abject from *Powers of Horror* (Kristeva 1982). The book had been translated in 1982 and was causing quite a stir. Liz is a great speaker and I was mesmerised. In the early 1980s, I had been teaching a new subject on the horror film with a particular focus on the female monster who had emerged as a new force in horror films of the 1970s. Think of the horror films released in that decade which featured a female monster. *Alien* – of course. *The Exorcist*, *Carrie*, *Rabid*, *The Brood*, and the rape revenge film, *I Spit on Your Grave*. And, of course, two great lesbian vampire films – *Vampire Lovers* with Ingrid Pitt and *Daughters of Darkness* starring Delphine Seyrig. Then Sam Riami's wonderful *Evil Dead* in 1981. Fantastic! These films were all to become central to different chapters in *The Monstrous Feminine*.

Inspired by the essays in E. Ann Kaplan's (1978) edited volume, *Women in Film Noir*, which argued for the power of the femme fatale, I found myself searching for a new female protagonist of horror. And suddenly here was Kristeva's theory of abjection that explained horror in terms of the dangerous feminine, borders, and the body. Although Kristeva does not refer to film, the application of her theory of abjection to the horror film made perfect sense. Then, in 1985, I received an invitation from *Screen* to write an article on Kristeva's *Powers of Horror* for an edition they were planning to publish on the horror film. Mandy Merck was the editor. I was thrilled. Writing this article (Creed 1986) helped me to crystallise my ideas and develop my argument. I remember I called the article: 'The Monstrous-Feminine in Film, an *Imaginary* Abjection', because I wanted to emphasise that these images of female monstrosity were first and foremost *imaginary* – patriarchal stereotypes, many of which were centuries old. The *Screen* edition of 1986 featured a fantastic image of female monstrosity on the cover – one of the witches from Sam Rami's *Evil Dead* whose terrifying face, her mouth oozing blood, is both disgusting and compelling. It's a very in-your-face image. A key aspect of the monstrous-feminine. She commenced life as a patriarchal stereotype but like Frankenstein's monster she embarked on a life of her own. Shortly after the *Screen* article came out, Tony Bennett and Graham Martin invited me to submit a book for their 'Popular Fiction Series'. Routledge published the book in 1993. And here we are – 25 years later, and the concept of the monstrous-feminine continues to stimulate debate and discussion. I think this is largely because her various 'faces' have evolved over time, adapting to changing social and ideological conditions. In many films and art works, particularly where the artists are female, she offers a clear and direct challenge to dominant patriarchal values.

NC: What had drawn you to psychoanalytic theory and work of Julia Kristeva, in particular, in the context of studying the horror film?

BC: I had always been interested in Freud and his theory of dreams, repression, and the unconscious. I was also reading other works such as Freud's (1985) *The Uncanny* as well as Briffault's (1931) *The Mothers* and Bachofen's (1967) *Myth, Religion and Mother-Right.* These all inspired my thinking about women, myth, and horror and the fact that patriarchal images of female monstrosity went right back to Greek myths and legends and no doubt earlier. As Freud wrote about the power of myth, the Medusa and male castration anxieties, and the story of Oedipus, his ideas seemed particularly relevant. Then, in 1975 Laura Mulvey's brilliant article, 'Visual Pleasure and Narrative Cinema' took all of us by storm. Mulvey's use of psychoanalytic theory in the interpretation of film suddenly went to a whole new level. I was particularly interested in her use of Lacan's mirror stage and Freud's theory of castration. Mulvey (1975) showed how the patriarchal unconscious influences not just meaning but also filmic structure, that is, structures of looking. This was completely new. The idea that the gaze could be gendered through unconscious structures of looking changed everything. It affected film form. On close analysis I could see that when the male character subjected the woman to his controlling gaze, he was almost always physically positioned to the left or right of the frame and in the foreground. The woman was to the centre in the middle ground. This structure applied to almost every film I watched across all genres with one exception – the horror genre. While the female monster does not necessarily 'control' the gaze in the same way as the male, she 'captures' the gaze in an aggressive manner because of her monstrous nature and appearance – particularly when she presents the threat of active castration. So Mulvey's theory opened up a new way of thinking about film and psychoanalytic theory for me. It showed how the patriarchal unconscious, or the unconscious full stop, structures representation and ideology. This is why I am still committed to psychoanalytic theory. By the time I read Kristeva's *Powers of Horror*, I was already drawn to psychoanalytic theory. Kristeva's theory of abjection and the abject feminine offered such a persuasive way of understanding the concept of woman as monster. It changed the way I viewed the horror film. Then around the same time. I read Elizabeth Cowie's (1984) impressive article, *Fantasia*, which appeared in *m/f*. She theorised that film could be viewed as fantasy and as a reworking of three major fantasies – the primal scene, and the fantasies of castration and seduction. She argued that the protagonist can occupy one, two or all three positions even if contradictory. Similarly the spectator can switch identification from male to female and even hold contradictory positions. Although she did not specifically discuss horror, her theory added a new dimension to my understanding of the horror film, particularly *Alien* and other science fiction horror films where primal scenes were key. I was drawn to the horror film because it offered narratives that featured a very different image of woman – woman as a terrifying monster, one whose main aim seemed to be to undermine or destroy the patriarchal symbolic order.

NC: Robin Wood (1978) argued something along these lines, didn't he?

BC: Yes, of course. Robin Wood presented a similar argument in his famous *Film Comment* article of 1978. It was called 'Return of the Repressed'. He did not write specifically of the female monster but of monsters in general. Very little of a serious nature had been written on horror in the seventies and eighties. I was particularly taken with Wood's discussion of Freud, the surrealists, and the unconscious. He held that the horror film was so very appealing because it spoke, through the figure of the monster, to our repressed desires to 'smash the norms that oppress us' – I think that was his phrase. Here he included the Church, State & Family as well as the Family. I wondered at the time if female spectators might have very specific norms they might like to see smashed. His argument seemed to make sense of the reasons why audiences found the monster such a sympathetic figure and why horror was so popular with younger people.

NC: What did your students think of the female monster? You said that you screened a number of 1970s films such as *The Exorcist* and *Carrie* which focussed on female monstrosity.

BC: They loved her! Particularly the female students. But not all students. When I screened *I Spit on Your Grave*, a group of male students came up after the lecture and told me they were shocked and offended and said I should have warned them first about the castration scene. The female students replied: 'Well, now you know how we feel. We are victims all the time. No-one warns us!'

I suggested we form a study group, meet monthly and watch horror films with female monsters. They loved the idea – they even had T-Shirts made, which were emblazoned with the logo: 'Savage Sisters'. We each agreed to raid our local video shop for promising titles. We watched so many films – many were totally blood and gore. It soon became obvious that women were just as likely to play the monster as the victim. The fact that she was uncontrollable, a horrifying female monster held great appeal. I think Kristeva describes her as a 'wily, uncontrollable' power – this is why she was so fascinating to us.

NC: Rereading *The Monstrous-Feminine* in the light of your more recent work informed by animal studies such as *Stray* (Creed 2017), I'm struck by how present the non-human animal already is as a theme in your first book. There you discuss boundary collapses between the human and animal and instances in which women are figured as animal. In what ways, if any, have your early readings of horror cinema informed your subsequent writings about animals and human-non-human animal relations?

BC: That is a great question. One of Kristeva's most powerful statements, which has always stayed with me is where she directly links woman's ability to procreate and give birth to the animal world and to what she describes as 'the great cycle of birth, decay and death'. I think this is why woman and animal are frequently aligned in fairy tales, horror, and science fiction. Think of *Beauty and the Beast*, *Little Red Riding Hood*, *King Kong*, and *Alien*. The female werewolf and female vampire are fascinating creatures. One horror film that makes this association between women, female animals and birth is David Cronenberg's *The Brood*. The scene that the censors found most offensive, and cut in many countries, including Australia, is not where the mutant creatures attack their human victims in a bloody frenzy but the scene where Nola, the mother, gives birth from her external womb sac and bites through the bloody umbilical cord with her teeth. This is what horrified the most – visible evidence the primal connection between human and non-human animals. The *Alien* quartet also draws compelling yet horrific comparisons. There is Ripley, on the one hand, a woman who 'adopts' Newt, her surrogate daughter, in a kind of clean birth, lined up against Mother Alien who gives birth in a completely animalistic way – laying eggs from her great slimy ovipositor. I see Mother Ripley and Mother Alien as opposite sides of the same human/animal being. In the end of course Ripley is impregnated and gives birth to an alien monster herself – one that she is forced to kill. She essentially morphs into Mother Alien – a terrifying form of the monstrous-feminine who confronts us with our worst nightmares about our animal origins.

NC: Is this a major aim of *Phallic Panic* – to explore the connection between human and animal?

BC: Yes. *Phallic Panic* is essentially a study of the monstrous masculine in which I argue that when man is made monstrous he is almost always assimilated into the feminine and the animal. This is the primal uncanny. He bleeds, gestates, gives birth, creates life (in test tubes), grows hair, and transforms into a creature. In order to become monstrous, to threaten the symbolic order, he must first abandon that order and cross over into the realm of the abject – to align himself with woman and animal. Despite his monstrous appearance, he is almost always a sympathetic figure from the Beast, the Wolfman, to the Creature from the Black Lagoon, and King Kong.

To return to your other question – Yes, these readings of the horror film have informed my recent work on human/animal because they confirm our animal origins – something that the Symbolic order is at pains to repress and deny. Think of the many discussions throughout the history of philosophy, from Aristotle to Descartes and Lacan whose main aim is to deny our animal origins –a connection championed by Charles Darwin. More recently, I explored the animal question and the influence of evolutionary theory on early film genres in *Darwin's Screens* (Creed 2009). The feminist philosopher, Kelly Oliver (2009), has written a fantastic book on the views of philosophers throughout history. *Animal Lessons: How They Teach us To Be Human.* Oliver challenges the belief that man is essentially different from the animal. She examines the writings of all the major philosophers to show how they go to great lengths to separate the two. Man is rational: animals are not. Man feels pain: animals do not. Man understands he will die: animals do not, etc. The horror film of course keeps this connection alive which I see as one of its more radical themes. It is essential that we do deny our kinship with the animal world – otherwise how could we even begin to justify the monstrous cruelty we inflict on our animal counterparts in scientific laboratories, factory farms, zoos, war, and sport. One of the very first documentary short films, which were made by Thomas Edison in 1903, is called *Electrocuting an Elephant.* A restored version is on YouTube. The elephant was Topsy. She had spent her life in circuses. Topsy was publicly electrocuted on Coney Island because she killed her trainer. Topsy was also fed poison in case the electrocution failed. It didn't. The film is a shocking testimony to human cruelty. The public were able to view the film on coin-operated kinetoscopes. Some great directors have made films about the human/animal relationship. Robert Bresson's wonderful *Au Hasard Balthazar* of 1966. Georges Franju's *Blood of Beasts.* Nicolas Philibert's *Nenette* and more recently Agnieszka Holland's *Spoor.* There are many, many more. Don't get me started .... I firmly believe that film theorists need to become more engaged with the animal question. This is what I attempted to do in *Stray*, which explores human-animal ethics in the Anthropocene. Although my focus is as much on other cultural forms such as photography and art as it is on film.

In *Stray* I have drawn on Kristeva's concept of the 'stray' to explore a state of being that human and animal share as well as the ways in which the stray is frequently rendered monstrous. In the context of abjection, Kristeva discusses human strays, beings who ceaselessly stray rather than establishing their bearings – as such the stray exists outside the symbolic order. The stray is a non-subject, what Kristeva (1982, p. 8) calls 'a deject'. I am interested in both human and animal strays, how they differ and what they share in common, such as a borderless, abject state of being. I think it is crucial to address the fact that in the period of the Anthropocene, through global warming, wars and the extinction of species, both human and animals are losing their homes/habitats and are in danger of living permanently in a state of exile. I think that animals who have been abandoned, ejected, and rendered homeless, understand – just as we do – how it feels to be othered, to live on the outside. I argue that in order to understand what is happening, and to act, we need to think from the outside, to develop a 'stray' ethics.

NC: In both *The Monstrous-Feminine* and *Phallic Panic* you discuss the importance of sound in horror films, from Regan's 'snarling, grunting voice' in *The Exorcist* as a form of semiotic upsurge in the former, to creaks and howls as signifiers of the uncanny in the latter. The complexity of sound in horror films is frequently 'underheard' but you clearly recognise it. Can you speak a little about the importance of sound as well as the visual in your research as a film scholar?

BC: Sound is a crucial dimension of the abject. Kristeva's semiotic proposes a pre-verbal dimension of language when the infant experiences itself through maternal sounds and the mother's tone of voice. The meanings contained therein do not relate to the symbolic order. Given that Kristeva's semiotic chora signifies a pre-lingual stage in which the infant is engulfed by a chaotic mix of emotions, feelings, and sounds, there is always the potential for the abject to irrupt through sound. Yes, definitely. Films about horror and the uncanny play on the power of sounds to unsettle the spectator. The rights sounds in horror can be very scary. Because the semiotic refers to the time of the mother-infant relationship, prior to entry into the symbolic and language, the maternal figure, particularly the monstrous-feminine, is associated directly with the irruption of abject sounds – grunts, howls, snarls and screams, and so on.

The scream, particularly woman's scream, is a staple of the horror genre – she seems to scream on behalf of all of the traumatised beings of the narrative. Sometimes, as in *Psycho*, her terror is also registered through her open mouth which forms an 'O' or a 'nothing' signifying the collapse of meaning in image and sound making way for the irruption of the abject. In films such as *Psycho* abject sounds can create a surplus of affect. Here the relationship between image and sound combines to bring about a collapse of the symbolic order. Sounds such as the 'snarling and grunting' in *The Exorcist* and, as you say the creaks and howls of the uncanny, cross the border between meaning and meaninglessness. The spectator may well take perverse pleasure in sounds that signify a tearing down of the patriarchal symbolic. There is a great article by Deborah Dixon (2011) called 'Scream: the sound of the monstrous' in which she explores sound, horror and the monstrous-feminine. There is another by Elizabeth Fairweather (2014) on Jerry Goldsmith and the sonification of the 'monstrous-feminine' in his science fiction scores. This is an area, which I would like to explore in more depth.

NC: As well as a key thinker on film, you are also a documentary film-maker. Your 1975 work *Homosexuality: A Film for Discussion* seems to demonstrate a belief in the potential of documentary to transform perceptions. Can you tell me about your own approach to film-making and your personal history as a film-maker?

BC: I take that as a compliment because I really did not make many films – only a few. I shot in super-8 and 16 mm. One is a documentary about my travels through China in 1978. This was just after the Cultural Revolution. It was an amazing experience. The other is the film you mention, which was on the beginnings of Gay Liberation and the daily lives and political activities of lesbians and gay men in Melbourne in the 1970s. Its focus is on two women and two men and their own personal histories. I also interview the general public on their views about same sex relationships. That was an eye-opener. I also made a short fiction film on a lesbian relationship. Yes, I still do believe in the power of the documentary film (and the fiction film) to change lives. I think this is particularly true for those of us who belong to marginalised groups in society. As a lesbian, I found film a powerful medium in helping me to understand the processes of othering and the workings of patriarchal ideology. Allowing for the way film can manipulate viewers, even in this age of fake news, film, assisted by the Internet, has the power to create what you might call 'a community of viewers'. I think this is most important. It enables the individual to see that they are not alone, that others share their values, and that collective action can bring about social change. My personal history as a film-maker was very short, but I keep thinking I should make a follow up to *Homosexuality* in which I would re-interview the four main participants. The interview was based on the structure of a 1970s conscious-raising group where the participants talk to each other about their childhoods, school, parents, and first relationships. It would be a kind of *LGBTI 40-UP* along the lines of the wonderful *7-UP* series directed by Michael Apted. It would be great to see where each one is now, what happened to them, their thoughts on gay marriage, the move into LGBTI politics, etc. I just need to find the time....

NC: The 1975 documentary foregrounds your important contribution to the Gay Liberation movement. In *The Monstrous-Feminine* there is clearly a strong feminist dimension to the work but would it be fair to say that sexuality is also, at times, a key concern?

BC: Yes, definitely. Sexuality is crucial. I wanted to convey the idea that the monstrous-feminine is very much in-your-face with her sexuality. During the period of Gay Liberation, we turned around the stereotypes, making 'Lesbians are Lovely' and 'Gay is Good' our new slogans. Other political liberation groups adopted similar strategies with: 'Black is Beautiful', 'The Personal Is Political', and 'I am Woman'. The monstrous-feminine is saying, in a similar fashion, 'The Monstrous Feminine is a Real Bitch'. 'Watch Out'! The monstrous-feminine has many faces given to her by patriarchal ideology – castrator, witch, lesbian, abject womb, mad mother, menstruating monster, etc. But as I have said, many artists and film-makers have turned that around. She also has her own history. Long before I theorised the concept in terms of the abject female body, female artists, for instance, such as Cindy Sherman were already creating images of the monstrous abject woman designed to shock the spectator. In relation to the horror film, the lesbian vampire held particular significance. Horror was virtually the only cultural form where you could see lesbians and lesbian desire albeit in a supernatural context.

NC: Have the psychic underpinnings of horror films changed significantly since the publication of *The Monstrous-Feminine* or do you feel the same kinds of anxiety about Woman and her phantasised body still regularly inform contemporary horror?

BC: Yes, I do think the nature of the genre has changed in relation to the representation of the monstrous-feminine. It has become more knowing, even satirical. A major reason is that an increasing number of women directors are making horror films – or are involved in some way, writing or having input into the script. Women use the phantasised or imaginary body of the monstrous-feminine in knowing ways. I am thinking of Ana Lily Amirpour's brilliant *A Girl Walks Home Alone at Night* in which the female vampire's body is shrouded in a burqa or Julia Ducournau's *Raw* in which becoming cannibal also means becoming liberated from all kinds of patriarchal norms of proper feminine behaviour. *Ginger Snaps*, which is co-scripted by Karen Walton, plays knowingly on the theme of menstruation as the heroine metamorphoses into a werewolf, while *Teeth*, a black comedy about the vagina dentata, thanks Camille Paglia in the credits for her inspiration. She introduced the director, Mitchell Lichtenstein to the ancient concept of the vagina dentata; his response was to make a comic female revenge horror film. I can think of a significant number of horror films which explore the monstrous-feminine and which women have directed since 2000. These include Jennifer Kent's *The Babadook*, Claire Denis'

Trouble Every Day, Julie Delpy's *The Countess*, and Karyn Kusama's *Jennifer's Body*. I think horror allows women film-makers and artists unusual freedom in which to push boundaries regarding gender, desire, and female agency.

An interesting and unexpected consequence of having proposed the idea of the monstrous feminine in the horror film is that women, and sometimes men, in a range of other disciplines, have subsequently taken up the concept. I did not expect that the idea would resonate so widely. I have come across articles on the monstrous-feminine in art and performance art, fashion, music, literature, medieval studies, the classics, women's health, religious studies, and research into new media technologies. One of the most unusual articles discussed the monstrous-feminine in relation to equality and inclusion in the workplace (Vacchani 2014). The majority of these did not regard her in a negative context at all, but rather used the concept to discuss how it might empower women. Sometimes I read works or see an exhibition, which somehow assume that the monstrous-feminine is a concept that has always existed, which I suppose it has in a way, well the idea of the female monster has, but some authors and artists use the term 'monstrous-feminine' without acknowledging its origin. I think it is important to understand that I developed the concept of the monstrous-feminine in the 1980s, which was a very political time, and in the visual arts, specifically in relation to the horror film and Kristeva's theory of the abject. The article first appeared in *Screen*, in an edition devoted to body horror at a time when feminist film theory was highly influential and women artists were exploring the nature and meaning of female sexuality in a patriarchal world.

NC: Given the insightful and compelling readings you provide of films from the Alien franchise in *The Monstrous-Feminine* and *Phallic Panic*, I'd very much like to hear your thoughts on Ridley Scott's recent efforts, *Prometheus* and *Alien Covenant*, and their re-visioning of the alien(s), which strike me as ultraconservative.

BC: I couldn't agree more. Ridley Scott re-works his original idea, which is about the primeval mother, in order to return to the *father* as the origin of life. Prometheus was the Greek God who created man from clay. Feeling sorry for his offspring, he stole fire from Zeus. Zeus punished him by creating the first woman – Pandora. We all know about Pandora. She opened the forbidden box and set loose all of the evils that befell the world. *Prometheus*, which is a pretty dull film, is all about man as the creator of life – the male mother. Mary Shelley made this very clear with her subtitle for Frankenstein – 'the Modern Prometheus'. I wrote about the male mothers of the horror film in *Phallic Panic* and they are all a lot more interesting than the duo in these two films. *Alien Covenant* is a better film but it simply continues the theme of male mothers starting right in the opening scene where Guy Pearce, as the mad scientist, and Michael Fassbinder, as his android son, David/Walter, establish the latter's origins. 'You are my creation' Pearce tells him, echoing *Frankenstein* and *Dr Jekyll and Mr Hyde* and all of those films from the mad-scientist sub-genre of horror films. There are some spectacular moments and genuinely scary scenes in *Alien Covenant* but nothing new. Certainly nothing to compete with the *Alien* franchise. And somehow I find it impossible to believe that the wonderfully monstrous cavern of fleshy pulsating eggs sprang first from the son's imagination, which is what these two films are arguing. Back to Zeus' noble forehead! The origin-of-life narrative of these films is very dull. In fact, neither *Prometheus* nor *Alien Covenant* seem to have much to do with the themes of the *Alien* franchise which offered a completely new take on origins, birth, maternity, cloning, alien-ness, sexuality and female power

NC: It seems fitting to end by asking you if there are any aspects of *The Monstrous-Feminine* you now wish you could revisit and, possibly, rethink. Do you disagree at all with your earlier self?

BC: Well, it is timely that you ask about revisiting *The Monstrous-Feminine* as Routledge have recently invited me to write an additional section of around three to four chapters, for a new edition of *The Monstrous Feminine.* This will explore developments over the past two decades. I am not planning to change my original argument in any way. Rather add to it – emphasise some aspects more. Although I am always ready to disagree with my earlier self as you put it. In the main, I will explore different or new representations of the monstrous-feminine in new contexts – queer, human/animal theory, the Anthropocene, the inhuman, and the #MeToo movement, for example. One thing I will emphasise more, however, is the notion of abjection and boundaries. Some theorists have criticised my argument for talking about the abject as if it were an object, rather than something that is produced when boundaries are traversed. I thought this was clear enough but I will emphasise this in more detail.

The thing that I do wish I had discussed more was Kristeva's argument about the radical potential of the abject. In the section on 'signs' she writes something along the lines of 'In abjection, revolt is completely within being or self'. She sees the abject self as creating new forms of culture. I do discuss the subversiveness of the monstrous feminine, and her espousal of the improper body and her black humour. Looking back, I should have emphasised this more – the fact that she has subverted her own stereotypes. But now I wish I had also explored possible outcomes of her revolt. This is what I will do in the new section. So, yes, it is a very relevant question you ask. Twenty-five years later, and there is still much to say. Like all true monsters, the monstrous-feminine is a tricky creature. She knows how to adapt to whatever comes her way.

References

Bachofen, J. J. (1967) *Myth, Religion and Mother Right.* Translated from the German by R. Manheim. New York: Bollingen Foundation.

Briffault, R. (1931) *The Mothers: The Matriarchal Theory of Social Origins.* New York: The Macmillan Company.

Cowie, B. (1984) 'Fantasia,' *m/f* 9, pp. 70–105.

Creed, B. (1986) 'Horror and the Monstrous-Feminine: An Imaginary Abjection,' *Screen* 27 (1), pp. 44–70.

Creed, B. (1993) *The Monstrous-Feminine: Film, Feminism, Psychoanalysis.* London: Routledge.

Creed, B. (2009) *Darwin's Screens: Evolutionary Aesthetics, Time and Sexual Display in Cinema.* Melbourne: Melbourne University Press.

Creed, B. (2017) *Stray: Human Animal Ethics in the Anthropocene.* Sydney: Power Publications.

Dixon, D. (2011) 'Scream: The Sound of the Monstrous,' *Cultural Geographies* 18 (1), pp. 435–455.

Fairweather, E. (2014) 'Jerry Goldsmith and the Sonification of the "Monstrous-Feminine" in his Science Fiction Scores,' *Divergence Press* 2 [online]. Available at http://divergencepress.net/articles/2016/11/3/jerry-goldsmith-and-the-sonification-of-the-monstrous-feminine-in-his-science-fiction-scores (Accessed: 15th March 2019).

Freud, S. (1985) 'The "Uncanny",' in *The Pelican Freud Library: Volume 14.* Translated from the German by James Strachey. London: Pelican, pp. 339–376.

Kaplan, E. A. (ed.) (1978) *Women in Film Noir.* London: BFI.

Kristeva, J. (1982) *Powers of Horror: An Essay on Abjection.* Translated from the French by L. S. Roudiez. New York: Columbia University Press.

Mulvey, L. (1975) 'Visual Pleasure and Narrative Cinema,' *Screen* 16 (3), pp. 6–18.

Oliver, K. (2009) *Animal Lessons: How They Teach Us to Be Human.* New York: Columbia University Press.

Vachhani, V. (2014) 'Always Different?: Exploring the Monstrous-Feminine and Maternal Embodiment in Organisation,' *Equality, Diversity and Inclusion: An International Journal* 33 (7), pp. 648–661.

Wood, R. (1978) 'Return of the Repressed,' *Film Comment* 14 (4), pp. 24–32.

6 Abjection beyond Tears

Ellyn Burstyn as Liminal (On Set) Mother in *The Exorcist*

Mark Nicholls

In her landmark analysis of William Friedkin's *The Exorcist* (dir. 1973), Barbara Creed writes of the way in which the film mobilises abject substances, such as blood, urine, excrement, and bile, in staging a clash between the worlds of the symbolic and the pre-symbolic. These substances become abject when they disturb our secure sense of borders, particularly those relating to the inside and outside of the body. The effect of this strategy of abject mobilisation in *The Exorcist* is to inscribe upon the audience the terrifying and compelling prospects of a highly fragile symbolic order (Creed 1993, pp. 32–42). The pervasive and enduring cultural impact of *The Exorcist* demonstrates both the power of this message and, indeed, the power of its method. Mediating the extremes of the symbolic and pre-symbolic in *The Exorcist* is the central character of Chris MacNeil. Played by Emmy, Tony, and Academy Award-winning actress, Ellyn Burstyn, Chris is a Hollywood actress who discovers her daughter, Regan (Linda Blair), is demonically possessed. Regan becomes subject to bodily levitation, 360-degree head-panning, and the involuntary production of an impressive range of the most abject substances and the most abject language imaginable. It is her mother Chris, however, who endures both the literal and the more damaging emotional soiling of the experience, situated, as she is, at the very border of this struggle between good and evil. This essay considers the way Ellen Burstyn created the role and conjured the emotional reality of its situation, central both to Friedkin's project as an established documentary film-maker and to the film's reception ever since. Analysing elements of Burstyn's performance and her significant personal reflections on the process, as well as those of her colleagues, particularly Linda Blair's, this essay provides a creative practice account which demonstrates Burstyn's creation of the abject mother of the liminal space. It also investigates the limits to which William Friedkin, as director, was prepared to push his cast, Burstyn and Blair in particular but not exclusively, in order to create a horrifying and convincing image of female monstrosity. This joint performance, I contend, is both central to Barbara Creed's groundbreaking analysis and, indeed, to the power of *The Exorcist* as one of the most influential films in cinema history.

The sadistic behaviour of male directors (Hitchcock, Tarantino) towards actresses has recently received detailed attention in the confessional female narratives of the #MeToo movement. I argue that this emerging feminist global discourse is relevant to the experiences of the two main actresses of *The Exorcist* in the context of their work with the film's director, William Friedkin. Creed's argument is that the monstrous feminine is essentially a creation of male fears and fantasies projected *onto* abject images that fill the screen. In this essay I go *behind* the screen to explore what took place on the set of *The Exorcist* and in particular to Ellyn Burstyn as Chris MacNeil, the mother charged with engaging with her teenage daughter as she metamorphosed into something both human and inhuman. In *The Exorcist*, off-screen events, desires and emotions were central to the construction of one of the most horrific – yet strangely compelling – female monsters of twentieth-century cinema.

Burstyn writes about her work on *The Exorcist* in over 30 pages of her revealing memoir, *Lessons in becoming myself* (2006). She has also been most forthcoming about this role in extensive interviews and Q&A sessions given to fellow actors and film festival audiences. Together with similar evidence provided by her colleagues who also worked on the film, this primary material provides a compelling and sometimes insightfully banal illustration of the film and Burstyn's significant role in its creation. Assembled in this way, the creative practice account stands as a useful method in understanding the somewhat obscure and under-theorised notion of social history within the creative arts. It engages interview material, memoirs, reflections, and auto-biography as primary evidence but, most importantly, assumes such texts to be relative, highly subjective and therefore not of unassailable authority. As any internet search will divulge, the history of *The Exorcist* is replete with myth and hype to almost absurd levels. Max von Sydow, who played Father Merrin in the film, has pointed out the almost-too-obvious publicity agenda behind the hype and clearly Burstyn's account contributes to this compromised authority (Jones dir. 1998). It is therefore important to point out that, looking at these texts together with the primary evidence of the film, the creative practice account does not aspire to create a definitive history of the performing arts event. In an industry saturated in fiction and creative logic, however, it does provide compelling insights into its operations which should not be ignored.

Nine Months in 1972 and 1973

The author of the original best-selling novel, William Peter Blatty, based the character of Chris MacNeil on his friend, Shirley MacLaine. Warner Bros. and William Friedkin considered MacLaine's future on-screen rival in *The Turning Point* (Ross dir. 1977), Anne Bancroft, for this much sought-after role early in 1972, but Burstyn was finally approached soon after her nomination for best supporting actress in Peter Bogdanovich's *The Last Picture Show* at the Academy Awards that year (Bustyn 2006, p. 247; Friedkin 2013, p. 241). Apart from some location shooting in Manhattan, Georgetown, in the autumn of 1972 and Baghdad the following spring, the film was shot at F&B Ceco Studios on West 55th Street and 10th Avenue in New York between August 1972 and May 1973. At that time, the US was concerning itself with the November Presidential Elections, the re-election of President Nixon, and largely ignoring the emerging news about the Watergate break-ins. The substantial backdrop to the production of *The Exorcist* for Burstyn, however, was the business of her divorce, the stalking, erratic, and violent behaviour of her estranged husband, Neil Burstyn, and the traumatic effect of this on her 11-year-old son, Jefferson (Bustyn 2006, pp. 247–254). The extraordinary nature of the material that Burstyn was dealing with in the film necessarily required a particular process. This process was designed to allow her to understand that material and place her work as an actor at a suitable distance from the obvious distractions of her personal life and, indeed, the series of deaths, fires, robberies, and accidents that plagued the production.

Burstyn's pre-production preparation for the role and her work during the shoot were, unsurprisingly, extensive. She prepared a character history for Chris MacNeil – a surname of shocking co-incidence, given Burstyn's marital crisis at the time – and worked to chart Chris' consciousness across the plot as she progresses towards deeper knowledge of the supernatural for which her character once had little concern (Bustyn 2006, pp. 255–260). To match her idea of the MacLain-esque 'movie star' persona of her character, she initiated a physical 'regimen' of dieting, yoga, ballet, tap classes, and swimming (Bustyn 2006, p. 256). In the context of this character study, she worked with Friedkin to select a costume designer, Oscar de la Renta, a collaboration which always required a great deal of fitting work in the lead-up to a shoot (Bustyn 2006, pp. 256–261). As the first actor cast in the production, she read with a number of other actors auditioning for various parts. This included particular work supporting the young girl who would eventually be cast to play her daughter, Linda Blair (Bustyn 2006, pp. 256–278; Friedkin 2013, pp. 242–245).

Once the company had moved into the studio in New York, Burstyn and Friedkin rehearsed extensively (Friedkin 2013, p. 285; DallasFilmSociety 2013). The relatively generous and leisurely rehearsal time allowed in those days, and the results it produced, also spread over into a work environment which encouraged significant improvisation during the shoot itself. Burstyn's improvisations around Chris' phone conversation with her estranged husband, who we never see in the film, provide a key example (Burstyn 2006, pp. 261–263; von Sivers dir. 2015). Burstyn and Friedkin also undertook extensive research for the production.

They explored intended visual aspects of the film in art galleries and museums. They also interrogated its psychological dimension through reading and discussing the writings of C.G. Jung as well as recent studies on the paranormal undertaken at Duke University by J.B. Rhine (Burstyn 2006, pp. 255–263; Friedkin 2013, p. 261). Clearly, Burstyn had great admiration for her director on this project and the collaboration with Friedkin is central to the rhetoric of her production account (Burstyn 2006, p. 263). Beyond this research and conscious of the potential psychological impact of the work itself, quite apart from her own personal circumstances at the time, Burstyn's account makes much of the work she did with her California-based 'spiritual teacher' Reshad Field. Field gave her special prayers and meditations to work on at the beginning of each day of the shoot (Burstyn 2006, pp. 260–261). She also explains the significant impact of reading Margaret Fuller and Gloria Steinem writing for *Ms.* magazine at that time, and contemplating the ideas of female equality and advancement that were finding purchase in contemporary discourse in the age of Germaine Greer and Betty Friedan (Burstyn 2006, p. 271; Stockholms 2015). The fruit of much of this reading would be Burstyn's next film *Alice Doesn't Live Here Anymore* (Scorsese dir. 1974), which she produced and which had a profound impact on feminist film discourse thereafter. Describing her own work on *The Exorcist* shoot itself, Burstyn places particular emphasis on the trauma and physical scars of her scenes with Linda Blair in the infamous bed-shaking and crucifix vaginal-stabbing scenes (Burstyn 2006, pp. 272–276).[1] Less sensationally, but equally revealing, she also offers a detailed account of her work with Jason Miller who played Father Karras, particularly in one Georgetown exterior scene, shot on location, where she has to convince the priest/psychiatrist that her 'little girl' is possessed (Burstyn 2006, pp. 270–276). An important piece of dialogue about the nature of good and evil at the end of the film, that she worked hard to change, also received a significant amount of her attention (Burstyn 2006, pp. 265–277).

Protecting the Father Image

Burstyn's account clearly emphasises the extent to which the psychodrama with her former husband Neil, and its effect on Jefferson, infiltrated her work on *The Exorcist*. As she begins to tell the story of the production and the back story of her character, Chris MacNeil, a show-biz history very much like her own, Burstyn pauses to write of Jefferson's encounter with a child psychologist, Jane Bauer. Jefferson, she writes, 'had put on a lot of weight during the past year and was beginning to be teased at school for being fat' (Burstyn 2006, p. 255). Intending to spend Jefferson's first 50-minute counselling session reading volume 9 of *The Collected Works of Carl Jung* dealing with archetypes and the collective unconscious, her study was interrupted after ten minutes when Jefferson emerged from Bauer's office in tears. At this point Burstyn spoke privately with Bauer, who advised her to inform Jefferson about the true mental condition of his father. Burstyn writes that she told Bauer that she had not done so before because she thought, from what she cites as 'a Jungian point of view', she should protect 'the father image' in her son's eyes. Having accepted Bauer's advice, Burstyn's narrative returns with almost shocking fluency to Chris MacNeil, her own physical 'regimen', the idea that to look like a movie star she needed to get thinner and the idea that her weight had always been her '*bête noire*' (Burstyn 2006, p. 256). The unfortunate overinvestment in this particular Hollywood 'shadow' archetype and the extent to which it influenced her work at the time could have been helped by the subsequent, deliberate non-casting of certain talented, young, and beautiful actors auditioning to play Chris' assistant. Burstyn realises the full implication of this dynamic at the time of writing, but it could have escaped at least some impact on her preparations while working on the film in 1972 (Burstyn 2006, pp. 255–263). In a diary entry which she quotes for December 7, 1972, her fortieth birthday, she writes:

> . . . The work is good. Better than good. I'm doing my best work. All is well with me. I'm not fat. I'm in love. My kid is doing good in school. I have money in the bank.
>
> (Burstyn 2006, p. 273)

Burstyn ends her discussion of *The Exorcist* with the story of a troubling and disturbing, attempted moment of death-bed *rapprochement* with her biological father (Burstyn 2006, pp. 280–281). Her previous, deliberate protection of 'the father image' in the eyes of her son and, more broadly, in her own, perhaps accidental and unreflecting general conduct haunts Burstyn's history of the film. Throughout the narrative, her estranged husband Neil keeps 'jumping out of the bushes' (Burstyn 2006, p. 257), quite literally on one occasion. Prior to her move from Los Angeles to New York, Neil violently smashed his way into her home early one morning, forcing her to flee and the police to be called to take him away (ibid.). Subsequently, she had to face Neil, and her own feelings of pity for his condition, in court over the question of his psychosis and potential custody of Jefferson. The result of this court date was that she received full custody but had to agree to give Neil half her royalties from *The Last Picture Show* (Burstyn 2006, pp. 258–259). Having left Los Angeles, partly to get away from Neil, she discovered that he was staying with family three blocks away from her building and that she would have to be constantly looking over her shoulder (Burstyn 2006, p. 261). Soon after shooting began, she learned that Neil had attacked his own father, had been hospitalised, and was receiving shock treatment (Burstyn 2006, pp. 268–269).

Considered in this context, we can see how the filming of *The Exorcist* presented Burstyn with very particular dilemmas of self-protection, let alone workplace professionalism, in relation to broader contemporary dilemmas of male authority, violence, and, indeed, the issues of the protection of children. Burstyn's emphasis that she took particular care that her initial negotiations with Friedkin and author Blatty should take place not in their offices but in neutral territory is important to note (Burstyn 2006, pp. 245–250, SAG-AFTRA 2013, Filmfest 2016). The fact that when he arrived in Los Angeles, Jason Miller seemed to think he had the right to demand Burstyn pick him up at his hotel, take him out to dinner and then, when she demurred, said 'Get your ass over here' (Burstyn 2006, p. 257) is clear evidence that her sensitivities about working with such men in the industry of that time were in no way unfounded. Only on reflection did she finally refuse Miller's dictates and this encounter did not stop him from making a pass at her when they finally met with Friedkin the very next day (ibid.).

Burstyn's collaboration with Billy Friedkin was, gratifyingly, more professionally conducted. Like her colleagues, Burstyn has always been at pains to stress her admiration for Friedkin and his work on the film (Burstyn 2006, pp. 262–279; Bouzereau dir. 2010; Jones dir. 1998; Stockholms 2015). She also relates the extent to which she was clearly 'spellbound' by him and eager that he should be pleased with her work (Burstyn 2006, 263–278). Reading her account, we realise that their mutual negotiation of issues of power and authority on set were far from simple. Key moments in the filming process clearly demonstrate the complexity of these issues. These moments demonstrate how subtle and challenging these working relationships can be in an industry where notions of professionalism and that concept's relationship to wider community standards is somewhat confused and, at times, highly tenuous.

Writing of her first scene in the movie, the first scene she shot, Burstyn tells of a delay caused by the colour of her satin pyjamas. Owen Roizman, director of photography, had them dyed from white to pink. This colour did not please Burstyn, who was justifiably concerned that the new shade was too close to her skin colour and made her looked washed out. Deliberating over the issue, trying, as she writes 'to be a good girl, as was my habit' (Bursytn 2006, p. 269), she finally took the problem to Friedkin who exploded, reduced her to tears and left her begging him not to cancel the day's shoot and not to blame anybody. Burstyn's appraisal of the situation is instructive:

> During this tearful plea, I saw Billy scrutinizing me, watching my nose and eyes turn red and blotchy and calculating that if this continued, he wouldn't be able to photograph my face. It was a many-layered exchange, and I say Billy decided that he couldn't yell at

> me. I cried too easily and ruined my face. He'd have to be careful. He never yelled at me again. Everyone else, to be sure, but if he was going to blow, he would actually tell me to leave the set and go to my dressing room.
>
> (Bursytn 2006, p. 269)

What is evident in this passage is an all too familiar element of handling. This reveals Friedkin as a subtle manipulator and as a director who can deploy aggression and turn it off at will, according to who he is dealing with at the time. The incident also points to a slightly placatory tendency in Burstyn, and a not unreasonable note of relief that she found personal exemption from the less savoury aspects of what, we can only really conclude, were nothing less than patent directorial tactics (Burstyn 2006, p. 269).

In shooting the infamous scene in which Regan repeatedly stabs her vagina with a crucifix, Burstyn was badly injured. Recounting the scene she extends the discussion of her collaboration with Friedkin and makes her director's deliberate use of violence, personal danger, and extreme manipulation abundantly clear. As Burstyn explains the incident, at the point where Regan was to hit Chris, the special-effects expert, Marcel Vercoutere, was required to pull a wire connected to a rig around Burstyn's midriff so that she would crash violently to the floor. On the first take she landed on her bottom and when Friedkin wanted to shoot again, she complained that she was being pulled too hard and that she feared injury. Friedkin insisted that the event needed to look real but agreed to her request. At this point he clearly instructed Vercoutere not to pull so hard, but Burstyn then writes that she 'felt an exchange between them behind my back' (Burstyn 2006, p. 275). Vercoutere confirms that Friedkin did, indeed, reverse his earlier instruction, telling him to "give it to her this time" (Jones 1998). According to Burstyn's account, this resulted in her being pulled 'much harder than the first time' (Burstyn 2006, p. 275), causing her to fall on her sacrum, injuring herself badly and screaming with 'the worst pain I ever felt' (ibid.). She then looked to Friedkin to cut, but he simply instructed cinematographer Owen Roizman to move the camera in closer, holding the shot to capture her pain, until Burstyn forced the cut but telling him to 'turn the fucking camera off' (Burstyn 2006, p. 276).

Burstyn's evaluation of the incident comes two pages later. It tells a great deal about levels of genuine ambivalence that confront actors, directors, and other creative professionals in such situations both immediately and upon later and mature reflection. The incident was clearly significant and had physical impact on her. She writes, 'this was the beginning of a long line of doctors and practitioners who would treat my back and the arthritis that developed in the scar tissue' (Burstyn 2006,

p. 278). Notably, however, she appraises Friedkin's performance with a level of generosity and an obvious sense of personal responsibility:

> Although I've been angry at Billy for this, I don't blame him. If I had to shoot the scene today, I would insist on padding on me *and* the floor. I would not allow anyone to yank me so hard. I would take care of myself. I didn't know how to do it then. That was not Billy's fault. Billy would do anything to 'get the shot'. That was his priority. I knew that about him. I just didn't know yet how to defend myself in the face of that fact. I do now.
>
> (ibid.)

Nevertheless, both in *Lessons* and in the broad spectrum of interviews on the making of the film, Burstyn gives a very clear indication that Friedkin's methods were 'way beyond what anyone needs to do to make a movie' (Jones dir. 1998).

"Father Karras, It's My Little Girl"

Quite apart from Burstyn's personal anxieties over the care of her son Jefferson at the time of shooting *The Exorcist*, there is nothing remarkable in her modest references to her specific, somewhat protective, work with the child actor playing Regan, Linda Blair. Creed's analysis of the film emphasises repressed sexual desires between mother and daughter, maternal authority over the mapping of the daughter's clean and proper body, the daughter's possessiveness over her mother, and the psychological and social energies at play working to disrupt this dyadic relationship (Creed 1993, pp. 35–40). In addition to the way we understand the relationship in this context, the particular nature of Burstyn's role as Regan's mother would necessarily bring them both into a close working relationship, as it would for two actors in almost any similar circumstances. Friedkin points out that, 'Ellen and Linda developed a rapport that allowed their scenes together to become effortless' (Friedkin 2013, p. 256). In *Lessons*, Burstyn points to her work with Blair in two important instances. In pre-production she indicates the way she worked with Blair to loosen up and improve her performance by intentionally moving away from the script and improvising during her initial readings and screen test (Burstyn 2006, p. 256; Friedkin 2013, p. 245). Pre-empting her own experience of on-set physical danger as discussed above, Burstyn tells the story of Blair's own back injury endured during the filming of the bed tossing scene when a strap which was to hold her securely in place came loose. Blair kept yelling 'stop' which was apparently too close to the script to alert anyone that she was no longer in character and Burstyn had to take her aside to advise her to yell 'Cut, Billy' (Burstyn 2006, p. 272).

In a film which is essentially about rescuing a child from significant harm, Burstyn's reference to Blair's incident demonstrates the full extent to which both actors had to confront the extremities of Friedkin's set and its particular incarnation of a type of theatre of cruelty. The general account of Blair's own experience as a child actor working with Friedkin demonstrates the extent to which the set housed an environment of anxiety which cannot but have impacted on the work of Burstyn and her colleagues. Beyond the extremity of the material they were working on, this anxiety was certainly about the relationship of that material to their own lives outside work – a familiar discourse for any actor trained in the Adler and Strasberg schools of acting, 'method' or otherwise. The fact that their work involved a child to such a great extent obviously extended this anxiety and their subsequent recollections of it. Beyond her account of the bed tossing scene, Burstyn's version of Friedkin's attempts to 'protect' Blair from the excesses of the material tells us more about Friedkin's relative lack of success in this. Hiring actor Eileen Dietz as Blair's body double, then later being forced to argue that Dietz had little more than 8 s of actual screen time in the film, confirms what any viewing of the film will demonstrate as to how much Blair did and did not have to do. It was certainly Mercedes McCambridge's voice which was later used to overdub 'some of the demon's lines', but any notion that Blair did not have to at least mouth expressions such as 'Fuck me. Fuck me', 'your cunting daughter' and 'let Jesus fuck you' while on set is naïve in the extreme (Burstyn 2006, pp. 272–273). As many of her adult colleagues have remarked, Blair was certainly called on to speak such lines regularly on set (Jones dir. 1998). According to Friedkin, whatever lines were overdubbed by McCambridge, he is quite definite about the fact that 'Linda Blair recorded everything' (Friedkin 2013, pp. 285–304).

Blair's own account of the shoot emphasises the extreme difficulties she encountered, but she is equally concerned to stress her own precocious professionalism. In relation to the bed-tossing scene, Blair contradicts Burstyn by making a point of the fact that she called 'stop it, really' rather than 'stop it Billy' and hence she boasts that she 'never broke character'(Jones 1998). In relation to the foul language, sexual gestures and concepts and extreme behaviour in which she was required to involve herself and contemplate, she repeatedly states that, as a 13-year-old child, she did not understand what any of it meant. Furthermore she emphasises that the processes she went through to deliver the lines and perform the business were thoroughly mechanical and simply the result of her carrying out her director's instructions exactly as he required. In this she clearly endorses Friedkin's view that their relationship was one of "mutual trust" and makes much of her consistency with the general cast tendency to ratify Friedkin's personal vision for the film however extreme. Clearly essential to Blair's mature vision of the shoot was the fact that she understood that Friedkin was convinced of her psychological stability and suitability for the job and that he had a developed understanding and consciousness of the full implications of working with a minor (Bouzereau dir. 2010; Jones dir. 1998). It is also important to remember that Blair was accompanied on set by one of her parents at all times.

As Burstyn makes clear, the dilemma was clearly a concern for the cast and crew as a whole. Highly aware of the situation, many of her elder colleagues on set have praised Blair's precocious professionalism and her ability to keep the line between her character and herself. This involves stressing both that she had a particular understanding of this line and that this understanding was demonstrated in her on-set behaviour and performance. It is important to also make the point that, for all their assertions of her professionalism, her colleagues were highly conscious of her as a child and the extent to which her 'professionalism' was really ignorance and innocence remains an open question (Burstyn 2006, pp. 272–273; Bouzereau, dir. 2010; Jones dir. 1998). The fact that Friedkin has totally contradicted Blair's statements about her own ignorance of, an innocence towards, the explicit material she encountered, further raises the question as to how much those around her were deluding themselves. More importantly, however, Friedkin's account of his first meeting with Blair and her mother – in which Blair told him she had read the novel and fully understood what, for example, masturbation was – may slightly detract from the tale of her precocious professionalism, but it does confirm her view that Friedkin felt assured of her sense of balance and that he knew she could handle the material. This is Friedkin's enduring view also (Friedkin 2013, pp. 243–245; DallasFilmSociety 2013; Jones dir. 1998; Maron 2016). Friedkin has said very little about these events and comparatively little about Burstyn and Blair, but he has repeatedly emphasised his opinion that Burstyn is 'supremely intelligent' (Friedkin 2013, p. 238; Jones dir. 1998), and that the primary quality he looks for in an actor is intelligence (Maron 2016).

With Burstyn, Roizman, make-up artist Dick Smith, and especially Blair expressing their understanding of these anxieties on set, particularly in relation to working with a minor, there is no direct complaint made by anyone. As in her own account of her own on-set trauma, Burstyn does not comment on Friedkin's work with Blair. Reading her account closely, however, leaves little room for doubt as to what was actually going on. In the 1988 interview, she makes her positive feelings for Friedkin clear, but has little reluctance in pronouncing him 'a maniac' (Jones dir. 1998). There are a great many personal and professional reasons for looking at these pronouncements by film-makers as questionable. In an environment where the principal protagonists of a shoot have no particular interest in calling out bad behaviour we can still learn a great deal about process and practice. In a context of extremity, but not clouded by accusation and enduring recrimination – at least as we can read it here through, largely, Burstyn's perspective – we can come to a less sensationalised understanding of practice. As Burstyn and her colleagues present it, we gain a strong sense of what actually happens on these shoots and how this can inform our understanding of the final film.

Artificial Stimulants

In Burstyn's account of the two back-injuring scenes of the film, we learn of Friedkin's drive towards making these scenes look real. We also note that on set, during one of these scenes, he played a recording of a real exorcism (Burstyn 2006, p. 274). Following the troubles with theft and fire on the set, we also learn that Friedkin brought in a priest, Father William O'Malley who played the character of Father Dyer, to bless the set (Jones dir. 1998). From these demonstrative gestures of questionable professionalism we understand how Friedkin was clearly concerned with creating an environment to induce suitable performances from his actors in response (DallasFilmSociety 2013). For Friedkin, 'acting is *reacting*', and by telling his actors to forget everything they had done in their extensive rehearsal period Friedkin demonstrates the way in which he was clearly interested in what they produced in the environment and in the moment he had created for them on set (Friedkin 2013, pp. 253–265). This is also emphasised by Burstyn's colleagues discussing the problems associated with freezing Regan's bedroom set to below-zero temperatures in order to achieve the effect of visible breath during the climactic exorcism scenes (Friedkin 2013, p. 267; Jones dir. 1998). In his 1988 interview, Jason Miller tells of his complaint that Friedkin undermined his professionalism as an actor by firing off guns and using other artificial stimulants to induce the sort of anxious performances he required (Jones dir. 1998). Friedkin confirms this but says he fired off blanks, not a gun (DallasFilmSociety 2013). Beyond this, Friedkin induced, and later highly praised, a performance from Miller in a key scene shot at the time of Miller's son's life-threatening injury and hospitalisation. He also created a similar performance from an apparently thankful Bill O'Malley (Fr. Dyer) by slapping him across the face just before he was to act the scene in which his character gives Fr. Karras a final blessing and absolution. From these examples, we can determine the extent to which such environmental stimulants are appealing to Friedkin as a director, and seemingly justifiable (Friedkin 2013, p. 258).

In his memoirs, Friedkin says nothing of the moments of on-set tension that Burstyn and Blair have discussed and which I have considered here. In fact, in discussing over 90 pages of his treatment of *The Exorcist*, his account of his work with these actors, as has been alluded to, is full of praise and places an emphasis on their intelligence but it is comparatively brief. Not commenting directly on these scenes, his does give some indication of his thoughts in terms of the potential criticism of his excessive measures. Of the O'Malley slap scene he writes:

> This is not a solution I recommend to aspiring directors, but there are times when you have to have *the* solution to whatever problems arise. Occasionally and rarely, the solution is as drastic as the one I've described, which I have used on only three occasions in a career spanning more than forty years.
>
> (Friedkin 2013, p. 265)

Actor's Studio Co-President (since 1995) and Artistic Director (New York, 1981–1988 & 2008–2017), Burstyn has expressed caution over the relationship between the artificialities of demonstrative technique and good acting. She has also expressed challenges to certain popular perceptions of the 'method' by making statements, for example in relation to the use of character make-up, which demonstrate her belief in the necessity to separate her work from the rest of her life (Stockholms 2015). In terms of her collaboration with directors, when recently asked about what she appreciates in a director, she has responded repeatedly, if a little churlishly, 'I look for a director that does not interfere with my process' (SAG-AFTRA 2013). Furthermore, Burstyn has indicated that she likes a director who leaves here alone and interferes only when strictly necessarily (SAG-AFTRA 2013; Stockholms 2015). Despite these statements, this essay has clearly indicated the extent to which Burstyn's essential lack of dogmatism on these points did not get in the way of her pursuit of the 'real', nor in the way of Friedkin's process to achieve this goal.

Outlining the notorious sound problems involved and the anticipated requirements of post-synchronisation, Burstyn makes much of her Georgetown exterior location scene with Jason Miller. In this she asserts her particular lack of compromise over the performance she achieved in this emotionally potent encounter in the film when she has to admit that she is asking the priest for an exorcism for 'my little girl' (Burstyn 2006, pp. 270–271). She also makes much of the debate with Friedkin and Blatty over her last lines in the film, essentially Chris MacNeil's conclusions as to her beliefs about God and the devil and what had, in fact, happened to her and her daughter (Burstyn 2006, pp. 265–267). In both cases, Burstyn asserts the case for her character, which she has articulated in more recent interviews in general terms as 'about being real' (Filmfest 2016; Walsh 2018). For Burstyn, this comes from her training under Lee Strasberg at The Actors Studio. The idea of 'being real' is quite different from being 'natural', in the sense of what we might think of as a confident on camera/stage performance, of being at ease. What Strasberg taught her to articulate in this context of 'real', she explains, was 'to be present on the stage', in the moment and in character (Burstyn 2015; Filmfest 2016). Frequently she has acknowledged Peter Bogdanovich's direction when she was having difficulties with a dialogue-free scene on the set of *The Last Picture Show*, 'Think the thoughts of the character and the camera will read your mind' (Filmfest 2016; SAG-AFTRA 2013). In this context and despite her expressed reservations about Friedkin's maniacal tendencies, subscribing to such ideas, she can allow herself little room for disagreement with Friedkin's methods. Concluding that his approach was about building the film in such a way that audiences believed in the characters, particularly in the performance of a female child succumbing to possession by the devil, and their relationships, Burstyn can only really see these methods as substantially consistent with at least the essential aims of her own process (Stockholms 2015). Certainly this seems to be the conclusion of many of her colleagues who, like Max von Sydow, view Friedkin's methods on the film as stimulating but most unusual (Jones dir. 1998).

One of the most popular discourses about the making of *The Exorcist* is the cataloguing of accident, misfortune and even death that occurred during that time – the so-called '*Exorcist* Curse'. For all her intelligence, professional insight and broad-minded common sense, Burstyn is not exempt from indulging the audience's appetite for this type of delicious publicity hype and she carefully sets the fires and cast-related deaths out in an obvious list (Burstyn 2006, pp. 264–265; Jones dir. 1998).[2] Beyond the attractive fodder they provide the films on-going publicity, one reason for Burstyn's dedication to their significance lies in their essential validation of her Jung-inspired spirituality. In raising the idea of a film company exhibiting a 'collective shadow' and that shadow being potentially a manifestation of evil, like the 'collective shadow of Germany during World War II', she directly references one of Jung's most well-known and politically complex observations (Gellert 1998, p. 75). Continuing to highlight the extent of bad luck which fell on the cast and crew during the shoot simply operates to justify a largely harmless numinous curiosity in Burstyn. It also articulates a spiritual engagement which she has obviously found useful in the creation of her roles and, indeed, in the difficulties encountered in the more complex performance of self. Beyond this, however, there is a strong sense that in continuing to spin the tale, Burstyn is once again validating Friedkin's method of creating of an environment of extreme, artificial events and stimulants deemed necessary in constructing a convincing narrative of female metamorphosis, hysteria, and possession. Friedkin, she points out, was not pursuing a religious curiosity in making the film, but a psychological one (Stockholms 2015).

Friedkin himself sees no particular advantage in advancing or taking away from the narrative of *The Exorcist* Curse. He merely states that had he thought there was anything untoward happening at the time, he could not have continued with the project (DallasFilmSociety 2013; Maron 2016). The idea then that he brought in the priest, William O'Malley, to bless the set should thus be seen to be as artificial and tactical as his ability to turn his workplace rage off and on at will. In repeatedly emphasising the spooky story of the film's engagement with evil, Burstyn is doing the same thing. As Friedkin built an environment for his actors to elicit a certain emotional response Burstyn continues to build such an environment to play on the emotional sensibilities of the film's audience. This should not be reduced to the status of a necessarily commercially minded activity, nor is Burstyn's Jungian explanation of co-incidence in this case particularly convincing. Burstyn, like Friedkin, is essentially a storyteller. Whatever she may believe about the truth of the list of events that occurred in the lives of those she worked with over an nine-month production, we can easily excuse her the indulgence of reciting them in connection with her substantial work on the film. Everyone knows, ghost stories are always best heard and told very late at night with the lights turned out. As she observes in Friedkin's process, the surreal is achieved by convincing the audience of the extent and viability of the real, of characters and their relationships, and then taking them one step beyond it (Jones dir. 1998; Stockholms 2015). Convinced of this practice, Burstyn's recourse to the fabulous is not surprising. It works gradually to lure the spectator into an environment of doubt based on the presence of thoroughly believable but extraordinary incidents. It is up to the film's ever-increasing audience how much to insist on tightening the metaphorical restraining straps and laying down the protective padding. Nevertheless this still leaves the issue of Friedkin's maniacal method casting a dark shadow over the film. Given the new feminist stand of the #MeToo movement, which has impacted on the Hollywood scene, one wonders whether Burstyn, if asked, might not offer a different perspective on the extra-diegetic events which took place on the set of *The Exorcist.*

With thanks to Alison Wirtz and Terrie Waddell for their contributions to this essay.

Notes

1 Burstyn goes on to refer to this as 'the masturbation scene' (2006, p. 275), and the scene is commonly referred to in this way. Blatty and Friedkin use this term in interviews (Bouzereau dir. 2010; Jones dir. 1998; DallasFilmSociety 2013). In the novel Blatty writes 'she thrust down down the crucifix into her vagina and began to masturbate ferociously' (1973, p. 183).

2 These accidents include the near death of Jason Miller's son when hit by a motorcycle while playing on a beach, the unexplained fire which destroyed the Regan bedroom set, and the deaths of cast member Jack MacGowran, Max von Sydow's brother, Linda Blair's grandfather, the assistant cameraman's new born child, the designer of the Regan bedroom set, and one of the production's security guards who was accidentally shot by a New York policeman who believed him to be carrying a gun (Burstyn 2006, pp. 263–265).

References

Blatty, W. 1973, *The Exorcist*, Corgi: London.
Bouzereau, L. (dir.) 2010, *Raising Hell: Filming* The Exorcist, videorecording, Warner Brothers, USA.
Burstyn, E. 2006, *Lessons in Becoming Myself*, Riverhead Books, New York.
Creed, B. 1993, *The Monstrous-feminine: Film, Feminism, Psychoanalysis*, Routledge, London.
DallasFilmSociety. 2013, *William Friedkin at 2013 Dallas International Film Festival*, viewed 2 March 2019, www.youtube.com/watch?v=xP2M4Gsp-rQ
Filmfest München. 2016, *Film Makers Live! Ellen Burstyn*, viewed 2 March 2019, www.youtube.com/watch?v=3AsTwAjd9GQ
Friedkin, W (dir.) 1973, *The Exorcist*, motion picture, Warner Brothers, USA.
Friedkin, W. 2013, *The Friedkin Connection: A Memoir*, HarperCollins, New York.
Gellert, M. 1998, 'The eruption of the shadow in Nazi Germany', *Psychological Perspectives: A Semiannual Journal of Jungian Thought*, vol. 37, no. 1, pp. 72–89.
Jones, N. (dir.) 1998, *The Fear of God: The Making of* The Exorcist, videorecording, BBC, United Kingdom.
Maron, M. 2016, '#684', *WTF Podcast with Marc Maron*, podcast, www.wtfpod.com/podcast/episodes/episode_684_-_william_friedkin?rq=684
Ross, H. (dir.) 1977, *The Turning Point*, motion picture, 20th Century Fox.
SAG-AFTRA Foundation. 2013, *Conversations with Ellen Burstyn*, viewed 2 March 2019, www.youtube.com/watch?v=z3E3ECle1bk
Scorsese, M. (dir.) 1974, *Alice Doesn't Live Here Anymore, motion picture, Warner Brothers, USA.*
Stockholms filmfestival. 2015, *Ellen Burstyn – Stockholm Achievement Award – Face2face*, viewed 2 March 2019, www.youtube.com/watch?v=hktV8lhVGGU
von Sivers, M. (dir.) 2015, *Skådespelaren Ellen Burstyn tar Kampen för Kvinnorollerna: Malou Efter tio, videorecording, TV4, Sweden.*
Walsh, K. 2018, *An Evening with Ellen Burstyn*, Florida Film Festival.

7 Carrie's Sisters

New Blood in Contemporary Female Horror Cinema

Patricia Pisters

> One evening I stood in the middle of my living room and I looked out at a blood-red sunset spreading out over the horizon of the Pacific. Suddenly [...] I saw a huge black centrifuge inside my head. I saw a tall figure in a floor-length evening gown approaching the centrifuge with a vase-sized glass tube of blood in her hand. [...] I watched as the figure carefully put the tube of blood into the centrifuge, closed the lid, and pushed a button on the front of the machine. The centrifuge began to whirl. [...] Blood was everywhere. [...] I looked out toward the ocean and saw the blood on the window had merged into the sunset; I couldn't tell where one ended and the other began.
>
> (Jamison 2016, pp. 79–80)

A hallucinatory scarlet moment, full of images of blood. In the quote above, clinical psychologist Kay Redfield Jamison vividly describes her own experiences of bipolarity. When the gowned shape turns around, to Jamison's great horror, the figure appears to be herself. Her dress, cape, and long white gloves are covered in blood. The tube of blood splashing out centrifugally, leaving red splashes everywhere on the windowpane, on the walls and paintings, soaking into the carpet. Finally, inner and outer worlds fuse in the colour red. While this scene is not from a horror movie, it nevertheless brings together several elements that I want to explore in this essay: a female perspective and female agency (Jamison is both observant and observer) in horror aesthetics; the forms, affects, and meanings of the red/blood splashing, seeping, staining everywhere; and an intimate, inner perspective merging with perceptions of the outer world. These are all dimensions of the vein of 'new blood' in the contemporary horror cinema directed by women that will also run through the following pages.

In the 1970s and 1980s, the cinematographic horror genre reinvented itself, partly inspired by societal developments concerning sexual liberation and women's emancipation. While many of these developments found translations in generic images, the horror genre was nevertheless dominated by male directors, with the exception of a few female directors that confirmed the rule.[1] Barbara Creed's *The monstrous-feminine* made a tremendous contribution in understanding the deeper gendered psychology of these popular horror films.[2] Beyond the classical idea of the male monster and the female victim as 'damsel in distress', Creed adapted Julia Kristeva's notion of abjection to identify the feminine, and especially its reproductive functions, as monstrous. And beyond Freud's classical idea of the woman as castrated, she, rereading Freud's case study Little Hans, made an argument for the dangerous 'castrating' woman. By referring to a large spectrum of horror subgenres, Creed demonstrated how monstrous femininity takes shape in these films that are by and large inspired by male phantasies and anxieties about the other sex.

Since the new millennium, a striking number of women have started to adopt and adapt formal and thematic elements from horror cinema.[3] In this essay, I will look at some of interesting horror films directed by woman, asking how these films are indebted to Creed's psychoanalytic concepts, and investigating if and how they might open new perspectives on 'female monstrosity' as abject or/and castrating. By following a common red thread of blood in the aesthetics (as form, affect and meaning) of contemporary horror cinema, I focus my arguments around Jane Campion's *In the Cut* (dir. 2003) and Lucille Hadzihalilovic's *Evolution* (dir. 2015). But let's start by returning to Creed's work and one of the bloodiest heroines of the 1970s horror cinema, Brian de Palma's *Carrie* (dir. 1976), and its remake by Kimberly Pierce in 2013.

Carrie and the 'Curse of Blood' as Abjection and Castration

One of the most seminal images of popular horror cinema of the 1970s is that of a girl in a soft pink prom dress drenched in thick red gushes of pig's blood; the apotheosis of humiliation and shame that unleashes the shy (and bullied) heroine's hidden telekinetic powers in Brian de Palma's *Carrie* (1976). The film is based on the novel by Stephen King (1974), featuring Sissy Spacek as Carrie. Barbara Creed argues in the opening of *The monstrous-feminine* this scene symbolises one of the most striking images of abjection in the modern horror film: the association of pig's blood with menstrual blood. As insisted by the film, girls 'bleed like pigs' when their bodies are ready for reproduction. The bloody alliance of the nonhuman and human, combined with the procreative and maternal function of the female body, summarises the monstrous feminine as confrontation with 'the abject'. Creed transposes Julia Kristeva's psychoanalytic notion of the abject as that 'which signifies the place where meaning collapses, the place where "I" am not' (p. 8) to themes and images in the horror genre. The abject is related to any notion of an ambiguous border: between inside and outside of the body such as blood, wounds, retch and excrement; between mother and child; between human and nonhuman; and ultimately between life and death.

Creed convincingly argues that the horror film can be seen as a 'modern defilement rite' that 'attempts to separate out the symbolic order from all that threatens its stability, particularly the mother and all that her universe signifies' (p. 14). It is the 'impure' feminine body that signifies the abject par excellence: menstrual blood, intra-uterine spaces as monstrous wombs, and terrifying mothers as obsessed and mad creatures that cannot let go of their bodily offspring are all images that find many translations in horror figures such as alien monsters, possessed women, lesbian vampires, and scary witches. In de Palma's film, Carrie White's own mother, who suffers from theomania, is the first to declare this abjection of the feminine body as she lectures Carrie on the 'sin and weakness of women' (the first sin being intercourse and sexual pleasure) and God's punishment as 'the curse of blood'. This curse of blood is first of all translated in another curse, the curse of childbearing. Blood signifies the abject as it defies the inside and the outside of the body (at least once a month for fertile women, and mothers in labour).

Does it make a difference when these female issues are presented from a woman's perspective? The question as to whether a feminine directorial gaze makes all the difference is a thorny one to which I will return at the end of this essay. For now, I just want to observe two differences between the versions of *Carrie* that provide us with a starting point. First of all, Kimberly Pierce's *Carrie* (dir. 2013) has added a prologue and changed the epilogue. Contrary to de Palma's version that starts with the gym lesson and Carrie's showering body erotically filmed in slow-motion and soft-focus (until she discovers the blood running down her legs), the new *Carrie* starts with a flashback of Carrie's panicked mother crawling up the stairs in the throes of giving birth, leaving a trail of blood, asking God for forgiveness, thinking she is dying, in shock discovering that she has delivered a baby, trying to kill her offspring with a knife, but finding herself unable to do so. The film also ends with a nightmarish image of a female body in labour. Now it is Sue, Carrie's only friend who survives the prom massacre, who finds herself pregnant in Pierce's version of the story. We see her body struggling with contractions, when suddenly Carrie's bloody hand shoots out of her body. As in de Palma's version (where Carrie's hand grabs Sue from the grave) this then appears to be a horrific nightmare indeed. The 'curse of childbearing' is literalised in this new prologue and epilogue and clearly resonates with Creed's notion of abjection. Nevertheless, these scenes seem to translate more the fears and anxieties from a woman's perspective, whose experience of having something growing inside her own body can be scary and alienating for herself as well.

Moreover, Pierce's version emphasises the necessity of knowledge for women to understand their own bodies, desires, feelings, and social and religious doctrines. A second difference is that the new Carrie, now embodied by Chloë Grace Moretz, has much more knowledge, agency, and control than her 'twin sister' from De Palma's film. For instance, this Carrie counters her mother's biblical dogma that all women are sinful ('I am not Eve, mother!'). And when she discovers her powers to break glass or move things by her mental energy, she starts to read about telekinesis and practises her skills in her bedroom. In this way Carrie's feminine powers are not just wild, uncontrollable forces of nature that just unleash under great (social) pressure, but can be learned and practised.[4] Both the internal, subjective female perspective and feminine knowledge agency and control seem important elements in female-directed blood-filled stories, to which I will return in the next sections as well.

Creed connects female monstrosity also in another way to 'the curse of blood', namely the blood of violence provoked by women as fearsome castrating figures, possessed by 'the curse of murder' as proclaimed by Carrie's mad mother. In the second part of *The monstrous-feminine*, Creed rereads Freud's case of Little Hans, insisting that 'Hans's various phobias and fears all stem from his original anxiety concerning his mother's genitals ...[which] ultimately represent castration, suffocation, death, the void – themes also common to the representation of the monstrous-feminine in the horror film' (Creed 1993, p. 102) Creed explains further that 'not knowing anything about the true nature of the female genitals, coition, and the origin of babies [...] he constructs a series of phantasies [...] in which he is almost always the passive victim of his mother's frightening sexuality'(p. 103). Creed discusses Carrie's witchcraft as a dimension of abjection and the ambiguous borders between the natural and the supernatural. Clearly, the unleashing of her uncontrollable, avenging, and murderous powers that turn the happy prom night into a blood flooded massacre colouring the entire lighting and mise-en-scène red, turns Carrie also into a dangerous, violent, and murderous femme castratrice, leaving no one alive, except Sue, the one schoolmate who was kind to her.

In de Palma's *Sisters* (1972), we also see this combination of monstrous femininity both as abject (the film opening with intra-uterine images of a Siamese twin) and as castrating (one of the twins embodying all the dark and murderous powers of the other). Like the images of abject femininity, the idea of the castrating woman takes many different forms, especially in the modern slasher film. It most prominently features in the subgenre of the rape-revenge movies of the 1970s and 1980s, one of the most controversial ones being Meir Zarchi's *I Spit on Your Grave* (1978).[5] As Creed explains, the slasher film deals specifically with castration anxieties. Among the group of youngsters who become sexually active and who typically are one by one killed with primitive weapons (axes, saws, knives) by an anonymous murderer, there is always one girl who survives. In her book *Men, Women, and Chainsaws*, Carol Clover called these resourceful and surviving heroines who are usually brown-haired and rather boyish (think of Laurie in *Halloween* [Carpenter dir.

1978]) 'final girls' (p. 201). The final girl allows cross-gender identification, and could be called the more innocent, that is sexually non-active, sister of the avenging castrating women of the rape-revenge films. The castrating woman in this more feminist subgenre takes revenge after a sexual assault and makes sure all of her perpetrators end in a bloodbath.

However, in spite of the gruesomeness of the heroine's revenge that is always justified by the rape at the beginning of the plot, Creed observes that there is still a gender misbalance if one compares the utter humiliation of the rape sequences of the woman, to the masochistic pleasures of the men who often die lured by the prospect of intercourse as they are first seduced before being murdered. Which makes her conclude that *I Spit on Your Grave* is 'still misogynistic in its representation of women' (Creed 1993, p. 129). Coralie Fargeat's over-the-top bloody *Revenge* (dir. 2017) presents a femme castratrice of the #MeToo-epoch with cult potential. *Revenge*'s empowered castratrice shows that it does make a difference when a female director films the same plot but with less masochistic pleasure for the men involved. Just like Anna Biller's *The Love Witch* (dir. 2016) offers a feminist pastiche on witchcraft, presenting a smashing modern-day sorceress who puts men under her deadly spell. These films offer new appropriations of typical horror elements described by Creed that nevertheless stay close to the genre formulas and all seem to confirm male anxieties, albeit from a female perspective and with certain feminist twists.

The 'Curse of Murder' of a Poetic Final Girl in *In the Cut*

Jane Campion's film *In the Cut* (2003) offers an interesting case with which to reconsider a feminine perspective and agency more radically but also more ambiguously. Usually described as an erotic thriller, I think it is defendable to consider Campion's female lead character as an atypical slasher or rape-revenge heroine. The film is about Frannie Avery, a high school literature teacher who gets involved with the detective that investigates a series of brutal murders of women in her Manhattan neighbourhood. In the space of this article I will not be able to do justice to all of the film's rich complexity, but I will highlight a few salient elements that indicate a different take on gendered violence through horror aesthetics.[6]

Let me start with images from towards the end of the film where we see Frannie (Meg Ryan) in a red dress, smeared with blood walking barefoot on the roadside. She has just killed the man who raped and dismembered her sister Pauline (Jennifer Jason Leigh); a fate of several other girls in her neighbourhood, all 'disarticulated' in particular violent ways. We see bloody body parts being pulled out of a bathtub, a washing machine, and on graphic evidential photos – all images that we are familiar with from the slasher genre (and unfortunately also still resonate with socially gendered violence). This gruesome fate was almost Frannie's as well. By escaping from the murderer she is a 'final girl' and by avenging her sister's assaulter she could classify as a 'castrating woman' of the rape-revenge plot (even though she uses a gun rather than a knife). In some respects, the typical gender roles of the slasher plot are reversed. Where in De Palma's *Sisters*, for instance, the twin sisters Danielle and Dominique (both played by Margot Kidder), symbolise the docile 'good girl' and the terrifying 'bad girl' Campion presents us with a perverse version of a 'good cop/bad cop' embodied by detective Giovanni Malloy (Marc Ruffalo) and his partner Richard Rodriguez (Nick Damici). Frannie gets sexually involved with Malloy and throughout the film there is a constant ambiguity whether or not he'd be a 'homme fatale'. In the final scenes, she finds out it was Rodriguez who is the murderer, and the film ends when she returns to Malloy whom she tied to the water pipe of her apartment.

Even if this role-reversal could be considered as a feminist perspective that the film offers, Campion does not just reverse plot roles. To understand why Campion's heroine gets involved in this potentially dangerous situation, it is important to take into consideration how the aesthetics of the film create a fusion between inner spaces and the outside world. From the beginning the film sets up a whole range of ambiguities. Over the opening credit sequence, for instance, we hear a sweet women's voice singing 'Que sera sera', while the accompanying piano music has threatening disharmonious tones. Images of a sleazy New York neighbourhood reveal garbage in the streets, filtered through a soft morning sunlight, a red flower painted on the pavement vaguely resembles the body contour of a crime scene; a courtyard garden is full of lush plants, some scarlet red flowers breaking the harmony and at the same time adding a lively dimension. Pauline, wearing a vermillion orange-red dress, is in the garden, drinking a coffee, observing the plants, the sky; suddenly white petals drop from the sky, dotting the summer scenery like a snowstorm. An interior shot shows the 'snowstorm' through the window, while a red Chinese wind chime in front of the window reveals a small cozy apartment. Frannie, still in bed half-awake, sees the white dots and dozes off again; the petals merging with snow-flakes of dreamy sepia black-and-white images of a winter landscape, a woman making pirouettes in ice, a man's hand forming a fist in close-up as if he is about to hit out but then he just skates away from the camera. When he returns towards the camera, his skate carves a deep black cut into the white ice. The cut slowly turns red, the title of the film appears, the letters seem to start bleeding.

Dream and reality merge in the mise-en-scène of this opening sequence, bringing us closely into Fran's private space and mental world. Fran and Pauline (who stayed the night with her sister) leave the apartment, talking about slang words and their meanings, slang words that are 'either sexual or violent, or both' as they comment in their dialogue.

Fran has sticky notes with expressions and poetic phrases everywhere in her apartment. Soon it becomes clear that she is writing a book on slang, loves poetry, and teaches literature at a high school. Throughout the film we see her looking, noting down poetic lines on display in public spaces, savouring the words and expressions, enjoying language, and talking with her sister about lovers and sexuality. Back to the beginning of the film, by the time the sisters walk outside, the fluid frames of the camera work and frames within frames in the mise-en-scène have rendered all spaces small and intimate. The warm yellow-brown colour palette is covered in almost every scene with flecks of bright red (a dress, a chime, a curtain, a cap, a cup, a couch, a notebook, a flower, flecks of red light, bloodstains), and the soft summer light combined with the hints of violence in the music, the icy snow, the title design, and the words has established a familiar world that feels safe, and at the same time has a threatening undertone. The colour red that pops up consistently as flecks, dots, specks, and spots in the mise-en-scène indicates this ambiguity, perhaps even creates the double affective quality of violence and sexuality that runs throughout the entire film.

As Creed and Clover demonstrate, the combination of sex and violence is characteristic of the horror genre, but the differences in Campion's aesthetics are striking. Instead of a lonely girl in a terribly deserted house, there is confidentiality in an urban setting, an intimate bond between two sisters who talk about relationships, sex, work, and daily life; Campion presents us Frannie's private world, where dreams, memories, poetry, imagination, daily life and harsh reality of gendered violence all blend together. *In the Cut* explores the female psyche through eroticism and sexual desire (Benoit) but also through language and poetry, and through the female look (Frannie secretly observing a man receiving fellatio in the basement of a café being one of the most salient acts of looking). All this creates a deeply twisted appropriation of genre conventions of the horror film. Campion's film addresses something beyond the expression of male anxiety for the monstrous-feminine and the thrilling disgust that usually is the affect that the genre calls for.[7] Rather, *In the Cut* stylistically constructs affective relations that open up the range of affects that the horror genre can reach for, thereby creating space for new perspectives. Here it is useful to make reference to Eugenie Brinkema, who argues for a more formal approach to the horror genre, emphasising that horror is a question of design and componentry that

> opens up fields of possibility for thinking horror in unexpected places, within unexpected juxtapositions [...] horror as a problematics of aesthetics, form, design, element, and composition [...] insisting that textual structures and components are not incidental to affective charge but are indeed responsible for it.
>
> (Brinkema 2015, p. 265; See also Brinkema 2014).

While I am not sure if form is responsible for affect and meaning (as I think all formal innovations are always connected to content and resonate with wider social developments), I do think that paying attention to the formal aspects of horror aesthetics, and especially thinking horror beyond the genre conventions, is helpful to rethink its affective meaning beyond gender conventions as well. I will just highlight one more element of *In the Cut* that speaks to this point. A central image in the film is the lighthouse. To the lighthouse is where the murderer takes his victims and where Fran is taken at the end of the film as well. It is here that she realises the truth, and where she kills her assaulter the moment he asks to marry her, offering her a blood-covered ring that all his victims wore when they were raped and killed. Obviously the lighthouse also refers to Virginia Woolf's famous novel *To the lighthouse*. Fran teaches the novel to her students, and in a scene at the beginning of the film we see her in class, a red lighthouse drawn on the blackboard, while she refers to Woolf's stream-of-consciousness style. One of her students complains that nothing happens in the novel, 'just an old lady who dies'. When Fran asks how many ladies have to die to make it good, the student replies 'at least three'. One cannot help to see this as a self-referential wink to the plot of the film, where indeed three women are brutally killed, perhaps as a formal reference to popular genre conventions, while at the same time the entire film is much closer to a subjective and meandering consciousness.

Virginia Woolf herself had a purely formal conception of the image of the lighthouse, as she stated: 'I mean nothing by the lighthouse, one has to have a central line down the middle of the book to hold the design together' (Woolf 2004, p. xiii). I'd like to suggest that the colour red in *In the Cut* functions in a similar compositional way as the lighthouse in Woolf's novel. The lighthouse functions as a beacon in the subjective worlds of Woolf's characters, such as Mrs Ramsay:

> She saw the light again. With some irony in her interrogation, for when one woke at all, one's relation changes, she looked at the steady light, the pitiless, the remorseless, which was so much her, so little her [...] but for all that, she thought, watching it with fascination, hypnotized, as if it were stroking with its silver fingers some sealed vessel in the brain whose bursting would flood her with delight.
>
> (2004, p. xiv)

Similarly, the composition of the images, sounds, and words in *In the Cut* create a stream-of-consciousness, create a subjective sphere of intimate relationships, of female sexuality as personal experience rather than display, of poetry, vulnerability and sexual pleasure, of trust and fear – and above all of creative agency.[8]

Maud Ellmann argues in her introduction to *To the lighthouse* that 'if the lighthouse is the "central line" it stands for all dividing lines that holds design together, for division as a principle of creativity. [...] *To the lighthouse* intimates that art is necessarily ambivalent, destructive and reparative by turns' (in Woolf 2004, p. xxii). As an element of composition, the redness of her lighthouse (and of all the other red splashes in the settings) stands for the poetry and erotic love that Frannie is quietly looking for, writing down lines of poetry in the metro, sticking them on the walls of her apartment. 'I want to do with you what spring does with the cherry trees', Malloy reads one of her notes when he visits her apartment for the first time. The metaphor is strong, connects to the summery petal storm at the beginning of the film, and starts to do its creative subconscious work in the aesthetics of the film, where the destructive physical violence afflicted on women's bodies is countered with reparative happiness of intimate pleasure; where the love for a potentially dangerous man has nothing to do with masochistic thrill-seeking but with a search between trust and distrust; and where reality merges with subjective perceptions, ambiguous feelings and thoughts in the composition of images and sounds. In short, if we can consider *In the Cut* as a feminine take on the horror film, it renders the notion of the monstrous-feminine itself ambiguous, presenting us with a 'dreamy final girl'. The abject as an ambiguous notion or border, cut and extended into creative abjection reaches beyond the typical horror emotions of fear, disgust, and other negative emotions infusing it with notions of poetry and feminine desire.

Posthuman Evolution and the 'Curse of Childbearing'

Let me return now to the curse of blood in relation to the curse of childbearing to see if, here too, we find new perspectives. As Creed observed, one of the most salient features of monstrous femininity is related to 'the fear of her generative power'(1993, p. 16), Ridley Scott's *Alien* (1979) contains not only a reworking of Freud's primal scene (where the child sees the parents have intercourse and phantasies about the question: where do babies come from?) as a scene of birth, but also the idea of the archaic parthenogenetic mother, the mother who can give birth without the help of a male counterpart. Creed analyses several different variations of birth scenes inside the mother-ship of *Alien*, all staged by the invisible alien archaic mother. Moreover, *Alien* is also an example of a horror film that contains 'monstrous wombs ...intra-uterine settings that consist of dark, narrow, winding passages leading to a central room, cellar or other symbolic place of birth' (Creed 1993, p. 53). Other horror films refer to the monstrosity of the womb belonging to a woman who usually gives birth to some kind of terrifying creature; see David Cronenberg's *The Brood* (dir. 1979) as case in point. Again, the point of view on the terrifying 'curse of child bearing' in 1970s horror cinema is presented from the point of view of male anxiety.[9]

In spite of its gendered specificity, it took quite a while before female directors picked up the question of pregnancy and childbearing themselves. Petra Costa and Lea Glob recently translated the anxieties about and changes caused by pregnancy in their beautiful docufiction *Olmo and the Seagull* (2015). While not a horror film, the inner experiences and uncertainties involved in this feminine life changing experience are nevertheless powerful and terrifying. Considering the transformative bodily experience that pregnancy is, Alice Lowe, who directed herself in *Prevenge* (2016) while being pregnant, indicates that 'pregnancy is the perfect time to make a horror movie' (in Miller 2017) As Harriet Cooper indicates, '*Prevenge* is a black-comedic slasher film about a pregnant woman turned serial killer working on the instructions of her fetus' (Cooper 2017, p. 1) that explores the status of pregnant women 'with a marvelous and hilarious directness' (ibid.). However interesting these films are, I will focus again on another female-directed film that addresses the questions of alien, alienating, and archaic motherhood and primal birth scenes, in more oblique and obtuse ways. *Evolution* (2015), directed by Lucille Hadzihalilovic addresses monstrosity in terms of striking and strange horror aesthetics. In 2004, Hadzihalilovic made *Innocence*, a film about girls growing up in a secluded boarding school deep in the woods who at the age of seven arrive in a coffin, all dressed in white, the colour of the ribbons in their hair indicating their age stages in becoming a proper woman. It is a film about the education of girls. Hadzihalilovich's soft use of horror elements in the mise-en-scène and narration creates feelings of unease, as Nikolaj Lübecker analyses in his book *The feel-bad film* (2015). *Evolution* also contains elements of mystery, mythology, and menace and striking formal elements that infuse Creed's notions of motherhood with new elements of ambiguity and ambivalence, addressing the feminine and female consciousness in a comparable yet different way than *In the Cut*.

Evolution is set in a remote microcosmos, a seaside village, filmed at the rocky shores of the Canary island Lanzarote. The village is uniquely populated by pre-adolescent boys, each of them living with a mother that might not be their biological mom. The women have a special connection to the sea, all alike in a sober, skin-coloured light-brown dress, wet hair worn in a tight tail, something alien in their black 'vaguely cetacean' eyes (Combs 2016, p. 71). At the beginning of the film, Nicolas (Max Brebant) is swimming in the sea when he sees among the waving corals a glimpse of a drowned body of a boy, a starfish on his body. Frightened, he runs home where his mother (Julie-Marie Parmentier) tells him that 'the sea makes you see strange things'. A little later, she swims to the surface with a huge and bright red starfish as proof that he imagined things. She feeds him with slimy black-green seaweed and makes him swallow a black substance that is his medication 'because at your age your body is changing and weakening like lizards or crabs'.

The eerie qualities of the setting and figures that populate this coastal commune, evoke horror scenarios in our mind but fail to fit any well-known template or affective response.

The starfish is an important and recurrent figure in the film. Besides its compositional bright red colour (to which I will return) it represents among others the Virgin Mary as Stella Maris (Star of the Sea), and as protector and guarantor of safe conduct over troubled waters (Combs 2016, p. 71). Connecting thus the sea (*la mer* in French) to motherhood (Virgin Mary, *la mère* in French) and to the language of the unconscious (the sea being a powerful force of nature and symbol for unconscious imagination). If Marguerite Duras, who was a master in describing *la mer/la mère* in poetic connection to the unconscious of her abstract characters, would ever have made a horror movie, she could have made *Evolution*. The starfish, however, also indicates a more posthuman conception of the unconscious, reproduction, and sexuality. One of the characteristics of starfish is that they can reproduce both sexually (by spawning, releasing sex cells into the water, usually in groups) and asexually (by breaking in two and regenerating the missing parts). And Hadzihalilovic has indicated in an interview that the film does not deal with sexuality, rather addresses a pre-sexual unconscious (in Prigge 2016).

Therefore, while the images that raise 'archaic motherhood' in first instance are more poetic and less horrific (the sea the starfish rather than an alien monstrous creature) Creed's notion of monstrous femininity is still relevant, albeit with another twist. As already indicated, the boys get some kind of medication to prepare them for 'changes in their body'. After the starfish incident, Nicolas becomes suspicious of his mother and follows her when she leaves the house at night. From behind a rock, he observes how the women of the village have grouped their naked bodies in a star-like pattern, crawling on the rocks like fish on dry land, seemingly giving birth to strange small creatures, or perhaps they are spawning. Definitely there is some form of nonhuman sexuality and reproduction going on; the women groan and cry, almost like a siren or mermaid call. Shocked and horrified, Nicolas runs back home. When he sees his mother later taking a shower, he notices strange suction cups on her back. Nicolas starts to rebel (drawing pictures, asking questions about the medication, openly doubting whether his mother truly is his mother). As a punishment he is brought to a gloomy hospital where all the doctors and nurses are also women. Here he undergoes an operation on his belly and is impregnated. The boys in the clinic, not all of whom survive, give birth either on the operating table or in some kind of water tank.

Here, we are in the full nightmare of phantasies about the monstrous feminine, archaic and parthenogenetic motherhood, and fearsome powerful women. While the operations on the boys' bellies and their giving birth to some kind of creature certainly has a Cronenbergian touch to it, the body horror is all rendered in a very quiet way, subdued by the unmoved faces of the nurses who are watching the operation. And by the boys who are afraid but also very calm. There is no screaming that could invite the audience to do likewise. At the same time, also contrary to the male horror films about scary motherhood and primal birthing phantasies, it's a boy's body that undergoes the scary transformation. While for Hadzilalilovic the choice of young boys has more to do with a pre-pubescent gender-neutral perspective that she wanted to convey, she realised that choosing a girl would have brought in all the cultural connotations there are (in Prigge 2016). However, in spite of this neutral sexuality she intends, the fact that these are all boys in the hands of scary mother figures who, moreover, seem to undergo typical female experiences, does address a man's worst nightmare embodying monstrous femininity. But there is also more.

The boys regain strength on the ward. Here one of the nurses who takes care of Nicolas (Roxane Duran) is kind and protective of him and helps him to escape from the hospital and from the island, using her own cetacean mermaid body as his oxygen tank they swim underwater, in an ambiguous embrace, an 'underwater odyssey that is also a kind of mating' (Combs 2016, p. 71). Perhaps we could even argue that *Evolution* presents us with a thwarted tale of a 'final boy' who manages to escape, if only with the help of a not-completely-human friend. The nurse takes Nicolas to a boat far from the shore, where she dives back into the water, leaving him behind. It is only at this moment, at the end of the film, that he shouts her name and we learn that she is called Stella. Thereby recalling the starfish from the beginning of the film and closing the dreamlike, nightmarish loop. Hadzihalilovic comments in an interview that *Evolution* is an 'intimate and psychological story' (in Prigge 2016). So even if the film addresses something that we could call a collective unconscious, raising the symbolic images of the sea and the starfish, just like Campion did in *In the Cut*, Hadzihalilovic constructs a dreamy (nightmarish) world, borrowing some elements from the horror genre, but also completely transforming its aesthetics, opening to a wider array of emotions and an ambiguous open-ended meaning.

As in in Campion's film, the colour red is the formal element in the mise-en-scène that constructs all these layered and ambivalent meanings. Godard's famous 'not blood, just red' and 'not red, just blood' comes to mind (Barry 2012, p. 4).[10] In *Evolution*, most of the settings are in dark or bleak colours: the black volcanic rocks of the island; the sand or skin-coloured dresses of the mothers; the white houses of the village at night covered in yellowish light points; and the green of the walls in the hospital matching the colour of the sea water in the deep sea scenes, sometimes filtered with some yellow sunlight, rendering the hospital like an underwater space of the unconscious (this also created the impression that the scene where Nicolas gives birth in a water tank could also be a dream). And in these monochromatic fields, red speckles, dots, and splashes stand out. The red starfish in close-up at the beginning of the film covers almost the entire scene, like a gigantic and almost hallucinatory pool of red. Nicolas is the only boy who wears red swimming trousers, and when he runs on the rocks in a long shot, his body is seen almost a moving red blood drop. In the hospital, the boys are covered by a dark red blanket, drenching their bodies in the subdued but violent redness of dried blood. Nicolas has a brown notebook and charcoal pencils to make his drawings, but Stella gives him a red pencil which he uses to colour the starfish on the belly of the boy in his drawings, and the curly vermillion hair of a female figure that he draws, and that seems to be inspired by the trails of wavy coral plants that he has seen in the deep sea.

All these formal elements in the mise-en-scène, and especially the construction of colour as both dangerous and trivial, nightmarishly mythical and mundane, add to the intimate, dreamlike, private unconscious dimensions of the film where the inner world and outer world seem to merge and where the nonhuman and human seem to combine in a posthuman universe.[11] This creates new dimensions of the monstrous-feminine where perhaps not everything is negative, and not every story needs to end in a gush of violence. The construction of colour red creates a psychological inner environment that invokes both danger and wonder. We see here how the notion of abjection as a liminal space between dream and reality, between the human and nonhuman, moves beyond Freudian psychoanalysis, perhaps into a posthuman mythical collective consciousness that is lurking below sea level.

A Trail of Red Transfusions

In talking about 'new blood', I cannot avoid one of the most notorious blood-sucking human/nonhuman abject figures of the horror genre: the vampire. Within the space of this article, I can only conclude by gesturing towards this bloodletting subgenre that prominently features in *The monstrous-feminine*. As Creed argued, the vampire, especially the female vampire, signifies the 'menstrual monster' par excellence (1993, pp. 59–72). Moreover, she is also an archaic mother-figure, giving and taking life, living for eternity herself as in *Daughters of Darkness* (Kümel dir. 1971) and *The Hunger* (Scott dir. 1983) One of the most striking new vampire films directed by a woman is *A Girl Walks Home Alone at Night* by Ana Lily Amirpour (dir. 2014). While the girl-vampire in Kathryn Bigelow's earlier take on the genre in *Near Dark* (dir. 1987) is brought back to a 'normal human life via a blood transfusion, leaving the question whether or not she is happy with that confirmation of the status quo at the end of the film dubious' (Schneider 2003,

p. 87), Amirpour's vampire girl is the first Iranian-American vampire that does not return to humanity. She is lonely, roams the streets of 'Bad City', her black *hijab* floating around her like a bat cloak. She feeds on bad guys and spares those who are good. The film is filmed in beautiful black -and-white cinematography. Red appears only in the posters but is absent from the mise-en-scène of the film. And yet, as Richard Misek has pointed out, in black-and-white film, blood is an example of an 'absent colour, that trace of colour reality that underlies black-and-white-images' (2010, p. 83). And so, also in this vampire film, there is a construction of 'red' at certain pointed (or rather 'fanged') moments in the film. Like Campion and Hadzihalilovic, Amirpour has created an inner space by using elements of horror aesthetics, in particular a formal and new red/blood. It is 'the Iranian environment in my brain' she explains in an interview, where she also talks about her interest in Jung's archetypes and Jodorowsky's dream logic (Juzwiak 2014).

And so, in concluding, I argue that the increase of female directors who have appropriated the elements of horror aesthetics, indicates that the monstrous-feminine as a figure signifying bloody abjection and violence, is still incredibly valuable. At the same time the strictly Freudian psychoanalytic interpretations of the monstrous-feminine have opened up to other perspectives where female empowerment, agency and creativity create different kinds of ambiguities, different kind of affects, especially between inner streams of consciousness and outer perspectives on social injustice, power balances, and our relation to the world. Granted, the extension of horror aesthetics beyond fear and disgust, and across other genres in appropriating formal elements to address the notion of the abject in new ways, is also happening in male-directed films. Think of the friendship between a bullied young boy and a girl-vampire (who is a victim of child abuse) in Thomas Alfredson's *Let the Right One In* (dir. 2008). But then again, this 'gender neutrality' can only happen by working through the notions of the monstrous-feminine, by transfusing the fresh blood of the multiple feminine perspectives of Carrie's sisters with other human and nonhuman, natural and supernatural consanguineous relationships central to the horror film.

Notes

1 Stephanie Rothman directed *Blood Bath* (1966) and *The Velvet Vampire* (1971); Amy Holden Jones made *The Slumber Party Massacre* (1982). Deborah Brock and Sally Matison directied the second and third part of this trilogy, all made within Roger Corman's production company. Katherine Bigelow co-wrote and directed the vampire-western *Near Dark* (1987). Other female directors in the 1980s are Jackie Kong (*Blood Diner*, 1987), Mary Lambert (*Pet Semetary*, 1989) and Katt Shea (*Dance of the Damned*, 1989). I also should mention here from the art world the short 8 mm films by Ana Mendieta such as *Sweating Blood* (1973), *Blood Writing* (1974), *Blood Sign* (1974), *Blood and Feathers* (1974), *Blood Inside Outside* (1975), *Silueta Sangrienta* (1975) and *Corazón de Roca con Sangre* (1975).

2 Carol Clover's *Men, women and chainsaws* (1992) and Rohna Berenstein's *Attack of the leading ladies* (1996) are other important studies on horror and gender from the same period.

3 Between 2000 and 2018 the list of female directors who have appropriated the horror genre has become quite impressive and this essay is part of a book length study on female authored horror cinema. Among the directors that have used the language and tropes of horror cinema in one or more films are Mary Harron, Claire Denis, Marina de Van, Jane Campion, Lucille Hadzihalilovic, Kerry Ann Mullany, Julie Delpy, Karen Kusama, Emily Hagins, Andrea Arnold, Lynne Ramsey, Jen and Sylvia Soska, Kimberly Pierce, Axelle Carolyn, Helene Cattet, Ana Lily Amirpour, Leigh Janiak, Carol Morley, Jennifer Kent, Veronika Franz & Severin Fiala, Ruth Plath, Karyn Kusama, Kate Shenton, Anna Biller, Julia Ducournau, Alice Lowe, Jovanka Vuchovic, Annie Clark, Roxanne Benjamin, Lisa Bruhlman, Issa Lopez, Coralie Fargeat, and Shin Su-Won.

4 Pierce's *Carrie* thus resembles one of the heroines in Naomi Alderman's novel *The Power* (2016), who discover they have electrical superpowers that they can use (and abuse) to change the gender balance in the world.

5 See David Maguire's 'cultography' (2018) on this film (originally called *Day of the Woman*) and its remake and sequel by Steven Monroe (in 2010 and 2013) for its historical and political contexts and its polemic status as 'ground zero' for the rape-revenge genre and its countless imitators.

6 The film received mixed reviews, especially from male critics. Philip French, for instance, after wittily but flatly summarising the plot, remarks that the film just repeats the plot of *The Eyes of Laura Mars* (Kershner dir. 1978) to conclude rather condescendingly that of course the difference is that now, 25 years after male directors broke the taboo subject (a woman falling in love with a murderer), a feminist director changes the style, singing 'non, je ne regretted Ryan' (French 2003). See for an overview of *In the Cut*'s critical reception Lucy Butler (2014). See for an extended analysis of Campion's film Gozde Onaran's *Escaping entrapment* (Onaran 2017, pp. 117–157) and Catherine Benoit, 'Sex and violence as phantasm: eros and thanatos in Campion's *In the Cut*' (Benoit 2006).

7 See also Linda Williams, 'Film bodies: gender, genre, and excess' (1991).

8 See for the international reception of *In the Cut* Lucy Butler (2014).

9 Another worthwhile example to mention here is David Lynch's *Eraserhead* (dir. 1977), a film filled with anxieties about pregnancy and a monstrous brood that was inspired by his own experiences of becoming a parent.

10 'Not blood, just red' was Godard's commentary on the colour scheme of *Pierrot le Fou* (1965); 'Not red, just blood' was what he noted about *La Chinoise* (1967).

11 In Horror film: a critical introduction, Murray Leeder recalls H.P. Lovecraft's short story 'The colour out of space' in which Lovecraft describes the polluted consequences of an alien meteorite as a 'colour that was almost impossible to describe' (Leeder 2018, p. 186). Lovecraft's story then is the starting point for reflections on chromophobia and chromophilia in relation to the construction of fear through colour in horror cinema.

Works Cited

Alderman, N 2016, *The Power*, Back Bay Books, London.

Alfredson, T (dir.) 2008, *Let the Right One In*, Motion Picture, EFTI, Sweden.

Amirpour, A (dir.) 2014, *A Girl Walks Home Alone at Night*, Motion Picture, Vice Films, Persia.

Barry, R 2012, "It's not blood, it's red: colours of Jean-Luc Godard", *Vertigo*, vol. 30, pp. 1–4.

Benoit, C 2006, "Sex and violence as phantasm: eros and thanatos in Campion's *In the Cut*", *Offscreen*, vol. 10, no. 4, viewed 1 March 2019, https://offscreen.com/view/in_the_cut

Berenstein, R 1996, *Attack of the Leading Ladies*, Columbia UP, New York.

Bigelow, K (dir.) 1987, *Near Dark*, Motion Picture, F/M Entertainment, USA.

Biller, A (dir.) 2016, *The Love Witch*, Motion Picture, Anna Biller Productions, USA.

Brinkema, E 2014, *The Forms of the Affects*, Duke University Press, Durham and London.

Brinkema, E 2015, "Introduction: A Genreless Horror", *Journal of Visual Culture*, vol. 14, no. 3, pp. 263–266.

Butler, L 2014, "Too close to the bone: the international critical reception of Jane Campion's *In the Cut*," *Studies in Autralasian Cinema*, vol. 7, no. 1, pp. 9–22.

Campion, J (dir.) 2003, *In the Cut*, Motion Picture, Sony-Pathe, France and USA.

Carpenter, J (dir.) 1978, *Halloween*, Motion Picture, Compass International Pictures, USA.

Clover, C 1992, *Men, Women, and Chainsaws*, Princeton UP, Princeton.

Combs, R 2016, "Evolution", *Sight and Sound*, vol. 26, no. 6, p. 71.

Cooper, H 2017, "Alice Lowe's *Prevenge*: a response", *Studies in the Maternal*, vol. 9, no. 1, pp 1–6.

Costa, P & Glob, L (dir.) 2015, *Olmo and the Seagull*, Motion Picture, Taskovski Films, Denmark.

Creed, B 1993, *The Monstrous-feminine: Film, Feminism, Psychoanalysis*, Routledge, London.

Cronenburg, D (dir.) 1979, *The Brood*, Motion Picture, New World Pictures, Toronto.

de Palma, B (dir.) 1972, *Sisters*, Motion Picture, American International Pictures, USA.

de Palma, B (dir.) 1976, *Carrie*, Motion Picture, MGM, USA.

Fargeat, C (dir.) 2017, *Revenge*, Motion Picture, MES Productions, France.

French, P 2003, "In the cut", *The Guardian*, 2 November.

Godard, J-L (dir.) 1965, *Pierrot le Fou*, Motion Picture, Films Georges de Beauregard, France.

Godard, J-L (dir.) 1967, *La Chiniose*, Motion Picture, Athos Films, France.

Hadzihalilovic, L (dir.) 2004, *Innocence*, Motion Picture, UK Film Council, Britain and France.

Hadzihalilovic, L (dir.) 2015, *Evolution*, Motion Picture, Potemkine Films, France.

Jamison, K 1996, *An Unquiet Mind: A Memoir of Moods and Madness*. New York, Vintage.

Jones, A (dir.) 1982, *The Slumber Party Massacre*, Motion Picture, Santa Fe Productions, USA.

Juzviak, R 2014, "The Iranian vampire tale of *A Girl Walks Home Alone at Night*", *Gawker*, 21 November, viewed 01 March 2019, https://gawker.com/the-iranian-vampire-tale-of-a-girl-walks-home-alone-at-1661607676

Kershner, I (dir.) 1978, *The Eyes of Laura Mars*, Columbia Pictures, USA.
King, S 1974, *Carrie*, Doubleday, New York.
Kong, J (dir.) 1987, *Blood Diner*, Motion Picture, Vestromn Pictures, USA.
Kümel, H (dir.) 1971, *Daughters of Darkness*, Motion Picture, Showking Films, France.
Lambert, M (dir.) 1989, *Pet Semetary*, Motion Picture, Paramount Pictures, USA.
Leeder, M 2018, *Horror Film: A Critical Introduction*, Bloomsbury, London.
Lowe, A (dir.) 2016, *Prevenge*, Motion Picture, Western Edge Pictures, UK.
Lübecker, N 2015, *The Feel-bad Film*, Edinburgh UP, Edinburgh.
Lynch, D (dir.) 1977, *Eraserhead*, Motion Picture, American Film Institute, USA.
Maguire, D 2018, *I Spit on Your Grave*, Wallflower Press, London.
Mendieta, A (dir.) 1973, *Sweating Blood*, super 8 film, collection Isabel and Augustin Coppel, USA.
Miller, J 2017, "Pregnancy is the best time to make a horror movie", *The Cut*, 24 March.
Misek, R 2010, *Chromatic Cinema. A History of Screen Color*, Wiley-Blackwell, Malded, Oxford.
Onaran, G 2017, *Escaping Entrapment: Gothic Heroines in Contemporary Film*, doctoral thesis, University of Amsterdam, Netherlands.
Pierce, K (dir.) 2013, *Carrie*, Motion Picture, MGM, USA.
Prigge, M 2016, Lucile Hadzihalilovic doesn't want to classify her film *Evolution*", *Metro*, 24 November.
Rothman, S (dir.) 1966, *Blood Bath*, Avala Film, Yugoslavia.
Rothman, S (dir.) 1971, *The Velvet Vampire*, New World Pictures, The Philippines.
Schneider, S 2003, "Suck...don't suck: framing ideology in Kathryn Bigelow's *Near Dark*", D Jermyn & S Redmond, eds. *The Cinema of Kathryn Bigelow – Hollywood Transgressor,* Wallflower Press, London, pp. 72–90.
Scott, R (dir.) 1979, *Alien*, Motion Picture, 20th Century Fox, USA.
Scott, T (dir.) 1983, *The Hunger*, Motion Picture, MGM, USA.
Shea, K (dir.) 1989, *Dance of the Damned*, videocassette, Virgin Home Media, USA.
Williams, L 1991, "Film bodies: gender, genre, and excess", *Film Quarterly*, vol. 44, no. 4, pp. 2–13.
Woolf, V 2004, *To the Lighthouse*, Hogarth, London.
Zarchi, M (dir.) 1978, *I Spit on Your Grave*, Motion Picture, The Jerry Gross Organisation, USA.

Part III

Introduction

Reproductive and Post-Reproductive Bodies and the Monstrous-Feminine

Nicholas Chare, Jeanette Hoorn, and Audrey Yue

In this section, Tara Brabazon, Sneja Gunew, and E. Ann Kaplan each explore the monstrous-feminine in relation to biological themes and also as it intersects with resistance to patriarchy. In '"I will not be that girl in the box"', Brabazon reflects on the popularity of Bruce Miller's television adaptation of Canadian author Margaret Atwood's 1985 novel *The Handmaid's Tale*. The essay takes its title from words uttered by the central character, the handmaid Offred/Jane. As Brabazon observes, Atwood's feminist novel was influenced by the political situation in North American in the early 1980s, particularly Ronald Reagan's presidency and policies. She therefore poses the question why this story, a story which centres on women's subjugation in a fictional, patriarchal, totalitarian state known as the Republic of Gilead (a state which has replaced the US), is now of current interest. Brabazon suggests that the dystopian vision of oppression that is *The Handmaid's Tale* seemed unthinkable as a reality in 1985 but now appears painfully close to becoming prophetic. Brabazon believes efforts to make connections between *The Handmaid's Tale* and America as Trump envisions it are well founded. The ongoing television adaptation can justifiably be read as re-visioning the novel in the light of Donald Trump's presidency.

In the screen version of *The Handmaid's Tale*, the abject dimensions of the novel are graphically realised. Brabazon views the television show, with its vivid depictions of 'biological slavery', as 'more explicit and more violently ruthless' than the novel. The abject aspects of the show often revolve around bodies, particularly the female body viewed as a reproductive body, one regularly subject to violence. Due to the abject content, Brabazon finds the monstrous-feminine (as a way of thinking about anxieties towards women's bodies) a particularly valuable explanatory framework. She is also indebted to Creed for pioneering serious analysis of popular screen culture. Although Creed focusses in significant part on horror films, Brabazon here turns to television foregrounding the significant potential of the monstrous-feminine for transmedial approaches to the study of culture. For Brabazon, popular cultural forms such as the science fiction novel and science fiction television series should be viewed as providing crucial spaces for thinking the political.

A recurring theme in Brabazon's essay is what she sees as the need to re-energise cultural studies as a means to make sense of the contemporary political situation in the US. Brabazon does not believe cultural studies in its current form is capable of analysing and understanding creative responses to cultural phenomena like *The Handmaid's Tale* such as the fandom it has generated evolving around the relationship between the central character, the handmaid, Offred/June and a servant called Nick. For Brabazon, phenomena such as the 'shipping' of Offred and Nick, the desire which fans have manifested for that particular relationship within the show, must not be celebrated and efforts (inspired by readers of thinkers such as John Fiske) to read such occurrences as evidence of resistance are misplaced. Kristen Warner (2018, p. 200) reads the 'shipping' of Offred and Nick as therapeutic with 'the fantasy of passionate, unrelenting sexual desire in the midst of a hellscape' granting sanity 'in a time of need'. For Brabazon, however, as a mode of reception to the show it is essentially a leisure activity. She seeks to lay out examples of more politically engaged forms of reception for fans citing feminist responses to the show that openly speak resistance to its dystopian worldview. In this sense, Brabazon argues for more disruptive practices of reading. In a fan fiction context, Ika Willis (2006) has noted the value of supplementation in readings of texts, a coaxing into being of something lacking in a cultural text. For Brabazon, what *The Handmaid's Tale* lacks but holds the potential to spur into being through particular practices of reading, specifically ones informed by the concept of the monstrous-feminine, is a feminist politics for our times.

The next essay, Sneja Gunew's '"From a speculative point of view I wondered which of us I was"', again uses a quotation for its title but this time from Leonora Carrington's (2005) *The Hearing Trumpet*. In an exquisite essay, Gunew weaves together reflections on ageing and readings of the paintings and writings of Carrington and the recent Bulgarian films *Letter to America* (Dir. Iglika Trifonova, Bulgaria, 2001) and *Mila from Mars* (Dir. Zornitsa Sophia, Bulgaria, 2004). The effects of ageing are often described in terms that connote the abject. In his angry meditation on growing old, *On Aging*, Jean Améry, for example, tells of a woman's (presumably his wife, Maria) aversion to her yellowing complexion (Améry 1994, p. 28). The woman experiences ageing as an existential crisis, one causing her disgust and horror when she looks in the mirror (p. 29). Gunew notes that the ageing female body has traditionally been linked to the monstrous-feminine by way of the figure of the wizened crone, the witch. Griselda Pollock (2007, p. 47) has similarly noted in the context of art history that '[o]ld women represented by men [...] are there to terrify us as a *memento mori*; juxtaposed as scary witches, hags, old bags to the soft fullness of the one moment of feminine desirability: youth'. In the context of the monstrous-feminine, Jane Ussher (2006, p. 118) likewise observes that 'the post-menopausal women are represented primarily as the crone, the hag, or the dried-up grandmother figure, her body covered and her sexuality long left behind'. Additionally, Vivian Sobchack (1999, p. 202) has reflected on ageing women in relation to horror films such as *Attack of the 50 Foot Woman* (Dir. Nathan Juran, USA, 1958) and *The Wasp Woman* (Dirs, Roger Corman & Jack Hill, USA, 1959), suggesting middle-aged female characters are sometimes 'figured as more horrible in [...] their own middle-aged bodies than in or by the bodies of the "unnatural" and deadly monsters they become'. Gunew argues, however, that contemporary culture offers a more expansive iconography for representing female ageing, one that sometimes breaks with conventional negative imagery of this kind.

The essay begins with a description of Gunew's visit to Plovdiv National Archaeological Museum where she surveys the museum's extensive collection of prehistoric figurines. To Gunew, the figurines appear to be portrayals of the female body yet the gender is left indeterminate in the labelling of the exhibits. She speculates this reluctance to sex the artefacts is related to backlash against archaeologists such as Marija Gimbutas who linked such figurines with an ancient society of goddess worshippers in what she termed Old Europe (Gimbutas 1982). Mother Goddess interpretations of figurines have increasingly been challenged within archaeology (Bailey 2005, p. 12). Writing of Palaeolithic figurines in her history of art by women, Helen Rosenau (1944, p. 22) also urged caution noting that it is unclear whether the sculptures portray human beings or goddesses but she nonetheless suggested they 'express a subconscious notion of the potential powers of women'. For Gunew, continuing to read the figurines as goddesses offers a valuable 'alternative representational grammar' of the feminine. This grammar is at work in Carrington's art. Carrington was a leading exponent of Surrealism who employed the goddess as a motif in her work. In 1981, Rozsika Parker and Griselda Pollock signalled how the contribution of women such as Carrington and others including Leonor Fini and Remedios Varo to the Surrealist movement had 'been masked by male attitudes' (p. 137). Writing over 30 years later, Gunew contributes to resisting this neglect while examining the theme of ageing femininity as it manifests in Carrington's work.

Gunew then moves to a consideration of femininities in Bulgaria. She perceives Bulgarian women as sharing geographical kinship with goddess figurines of the kind displayed in Plovdiv. This may explain why, in Bulgaria, ageing women are not always viewed in negative terms, the figure of the 'granny' is venerated and valued. Gunew's analysis of

Letter to America attends carefully to the significance of sound, of song and also of silence, in the film. Song functions as a crucial vehicle of folk wisdom with grannies transmitting important knowledge by way of their lyrics. In *Mila from Mars*, grannies are portrayed as caring, as 'guardians of continuing life', and also as strongly communitarian. The two films present different but positive visions of ageing femininity that resist negative tropes.

Returning to prehistoric figurines in her conclusion, Gunew calls for a reconsideration of the archaeological record not in terms of what it reveals about the actual past but as a resource from out of which each age can construct its particular truths. Here the essay resonates with Brabazon's in that it calls for a shift in the reception of cultural artefacts. Gunew urges that we see the figures not simply or solely as evidence of a past culture but also as a resource for thinking our present and possible alternatives to it. In this context, she suggests the traces of a society of the mother goddess (real or imagined) embodied by the figurines help contribute to a different perception of women, including old women, that can form the basis for viewing post-menopausal women otherwise than as pitiful or terrifying. Gunew celebrates alternative articulations of the monstrous-feminine that emphasise wisdom and insight.

An alternative mode of re-articulating the monstrous-feminine is formulated by Joanna Frueh. In *Monster Beauty*, Frueh (2001, p. 100) writes of the stigma surrounding menopause with 'menopause discourse' sometimes producing 'an erotically exiled body'. Frueh, however, envisions post-menopausal women appropriating the monster as trope (through practices such as bodybuilding) as a means to counteract negative discourses and representation. Her concept of monster/beauty as a form of post-menopausal female embodiment is one that simultaneously attracts and repels, skirting the abject yet not embracing it. Gunew's re-visioning of ageing femininity is not reliant upon bodily transformations of this kind but on transforming attitudes and outlooks (although, of course, body modifications can also potentially encourage perceptual transformations). This re-visioning can be fostered through art and film but also by way of scholarship such as Creed's.

The final essay in this section, E. Ann Kaplan's 'The "Monstrous-Feminine": Dementia, Psychoanalysis and Mother-Daughter Relations in Dana Walrath's *Aliceheimer's*' offers a compelling analysis of the artist and writer Dana Walrath's (2016) graphic novel exploring the impact of Alzheimer's on her mother and on her relationship with her mother. Kaplan, like Gunew, discusses the social abjection experienced by older women in society. As she notes, older women have often been linked with 'the image of the wicked witch'. Examining ageism alongside contemporary perceptions of female ageing has never been more important given that, as Kaplan notes, the ageing population is growing. Kaplan's specific focus is on perceptions of women with dementia. These women can be perceived as monstrous in the negative sense of 'no longer having a recognizable *subjectivity*'. Media portrayals of dementia often employ a rhetoric allied to the monstrous-feminine. Dementia is signified by the blank stare, the look that is not, with empty eyes called upon to index an absent subject.

Although Kaplan does not make the connection, the 'blank stare' sometimes features in a horror context. In Ambrose Bierce's (1964, p. 8) horror story 'The Death of Halpin Frayser', a vengeful ghost is described as possessing a 'blank stare' in which 'was neither love, nor pity, nor intelligence', indexing 'a body without a soul'. The blank stare is also a recurring trope in films featuring the living dead. Matthew Weise (2009, p. 252) has written of the zombie that it 'possesses no reason or higher intelligence'. Bernard Perron (2016, p. 308) similarly describes zombies as often depicted as having 'lost their higher intelligence'. Lucy Swanson (2014, p. 178) explains that 'across cultural traditions and generic boundaries', the figure of the zombie has been 'characterized by a key physical trait: the blank stare'. In *Gerontophilia* (Dir. Bruce LaBruce, Canada, 2013), the central character Lake describes the retirement home where he works as like 'Night of the Living Dead' although he seems to link this vacantness with excessive use of medication rather than dementia. The zombie as a living dead embodies the corpse as abomination (Creed 1993, p. 11).

Kaplan argues that Walrath's *Aliceheimer's: Alzheimer's Through the Looking Glass* offers a vital corrective to media depictions of dementia, one that resists the trope of the dead-eyed monster. Like Brabazon and Gunew, therefore, she thinks through questions of resistance in relation to dominant representational frameworks. The graphic novel also provides a sensitive exploration of changing mother-daughter relations in response to the effects of Alzheimer's. Kaplan's reading of these relations is partly inspired by Melanie Klein's ideas about guilt and reparation as they manifest in mother-child relations and partly by Creed's careful differentiation between 'maternal authority' and 'paternal law'. Maternal authority poses a threat to male dominance and links with woman as a castrating rather than castrated figure. The child's relation to the mother as a powerful agent is potentially ambivalent. Kaplan is interested in what happens to a daughter when her mother ceases to register as an authority figure because of dementia, becoming increasingly dependent on her daughter.

The textual and visual analyses of *Aliceheimer's* register different layers to the graphic novel, communicating both conscious and unconscious perceptions of events. Kaplan is attentive to the nuanced role of colour in the novel, the 'pallid palette' which renders images dreamy and spectral. Additionally, she notes how the collage technique employed at times potentially incarnates traces of unprocessed aggression towards the mother. Like Pisters' essay in the preceding section, Kaplan reads the novel not just in terms of its narrative but also as a vehicle of affect. In another link with Creed's work, she sees the novel as likely cathartic. The encounter with abjection that the mother's deepening dementia causes forms a spur to catharsis. As Walrath's mother, Alice, begins to forget her recent past earlier life experiences come to the fore. Dementia in the novel is therefore not read as a loss of self but revealed as process of unbidden self-refashioning. Alice had always sought to mask her Armenian ancestry but with the onset of Alzheimer's this aspect of her identity, for instance, attains prominence. Alice had also not always behaved kindly to her daughter, likely envious of her, causing feelings of resentment. Through the dementia, however, a space for forgiveness and reconciliation to occur is created. The complex account of Alzheimer's provided by the graphic novel contests the dominant narrative of loss of self that is associated with the condition. Kaplan, like Gunew, therefore explores abjection as it shapes perceptions of the post-reproductive body and also how such perceptions are contingent and open to change. Her emphasis on culture as a nodal point for resistance to oppressive representational practices also resonates strongly with Brabazon's essay. The analyses of all three essays are only made possible by Creed's psychoanalytic framework as it is advanced in *The Monstrous-Feminine*.

References

Améry, J. (1994) *On Aging: Revolt and Resignation*. Translated from the German by J.D. Barlow. Bloomington: Indiana University Press.

Atwood, M. (1985) *The Handmaid's Tale*. Toronto: McClelland & Stewart.

Bailey, D. (2005) *Prehistoric Figurines: Representations of Corporeality in the Neolithic*. London: Routledge.

Bierce, A. (1964) 'The Death of Halpin Frayser,' in *Ghost and Horror Stories of Ambrose Bierce*. New York: Dover, pp. 1–14.

Carrington, L. (2005) *The Hearing Trumpet*. London: Penguin.

Creed, B. (1993) *The Monstrous-Feminine: Film, Feminism, Psychoanalysis*. London: Routledge.

Frueh, J. (2001) *Monster/Beauty: Building the Body of Love*. Berkeley: University of California Press.

Gimbutas, M. (1982) *The Goddesses and Gods of Old Europe: Myths and Cult Images*. 2nd Edition. London: Thames & Hudson.

Parker, R. & Pollock, G. (1981) *Old Mistresses: Women, Art and Ideology*. London: Pandora.

Perron, B. (2016) 'Wandering the Panels, Walking through Media: Zombies, Comics and the Post-Apocalyptic World,' *Journal of Graphic Novels and Comics* 7(3), pp. 306–318.

Pollock, G. (2007) *Encounters in the Virtual Feminist Museum: Time, Space and the Archive*. London: Routledge.

Rosenau, H. (1944) *Woman in Art: From Type to Personality*. London: Isomorph Ltd.

Sobchack, V. (1999) 'Scary Women: Cinema, Surgery and Special Effects,' in K. Woodward (ed.), *Figuring Age: Women, Bodies, Generations*. Bloomington: Indiana University Press, pp. 200–211.

Swanson, L. (2014) 'Blankness, Alienation and the Zombie in Recent Francophone Fiction,' *International Journal of Francophone Studies* 17(2), pp. 177–197.

Ussher, J.M. (2006) *Managing the Monstrous Feminine: Regulating the Reproductive Body*. Hove: Routledge.

Walrath, D. (2016) *Aliceheimer's: Alzheimer's Through the Looking Glass*. University Park: Penn State University Press.

Warner, K. (2018) 'JunexNick: The Quietist Ship in the *Handmaid* Fandom,' *Communication Culture & Critique* 11, pp. 198–200.

Weise, M. (2009) 'The Rules of Horror: Procedural Adaptation in *Clock Tower*, *Resident Evil* and *Dead Rising*,' in B. Perron (ed.), *Horror Video Games: Essays on the Fusion of Fear and Play*. Jefferson: McFarland, pp. 238–266.

Willis (2006) 'Keeping Promises to Queer Children: Making Space (for Mary Sue) at Hogwarts,' in K. Hellekson & K. Busse (eds.), *Fan Fiction and Fan Communities in the Age of the Internet: New Essays*. Jefferson, NC: McFarland & Company, pp. 153–170.

8 'I Will Not Be That Girl in the Box'

The Handmaid's Tale, Monstrous Wombs and Trump's America

Tara Brabazon

> But abjection is not something of which the subject can ever feel free – it is always there, beckoning the self to take up its place, the place where meaning collapses. The subject, constructed in/through language, through a desire for meaning, is also spoken by the abject, the place of meaninglessness – thus, the subject is constantly beset by abjection which fascinates desire but which must be repelled for fear of self-annihilation. The crucial point is that abject is always ambiguous.
>
> (Creed 1986, p. 48)

Barbara Creed's career has been courageous. She stared down theoretical dogma with a light intellectual touch, but staunch political imperatives. Her most famous article, published in 1986 in *Screen*, identified the monstrous-feminine as a powerful entity overturning the myth of monstrosity as a specifically masculine entity. I return to this essay and her resolute attention to abjection in screen culture, but translate and migrate her focus and platform of enquiry. I interrogate *The Handmaid's Tale* (creat. Miller 2017). Originally written by Margaret Atwood in 1985 amidst Reagan's America, this narrative was refashioned and refocussed for Trump's America through a small screen re-visioning. I summon Creed's monstrous-feminine and explore what happens when misogyny fuses with fascistic militarism amid a theocratic regime. I probe the rationale for the programme's renewed popularity and re-purposing in an array of cultural forms, particularly through comedic presentations on YouTube. There is something beckoning to the self under those red dresses and cloaks. There is something repellent yet appealing about the Unwomen, the discarded 'runt' of femininity that refuses to fit into the system and are dumped in colonies to work with toxic waste until their death.

There is intent and will in the alignment of this theory and popular culture, following the example of Barbara Creed. The monstrous-feminine has travelled from Reagan's America into Trump's interregnum presidency. So has Margaret Atwood's *The Handmaid's Tale* (1985).

My chapter aligns this time travelling theory and fiction to reveal the brutalising patriarchy and the feminist resistances that fight it, even amidst a 'place of meaninglessness' (Creed 1993, p. 10). In an era in which a president was elected after describing how he 'grabs 'em by the pussy' (Trump 2016), it is no surprise that in difficult times, feminism retracts to the body. The vagina remains the last stand of feminism. Managing (even) this entrance and exit to the body was the misogynist goal of Gilead. The rare fertile women needed their legs open and their mouths shut. They also needed to be repressed and obedient. Their only value was procreative. The remaining majority of women were expendable,[1] useless and unhuman. The women of value – but without rights – were walking wombs carrying future citizens to be subjugated to this theocratic patriarchy. June, the protagonist of *The Handmaid's Tale*, affirmed 'I won't be the girl in the box' (Trope 2018, pp. 186–188). Yet that is her required role. Being released from the box creates phallic panic.

Phallic Panic

Barbara Creed is a trailblazer who – rare for Australian researchers – aligned high theory and popular culture with rigour and delight. Freud, feminism and horror films mashed with relish and precision. Her summoning of the monstrous-feminine and the monstrous mother in particular not only transformed the viewing of *Alien* (Scott dir. 1979) and *Carrie* (de Palma dir. 1976), but the theorisation of the diversity of women in popular culture (Creed 1993). While Creed's deployment of 'phallic panic' in her book of the same name shaped the interpretation of male monstrosity as a displacement of and debt to the monstrous mother, the fear created through lack and loss extended far beyond horror and science fiction as genres (Creed 2005).

The deep repression, the indentured servitude and slavery, conveyed in *The Handmaid's Tale* is shocking but confirms the fear of the feminine. The abject infiltrates: mutilated bodies, discarded body parts, severed fingers, congealed blood, gouging, and visible injuries are inflicted in the name of discipline and disobedience. But as Creed demonstrated, the maternal is also abjected. Shame and humiliation hook into a woman's body, tightly restricting movement, behaviour and freedoms. This is a symbolic corset. Being a woman means being a slave. No income. No property. Possessing a vagina creates life narratives of becoming an 'unwoman', cleaning toxic waste until death, or a household cook and cleaner, a prostitute, a wife without purpose beyond the ornamental, a violent bullying 'aunt', or a vagina for hire (without payment) as a handmaid.[2]

The monstrous-feminine is not real, or accurate. It is not an object or a representation. It does not reside in Baudrillard's simulacrum, hooking, and unhooking signifiers at speed. Instead, it is mobile, coalescing anxiety, confirming 'male fears ... about female desire or feminine subjectivity' (Creed 1993, p. 7). It manifests through panic and violence. The conditionality of relationships – between husband and wife, wife and wife, wife and handmaid, wife and servant – is visceral in its fickleness. The arbitrariness and meaninglessness add to the absolute power. There is no reason for the capricious clothes or haphazard and ferocious subsidence by powerful men in the social order they created. But the tight, callous semiotic and structural violence demonstrates the vulnerability of women whether they are able to have children, or not. Either way, the presence of a vagina dooms them to capricious cruelty and the acidic corrosion of human rights.

The Handmaid's Tale: The Travelling, Transforming Oppression

The Handmaid's Tale did not have the markings of saturatingly successful popular culture. Yet it became the first series on a streaming service to win an Emmy for Outstanding Series. Created for television by Bruce Miller and based on Margaret Atwood's novel, it was produced and distributed by Hulu for ten episodes. Production began in late 2016. Trump's election and presidency would provide the inevitable frame for the show, with the first episodes released in April 2017. By May 2017, it was clear that the success was propulsive and international and its un/predictable context had fired and disseminated its iconography beyond the programme. A second series was renewed and broadcast from April 25, 2018, with a third series commissioned in May 2018.

The plot is unusual, even for a dystopic speculative fiction series.[3] The dissonance occurs because the second civil war in the US, alongside environmental pollution and sexually transmitted diseases, led to the collapse of fertility rates. The response to this reality was Gilead, a theonomic government where men rule and women are brutalised, raped, and subjugated. Women cannot read, own property, or work. This was a 'simpler' time that allowed a blinkered, anachronistic nostalgia to repress and kill. These behaviours are then naturalised (Moosavinia & Yousefi 2018, pp. 162–174). The women are classed, and dressed to perform their status. The Handmaids wear red. Marthas – the servants – wear green, wives wear blue, and prison women – called Unwomen – are worked in the colonies until death. Aunts wear brown and train the Handmaids. Jezebels are the prostitutes in the secret brothels servicing the needs of the ruling class of men.

While much is made of Trump and *The Handmaid's Tale*, the original context for the novel was also strange. Anti-abortion, televangelists, is the foundation for the Christian Right, affirming, like Tammy Faye Bakker, 'traditional marriage'. Ronald Reagan publicly shook the hand of Jerry Falwell, Fundamental Christian leader of the political group Moral Majority, on January 30, 1984. Catharine MacKinnon and Andrea Dworkin argued that consent to sex was not possible in a patriarchy and pornography was rape-inducing. This was the odd jigsaw of sex, abortion, rape, and hypocrisy in the mid-1980s. A review at the time by Mary McCarthy in the *New York Times* demonstrated the scale of the dystopia: 'I just can't see the intolerance of the far right, presently directed not only at abortion clinics and homosexuals but also at high school libraries and small-town schoolteachers, as leading to a super-biblical puritanism by which procreation will be insisted on and reading of any kind banned' (1986). McCarthy was wrong. The resilience, momentum, and traction of the far right – fuelled by xenophobia, racism, sexism, and an unemployed and underemployed working class – have naturalised the language of intolerance. In over three decades, the dystopia has moved from unthinkably distanced from any possible reality to a legitimate warning and fear of the budding intolerance and misogyny emerging in daily life.

Such a change could have been predicted. Communities, even extreme communities, gain an audience for their ideas, enhanced through the deterritorialisation of the online environment. These communities dialogue and naturalise and normalise particular languages and behaviours. What may seem bizarre to those outside of the community is shared within it, and these shared ideas become more extreme. This is a technique of neutralisation, that justifies the unjustifiable through generalizations and patterns of language such as, 'everyone does this' or 'most people think this way' (Sykes & Matza 1957, pp. 664–670) Religion is a strong technique of neutralisation. Irrational and illogical behaviours become neutralised through community engagement and repetition. But politically, this is how populism disconnects from popular culture. Empty slogans like 'Make America Great Again' or 'Blessed be the Fruit' are repeated so often they are naturalised and neutralised. They block questions such as, Was America ever great? What is 'greatness' in a nation? Why is nationalism a functional model for social, economic or political organisation? Why is Jesus' mother Mary configured as a modern model for women? Why should a procreative woman be valued more than a non-procreative woman? Such questions (and doubts and critiques) are silenced. Therefore the techniques of neutralisation and digitised populism carry these extreme views, languages, and behaviours beyond a small, localised community and concurrently render them more extreme.

The othering of foreigners, migrants, women, citizens of colour, and gays and lesbians is a quick tactic to naturalise and neutralise a series of highly contextual identities and behaviours. Sara Ahmed argues that 'normativity is comfortable for those who can inhabit it' (2014, p. 147). This is a powerful realisation. That is why colonisation continues in the mind, long after the armies have vacated the territories. A white face, speaking a national language and fulfilling the expectations of a 'normal body' enables a comfort not granted to many. But what is remarkable in *The Handmaid's Tale* is Offred/June's capacity to adapt to bizarre rituals. The role of the Aunts in normalising rape and mistreatment is important in validating discomfort and suffering as the life path of the Handmaids. The Aunts implement techniques of neutralisation.

Besides Atwood's book being critiqued in its original context for not being even remotely possible and thereby not fulfilling the parameters of speculative fiction, it was also questioned for its popular cultural genre poaching, particularly from romance. Maria Dvorak argued that Atwood ridiculed popular culture – which she described as 'mass culture' – while working within it (2001, p. 143). This rigidity in thinking about literature, writing, and culture is not only stunningly stuffy, but theoretically and politically inelegant. It is also wrong. Although this chapter from Dvorak was published in the early 2000s, it is remarkable that once more scholars repeat the divisions and demarcations of high and low culture. Because of the television series, the book has been released from the suffocating grip of literary critiques that require 'quality' and earnest restatements of historical determinations of cultural value. It can be a part of a breathing popular culture and is freed from its earnest discussions in school and university curricula. It can be political. It can transcend genre. Like Creed's work with horror, it can create discomfort.

The iconography of the novel summons Puritanism from New England, but also American slavery and Eastern European surveillance (Reis 1995, pp. 15–36).[4] It quilts historical events. The bible is twisted, selectively quoted, and actioned on flesh, like a knife through butter. Gilead, the renamed US, is derived from a biblical narrative of Joseph, his two wives and two slaves. He had children with all of them, but the slaves relinquished their children to the wives. However, because of the pervasive infertility in the post-war US, the currency of the culture is reproduction, because of its scarcity. The handmaids are sexual slaves and the children they produce from this slavery return to the elite after birth. At the conclusion of this eugenicist intervention, the handmaids are then moved to the next household so that no intimacy or relationship is possible with their child.

The television iteration is tougher, nastier, more explicit, and more violently ruthless than the book. But as Emily Nussbaum confirmed, both are unified with the 'recognition of the futility of trying to separate the personal from the political' (2017). What is clear in both the book and the television series is the impact of misogyny, the cost and consequences of a systematic, brutalising undermining and unravelling of the feminine (Massanari & Chess 2018, pp. 525–542).[5] An array of disciplines has used the narratives in the novel and screen form to provoke debate and consciousness, including research on the ethics of surrogacy and the history of biology (Busby & Vun 2010, pp. 13–93; Tonn 2018, pp. 415–417).

Gilead is Atwood's imagining of a post-civil war theocracy. Significantly, the attack on human rights is first, foremost, and structurally focussed on women. While originally framed by the anti-abortion Christian Right in Reagan's America, the relationship to the alt-right, a loose collection of misogynist, white ethno-nationalists, is provocatively drawn in the screen version (Marghitu & Johnson 2018, pp. 183–185). This 'community' only existed in nascent form through Reagan. Neoliberalism ruled. Money ruled. Profit ruled. Other concerns lagged. After the Global Financial Crisis, neoliberalism failed, publicly and starkly. Therefore new enemies to justify inequality needed to be summoned. Women – the monstrous-feminine – were the clear target and decoy. The globalising infertility created the excuse for the enslavement of fertile women. They are each designated to a member of the ruling elite where they are repeatedly raped, justified as part of a ritual. Their biological slavery grants the theocracy a future (Gibson 2018, p. 36). The valued currency of Gilead is children. As Margaret Atwood has confirmed, 'the ruling class monopolizes valuable things, so the elite of the regime arrange to have fertile females assigned to them as Handmaids' (2017). The productive vagina is all that is of value. Then the woman is discarded.

The violent attacks on women's bodies through stonings, hangings, eye gouging, finger severing, and repetitive rapes in the name of theocratic order transcend the conventional parameters of brutality in popular culture. Certainly the 2010s has seen television series screen 'torture porn', particularly when pop literature is reinscribed for television. *Outlander* (creat. Moore 2014), *Game of Thrones* (creat. Benioff & Weiss 2011) and *The Handmaid's Tale* are clear examples where watching the intricacies of torture has become part of post-broadcasting popular culture. Netflix and iTunes reorder 'broadcasting standards' to create alternative ways of seeing. Yet this torture and the rituals of public death are not part of a popular cultural dystopia alone. Writers such as Kevin Williamson have called for the hanging of women who have abortions. That is not fiction or dystopia. That is a real, frightening public commentary (Johnson 2014). The point of hanging, as so clearly shown in Foucault's *Discipline and punish* (1977), is that its public nature offers a 'lesson' about crime to the wider society. As Margrit Shildrick and Janet Price confirmed, within the Cartesian tradition, the body is to be monitored and feared as it is a barrier to rational thought (1999, pp. 1–14). Pain and torture must be visible to be a 'lesson'. While *Fifty Shades of Grey*, the books (James 2011) and films (Johnson 2015), naturalised an odd rendering of bondage, discipline, and sado-masochism, *The Handmaid's Tale* only permitted pleasure in the spaces between the theocratic rituals. It is furtive, desperate, and illicit.

Trump Studies Does *The Handmaid's Tale*

Barbara Creed's research, arguments, and tropes became the punctuation of much of Cultural Studies. Her rigour, insight, and imagination were passionate propulsions for the field. Returning to her work, the fire and innovation remains, but it is also clear how Cultural Studies has lost its energy, focus, rationale, and momentum. Cultural Studies as a paradigm has been based on a single premise: context matters to culture. From the earliest interventions by Raymond Williams and Richard Hoggart, the purpose of Cultural Studies was to demonstrate that New Criticism was wrong, offensive, elitist, and unproductive, both politically and intellectually. While the paradigm has travelled away from its key political imperatives since the 2000s, losing its way through under-theorised sorties into creative industries and neoliberalism, the irrationality of Trump's Presidency and confused events like Brexit confirm that the time has emerged for its resurgence. What is required is a tough, rigorous, hard, passionate critique of irrationality, injustice, and ignorance. Trump Studies[6] can – and must – graft a new branch to the history of Cultural Studies.

Much has been made in the popular literature about the 'parallels' between Trump and *The Handmaid's Tale*. It is accurate to draw these connections: border crises (Gunduz 2010, pp. 35–47), religious fanaticism, hypocrisy from political leadership, repression of gay, lesbian, bisexual and transgender communities (Himberg 2018), and the rise of conservative populism, particularly from women (Waterhouse 2018). Significantly Margaret Atwood confronted this con/textual relationship: 'People woke up on the 9th of November, people in the show, and they said we're in a different show. Nothing about the show had changed. But ...the frame had changed' (2018). That is the Cultural Studies moment. That is the moment where culture becomes popular culture and text becomes context. That is the moment where popular memory disconnects from one frame and rehooks into another.

Yet 'the audience' – never singular – is disobedient. We still – as Ien Ang confirmed – desperately see it (1991). Even in the midst of rape, murder, and violence, fans pick a particular narrative and fetishise it. Cultural Studies scholars – at their best – probe these uncomfortable fandoms. The JunexNick fandom that burgeoned on Tumblr[7] was uncomfortable and configured as a guilty pleasure by followers. Kristen Warner's refereed article summoned this unpopular 'shipping' to academic visibility (2018). So amidst the death, fear, rape and brutality, a group of fans still manage to 'ship' two characters, offering an alternative pathway through this dehumanising popular cultural maze.

Such a focus is important to summon, log, recognise, and contextualise, but not to celebrate. Too much of cultural studies, spurred on by John Fiske's 'resistive readings' (1989) and Henry Jenkins and his Textual Poachers, celebrated fans for being fans (1992). It was part condescension and part, as I have described it, ventriloquist dummy (Brabazon 2017, pp. 274–286). Theorists used fans to perform a 'resistance', even when one appeared to not exist or – let's be frank – did not exist. In good times, that strategy may be benevolent. But with Donald Trump in power, there must remain a focus on the political economy, on social justice and citizenship. Love and romance are fine. Shipping fictional characters on Tumblr is a leisure activity to pass the time. But more is required of scholars and citizens. Much more. The key point to grasp and remember is that the majority of the voting public in the US voted for a misogynist to be the president – although he failed to win the popular vote. This misogyny was not hidden. It was in plain sight. It was not an accident. What it does confirm is that for a particular voting community, the rights of women are not important. Claiming sex – claiming a woman's vagina – is the right of men. As in *The Handmaid's Tale*, other women create the conditions for extreme misogyny. Women, such as Valerie Huber, from Trump's Department of Health and Human Services validated the rhythm method over birth control and argued that women abstaining were more important than sexual planning (Crary 2018). Once women lose control of their bodies and the narratives of sex and reproduction then their own cultural role is Creed's monstrous-feminine, the depository/repository of male fear, horror, loathing, and disgust.

The Enslaving of Women

> Men: if you want to know what women's nightmares look like, just watch *The Handmaid's Tale*.
>
> (Valenti 2018)

The Handmaid's Tale remains important for political and intellectual reasons. It reclaims and summons Barbara Creed's theories, demonstrating the fear and hatred of women and their monstrous wombs. This fear evolves into an ordered, organised repression and is controlled by a brutalising theocracy. The combination of Creed's theory and Atwood's book and screen-inspired manifestations demonstrates that women will be co-opted to attack and facilitate the rape of other women (Pratama 2018). One of the truly remarkable, sadistic, and devastating female characters in contemporary fiction and television is Aunt Lydia. Played by Ann Dowd, her violent re-education of women performs so clearly the maxim that a woman does not a feminist make. However, the programme also demonstrates the powerful fightback of feminism. Four of the five directors on *The Handmaid's Tale* were women (Ketterer 1989, pp. 209–217). The iconography of the programme was powerfully feminine. When this iconography entered the simulacrum, the signifiers – particularly the red cloaks – bounced and ricocheted and hooked and unhooked into a diversity of debates.[8] In this chapter I am not endeavouring to understand *The Handmaid's Tale* in Donna Haraway's 'situated knowledges' (1988, pp. 575–599). Instead, I am fascinated and summon Trump Studies (Barbazon et al. 2018), and the posthumous Baudrillard's 'double refusal' (2010, pp. 17–18), to embrace the chaotic, the trans-contextual, accelerated, bouncing meaning. There is no 'privilege' in the 'partial perspective'. Instead, the disempowerment from viewing, through multiple lenses, the scale of the systematic disempowerment, injustice, ignorance, and error is a productive horror. Haraway's validation of 'objectivity' 30 years on seems not only counterproductive and anti-intellectual, but facilitating the disconnection of research from Trump Studies.

> Objectivity turns out to be particular and specific embodiment and definitely not about the false vision promising transcendence of all limits and all responsibility. The moral is simple: only partial perspective promises objective vision ... Feminist objectivity is about limited location and situated knowledge, not about transcendence and splitting of subject and object. It allows us to become answerable for what we learn how to see.
>
> (Haraway 1988, p. 581)

This 'feminist objectivity' is accountable feminism. Yet the problem with empirical / empiricist science is that there is an assumption that the research questions matter. That the funding agencies are supporting research in the best interests of human development and that all knowledge systems should be 'answerable'. Yes, research integrity is based on repeatability, transparency, accountability, and verification. But theory – staunch, unapologetic, anti-empiricist theory – must be more. It must create discomfort. It must move. It must wedge into uncomfortable spaces. It is not answerable. It answers back.

For example, in March 2017, women, dressed in red with white bonnets, protested abortion restriction bills in Texas. During the Women's Marches in 2017 and 2018, thousands of women dressed as Handmaids (Marghitu & Johnson 2018). As Schwartz confirmed, 'Yes, *The Handmaid's Tale* is feminist' (2017). Of greater interest is the doubt about this designation. What type of feminism would question a female writer picking the scab of theocratic misogyny? Atwood has confirmed that life – particularly a writer's life – is 'complex and mysterious, with ironies and loose ends, not a tidy system of goodies and baddies usefully labelled' (Atwood 1990, p. 21). The basis of the doubt about its feminist credentials is dismissed by carefully working with Barbara Creed's theories. Instead, Lucy Freibert argued that while the book is feminist, women were complicit in their own oppression, as if this reality cancels or erases the feminist resistance (Friebert 1985, pp. 280–291). The feminine juts and jars. It has edges. It cuts. It is implicated in patriarchy. It is required by misogyny to add repulsion to the injustice. There is no clean feminism, just as there is no impenetrable patriarchy. Complicity may reinforce already existing power. It may also offer a pathway through repressive patriarchy until a resistive option presents itself. Offred's 'resistance' to Gilead is clear, if small and tenuous: 'I will not be the girl in the box'. Feminists may want her to be the woman on the barricades or swinging from the multiple ropes drawn by hangmen. Sometimes summoning desire, hope, identity, and consciousness from hopelessness is enough. Sometimes summoning a future when there is none is the resistive act. Feminism rarely presents clean and crisp victories. Barbara Creed's theorisation of the monstrous-feminine is a reminder of the repulsion and hatred that all things feminine summon within the oppressor. Mostly, it is a repulsion of difference, a fear of a loss or a lack. Through *The Handmaid's Tale*, the response to that fear is rape, persecution, violence and death.

Transcending the Academic Box

> Like other things now, thought must be rationed.
>
> (Atwood 1985, p. 17)

The Handmaid's Tale was filmed in Toronto, Mississauga, Hamilton, Oakville, and Cambridge in Ontario, Canada. Critical of the US, this series configures Canada as a site and source of freedom. Yet the claustropolitanism remains clear. Borders are everywhere. The US is a prison. This US is re-imagined within the borders of Canada. Similarly, the actors playing the key roles in *The Handmaid's Tale* carry their ambivalent popular cultural relationships and pasts with them. Elisabeth Moss re-assembles Peggy Olsen from *Mad Men* (creat. Weiner 2007) and Robin Griffin from *Top of the Lake* (dir. Campion 2013). She summons a tough woman that – regardless of the obstacles – does not wilt. Samira Wiley, playing Moira, gathers Poussey from *Orange is the New Black* (creat. Kohan 2013) to add rejection and confusion to sexual denial, refusal, and displacement. Ann Dowd, who performs the depressingly powerful and implicated Aunt Lydia, was the cult leader from *The Leftovers* (dir. Leder 2014).

These movements of ideas, ideologies, and iconographies are important and are crucial to creating a saturating – overwhelming – popular cultural intervention in normative expectations. Contextual dystopias matter to political debates (Ketterer 1989, pp. 209–217). They offer a confused and productive reshuffling of past, present and future. While Barbara Creed summoned and sucked the monstrous-feminine through horror films, there is something profoundly appropriate in re-presenting her theories through a book that has been recognised as high culture and worthy of school and university curriculum,[9] but then permeates popular culture through an array of screen-based platforms and interfaces.

How are women to understand their lives? More precisely, how are they meant to understand how and why the feminine is systematically marginalised, demeaned, refused, decentred, and ignored? Creed's monstrous feminine – as a theory, concept, and trope – captures the fear and disgust in men that women's bodies summon. These bodies leak. They grow other humans. They stand for difference. They stand for an alternative to the phallic punctuation of culture. The rise of the alt-right – and yes, that verb was intentional – with the attendant retraction to heteronormative, procreative femininity creates new challenges and opportunities for feminism. In response, we must hope for a tough feminism that does not shirk or shrink for the fear, the abuse, the repulsion, and the disgust.

The Handmaid's Tale – the novel – finishes unusually in the history of dystopian fiction. It is an academic ending of a fictional tale. Dystopias are warnings and most frequently finish – as with George Orwell's *1984* – with a boot to the face[10] rather than a gentle hand (up) to the future. But the final part of the novel is composed of 'Historical Notes' from a conference on Gileadean Studies at the University of Denay, Nunavit in 2195. Professor Pieixoto's commentary confirms that the Republic of Gilead had ceased and it remains – only – of historical interest. Through an academic intervention, the burning cruelty and relentlessness of *The Handmaid's Tale* is released. It is in the past. Resistance did triumph. The screen series is yet to release its account of this future. The consequence of the Donald Trump context for the narrative is that not only is the book transcended, but there is a sense that this story will not end well. An academic conference and Gileadean Studies will not discharge the pressure from this present.

And yet. And yet. *The Handmaid's Tale* – through screen-based media – is an inspirational source for another generation of feminist scholars. Perhaps the academic conference in Gileadean Studies was a disappointment to readers. It was certainly a fascinating twist in plot and writing. Yet this disappointment has not been seen in contemporary higher degrees that remain inspired by the book, the film and the television series. Gileadean Studies – or indeed Handmaid's Tale Studies – have proven resilient. As Hedvig Marx, from her thesis derived from the Master's Programme at Linkoping University, revealed:

> The Handmaid's Tale makes me feel things; it reminds me of how precarious my human rights and privileges are, and, somewhat despite itself, how abundant they still somehow are at the same time … I know it is fiction, but I also know that it isn't. In a way, its own history is part of what gives its dystopian threat such momentum in the now. The almost impossible future of 1985 is the seemingly imminent future of 2017, and both of them are already in the past.
>
> (Marx 2018, p. 4)

Marx, as part of the next generation of feminist scholars, took the dystopia and summoned a resistance to it to create her dissertation. Perhaps Gileadean Studies is not required. Feminism will do just fine. These Handmaids, like all of us, have Tales. It is up to feminist scholars to tell them.

Notes

1 For a discussion of the diversity of feminisms in the book, please refer to Elizabeth des Chenes, *Women's issues in Margaret Atwood's The Handmaid's Tale* (Farmington Hills, Greenhaven Press, 2012).

2 The handmaid is based on the biblical story in Genesis of Jacob and his two wives, Rachel and Leah. They had two handmaids. One man had four women to impregnate and produced 12 sons. But the handmaids could not claim their children because they 'belonged' to Rachel and Leah.

3 I am recognising and applying Margaret Atwood's distinction between science fiction and speculative fiction. She stated that, 'I like to make a distinction between science fiction proper – for me, this label denotes books with things in them we can't yet do or begin to do, talking beings we can never meet, and places we can't go – and speculative fiction, which employs the means already more or less to hand, and takes place on Planet Earth' (Atwood 2004, p. 153).

4 Significantly, Margaret Atwood started writing *The Handmaid's Tale* in West Berlin in 1984. Please refer to R. Setoodeh, "Margaret Atwood on how Donald Trump helped 'the Handmaid's Tale," *Variety*, April 10, 2018, https://variety.com/2018/tv/news/margaret-atwood-handmaids-tale-trump-feminism-1202748535/

5 Barbara Creed's theorisation of the monstrous feminine was deployed with profound effectiveness to understand the grammar of the post-alt-right online environment.

6 Trump Studies was first used as a phrase in the journal *Cultural Anthropology* in January 2017. Please refer to M. Taussig, "Trump Studies," *Cultural Anthropology*, January 18, 2017, https://culanth.org/fieldsights/1046-trump-studies. From this foundational work, Tara Brabazon, Steve Redhead, and Sunny Rue Chivaura wrote a monograph, demonstrating how Trump Studies can be a rebooting moment for Cultural Studies. Please refer to Brabazon, T, Redhead, S & Chivaura, S 2018, *Trump studies: an intellectual's guide to why citizens vote against their best interests*, Emerald, Bingley.

7 'Splitscreen' is a strong example of the genre: http://splitscreen.tumblr.com/post/175782336779

8 An array of parodies of *The Handmaid's Tale* are available on *YouTube*: https://www.youtube.com/results?search_query=handmaid+tale+parody

9 The curricula politics and the politics of reading *The Handmaid's Tale* was well explored in Heidi Laing's *The Right (Not) to Read 'The Handmaid's Tale' in School: Tensions with/in Conversations about Risky Texts* (Saarbrucken: LAP Lambert Academic Publishing, 2010).

10 This metaphor has been used intentionally. George Orwell in *1984* described a 'boot stamping on a human face – forever' (1984, p. 390).

Works Cited

Ahmed, S 2014, *The cultural politics of emotion*, Edinburgh University Press: Edinburgh.

Ang, I 1991, *Desperately seeking the audience*, Routledge: London.
Atwood, M 1985, *The handmaid's tale*, McClelland and Stewart: Toronto.
Atwood, M 1990, 'If you can't say anything nice, don't say anything at all', in Scheier, L, Sheard, S & Wachtel, E (eds.), *Language in her eye: views on writing and gender by Canadian women writing in English*, Coach House: Toronto, pp. 15–22.
Atwood, M 2004, '*The handmaid's tale* and *Oryx and Crake* "In Context"', *PMLA*, vol. 119, no. 3, pp. 513–517.
Atwood, M 2017, 'Margaret Atwood on what "The Handmaid's Tale" means in the age of Trump', *The New York Times*, 10 March, www.nytimes.com/2017/03/10/books/review/margaret-atwood-handmaids-tale-age-of-trump.html
Atwood, M 2018, '"The Handmaid's Tale" author Margaret Atwood on President Donald Trump's America', *ABC News*, May 1, 2018, https://abcnews.go.com/Entertainment/handmaids-tale-author-margaret-atwood-president-donald-trumps/story?id=54934101
Baudrillard, J 2010, *Carnival and cannibal*, Seagull Books: Chicago.
Benioff, D & Weiss, D 2011, *Game of Thrones*, television broadcast, HBO, USA.
Brabazon, T 2017, 'By any means necessary: new youth activism', *European Journal of Communication*, vol. 32, no. 3, pp. 274–286.
Brabazon, T, Redhead, S & Chivaura, S 2018, *Trump studies: an intellectual's guide to why citizens vote against their best interests*, Emerald: Bingley.
Busby, K & Vun, D 2010, 'Revisiting *The handmaid's tale*: feminist theory meets empirical research on surrogate mothers', *Canadian Journal of Family Law*, vol. 26, pp. 13–93.
Campion, J (dir.) 2013, *Top of the Lake*, television broadcast, See-Saw Films, New Zealand.
Crary, D 2018, 'Trump administration family planning strategy is under fire', *US News*, 27 February 2018, www.usnews.com/news/news/articles/2018-02-27/trump-administration-family-planning-strategy-is-under-fire
Creed, B 1986, 'Horror and the monstrous-feminine: an imaginary abjection', *Screen*, vol. 27, no.1, pp. 44–70.
Creed, B 1993, *The monstrous-feminine: film, feminism, psychoanalysis*, Routledge: London.
Creed, B 2005, *Phallic panic: film, horror and the primal uncanny*, Melbourne University Press: Melbourne.
de Palma, B (dir.) 1976, *Carrie*, MGM Productions, USA.
des Chenes, E 2012, *Women's issues in Margaret Atwood's* The Handmaid's Tale, Greenhaven Press: Farmingwood Hills.
Dvorak, M 2001, 'What is real/reel? Margaret Atwood's "Rearrangement of shapes on a flat surface", or narrative collage', in H. Bloom (ed.), *Margaret Atwood's* The handmaid's tale*: modern critical interpretations,* Chelsea House Publishers: Broomall, pp. 141–154.
Fiske, J 1989, *Understanding popular culture*, Unwin Hyman: New York.
Foucault, M 1977, *Discipline and punish: the birth of the prison*, Vintage Books: New York.
Freibert, L 1985, 'Control and creativity: the politics of risk in Margaret Atwood's *Handmaid's tale*', in J. McCombs (ed.), *Critical essays on Margaret Atwood*, Hall: Boston, pp. 280–291.

Gibson, S 2018, 'Familiar nightmares: the harrowing world of *The Handmaid's Tale*', *Screen Education*, no. 89, pp. 36–43.

Gunduz, Z 2010, 'The European Union at 50: xenophobia, Islamophobia and the rise of the radical right', *Journal of Muslim Minority Affairs*, vol. 30, no. 1, pp. 35–47.

Haraway, D 1988, 'Situated knowledges: the science question in feminism and the privilege of partial perspective', *Feminist Studies*, vol. 14, no. 3, pp. 575–599.

Himberg, J 2018, 'The lavender menace returns: reading gender & sexuality in *The Handmaid's Tale*', *Communication, Culture & Critique*, vol. 11, pp. 195–197.

James, E 2011, *Fifty shades of grey*, Vintage Books.

Jenkins, H 1992, *Textual poachers*, Routledge: London.

Johnson, C 2014, '*National Review*'s Kevin D. Williamson: women who have abortions should be hanged and so should doctors', *Little Green Footballs*, web log post, 28 September, viewed 5 March 2019, http://littlegreenfootballs.com/article/43891_National_Reviews_Kevin_D._Williamson-_Women_Who_Have_Abortions_Should_Be_Hanged_and_So_Should_Doctors

Johnson, S 2015, *Fifty Shades of Grey*, motion picture, Universal Pictures, USA.

Ketterer, D 1989, 'Margaret Atwood's *The handmaid's tale*: a contextual dystopia', *Science Fiction Studies*, vol. 16, no. 2, pp. 209–217.

Kohan, J (creator) 2013, *Orange is the New Black*, television broadcast, Lionsgate, USA.

Laing, H 2010, *The right (not) to read* The handmaid's tale *in school: tensions with/in conversations about risky texts*, LAP Lambert Academic Publishing: Saarbrucken.

Leder, M (2014), *The Leftovers*, television broadcast, HBO, USA.

Marghitu, S & Johnson, K 2018, 'Feminist online responses against the U.S. alt-right: using *The Handmaid's Tale* as a symbol and catalyst of resistance', *Communication, Culture & Critique*, vol. 11, pp. 183–185.

Marx, H 2018, Moira, take me with you! Utopian hope and queer horizons in three versions of *The Handmaid's Tale*, Masters Thesis, Linkoping University, Linkoping.

Massanari, A & Chess, S 2018, 'Attack of the 50-foot social justice warrior: the discursive construction of SJW memes as the monstrous feminine', *Feminist Media Studies*, vol. 18, no. 4, pp. 525–542.

McCarthy, M 1986, 'Book review', *New York Times*, 9 February, https://archive.nytimes.com/www.nytimes.com/books/00/03/26/specials/mccarthy-atwood.html?mcubz=1

Miller, B (creator) 2017, *The Handmaid's Tale*, television broadcast, Daniel Wilson Productions, Toronto.

Moore, R (creator) 2014, *Outlander*, television broadcast, Stars, United Kingdom.

Moosavinia, S & Yousefi, T 2018, 'New norms of gender and emergence of identity crisis in Margaret Atwood's *The handmaid's tale*', *The Southeast Asian Journal of English Language Studies*, vol. 21, no. 1, pp. 162–174.

Nussbaum, E 2017, 'A cunning adaptation of *The handmaid's tale*', *The New Yorker*, 22 May, www.newyorker.com/magazine/2017/05/22/a-cunning-adaptation-of-the-handmaids-tale

Orwell, G 1984, *1984*, Clarendon Press: Oxford.
Pratama, N 2018, Analysis of Marxist-feminism on the oppressed women as breeding apparatus in *The handmaid's tale* novel, Honours Thesis, Diponegoro University, Semarang.
Reis, E 1995 'The devil, the body, and the feminine soul in Puritan New England', *The Journal of American History*, vol. 82, no. 1, pp. 15–36.
Schwartz, A 2017 'Yes, 'The Handmaid's Tale' is feminist', *The New Yorker*, 22 April, www.newyorker.com/culture/cultural-comment/yes-the-handmaids-tale-is-feminist
Scott, R (dir.) 1979, *Alien*, motion picture, 20th Century Fox, USA.
Shildrick, M & Price, J 1999, 'Openings on the body: a critical introduction', in J Price & M Shildrick (eds.), *Feminist theory and the body*, Routledge: New York, pp. 1–14.
Sykes, G & Matza, D 1957, 'Techniques of neutralisation: a theory of delinquency', *American Sociological Review*, vol. 22, no. 6, pp. 664–670.
Taussig, M 2017, 'Trump studies', *Cultural Anthropology*, 18 January, viewed 5 March 2019, https://culanth.org/fieldsights/trump-studies
Tonn, J 2018, '*The Handmaid's Tale*', *Journal of the History of Biology*, vol. 51, pp. 415–417.
Trope, A 2018, 'The girl in the box', *Communication, Culture & Critique*, vol. 11, pp. 186–188.
Trump, D 2016, 'Donald Trump's taped comments about women', transcript, *The New York Times*, 8 October, viewed 5 March 2019, www.nytimes.com/2016/10/08/us/donald-trump-tape-transcript.html
Valenti, J 2018, 'Why *The Handmaid's Tale* is more relevant one year after the first season', *The Guardian*, April 28, www.theguardian.com/commentisfree/2018/apr/25/handmaids-tale-season-2-return-trump-america-2018?CMP=fb_gu
Warner, K 2018, 'JunexNick: the quietest ship in the Handmaid fandom', *Communication, Culture & Critique*, vol. 11, pp. 198–200.
Waterhouse, J 2018, 'The creepy ways Gilead in "The Handmaid's Tale" resembles Trump's America', *Elle Australia*, 29 June, viewed 5 March 2019, www.elle.com.au/culture/handmaids-tale-gilead-america-17941
Weiner, M (creator) 2007, *Mad Men*, television broadcast, Lionsgate Television, USA.

9 'From a Speculative Point of View I Wondered Which of Us I Was'

Re-reading Old Women[1]

Sneja Gunew

On a recent visit to Plovdiv, Bulgaria, I was perusing various cabinets of what looked like small female statues (triangles at the crotch and dots for breasts) dating back millennia, but the labels made no such attribution and stated merely that these were humanoid figurines found in particular locations. 'Why the caginess?', I wondered. It could, arguably, be construed as a transgender moment, but somehow I doubt it. I think it may well have been a legacy of the backlash against the work of archaeologists such as Marija Gimbutas who saw these figurines as proof of goddess worship in the area and concluded that this was linked, amongst other attributes, to societies from which warfare was absent. That body of research includes figures such as Mary Daly, Heide Göttner-Abendroth, Gloria Feman Orenstein, and many others, and perhaps this interpretation was being discouraged by museologists of the area. Looking back I realise I've been stalking the goddess (or goddess discourse) throughout my life in various contexts, but not because I'm searching for a religion or utopia in the past. I'm not capitalising the term *goddess*, because I think that would instantly evoke archetypes that are also stereotypes such as, for example, when it is coupled to the maternal, as in *Mother Goddess* or the *Great Mother*, combinations that are also confining in the sense that the stench of male fantasy intrudes immediately (Purkiss 1996, p. 32). Feminist cultural theorists have rightly been wary of this concept, because when we are mostly battling for gender equity goddess invocation may be perceived as a retreat from material circumstances into a la-la land of fantasy (or phantasy). Even if one perceives the goddess as a figure (in the sense of figurative) of rebellion against patriarchally based heuristic frameworks, that still reinstates patriarchal concepts and confirms the male-female binary that is rightly being interrogated today (with the collateral damage often attendant on such interrogations such as the demise of anything labelled women's studies). But how then to imagine otherwise, to escape those confining conceptual structures? Figures such as Hélène Cixous and Catherine Clément (1986) and the movement around *écriture féminine* generated a promising direction but were also (unfairly) confined to the binaries of essentialist sexual difference. The attempts to consider another reality continue.

Twenty-five years ago Barb Creed's book *The Monstrous-Feminine* effectively reversed the abject status the feminine had acquired after Freud by making a case for its proactive status: she claimed that the feminine might be considered as castrating rather than castrated. Not surprisingly this move branches out into many complex considerations of where else in the history of representation across the sensory field (visual, auditory, taste etc.), there had been those kinds of inspiring reversals. If we consider the rather dismal terrain of old age and women's place within it, we soon come across the crone and certainly, in mainstream theorising, the crone remains an abjected figure, a cautionary tale, a *memento mori*. But not always and everywhere. For instance, Ally Acker's recent documentary *The Flowering of the Crone: Leonora Carrington. Another Reality* (dir. 2014) is a spirited examination of precisely 'another reality' and of Carrington as an artist who still has to be assigned her rightful place within the history of Surrealism and the Avant-Garde more broadly. Whitney Chadwick's book *Women Artists and the Surrealist Movement* (1985) ushered in a new awareness of Surrealist women artists, including Carrington, and Chadwick is featured in Acker's film. The film celebrates Carrington's consistent interrogations of normativity, especially her wide-ranging intellectual enquiries into multiple mythologies, including those of the Great Mother/Goddess. Carrington depicts that figure in a range of incarnations, for example, as Mother Goose as in her paintings: *Grandmother Moorhead's Aromatic Kitchen* (1975)[2] or in *The Giantess* (1947). Carrington and her 'coven' of female friends variously and intermittently gathered in Mexico City (Remedios Varo, Kati Horna)[3] fed each other and nurtured each other's work and such meetings are often depicted as taking place in a demonic kitchen from Hell (but then Hell is another goddess figure). Acker's film shows such a gathering towards the latter part of Carrington's life, at a time when her longstanding friends (alas neither Varo nor Horna survived) clearly enjoy each other's company. Carrington's work comprises skewed realities within plain sight of mainstream representations – the philosopher's stone of alchemy linked, in turn, to that ultimate metamorphosing space, the womb.[4] Although what is transmuted into what form remains enigmatic, that has not prevented a number of critics from claiming to provide 'keys' to her iconography.[5]

Carrington is a rare figure whose art spans painting and writing. Acker's film uses the framing device of an early short story Carrington produced called 'The debutante' (Carrington 2017b). It is a scathing satire of early twentieth-century social rituals that launched young women of a certain class onto the marriage market. It also incorporates many of the themes and motifs that subsequently permeated her art. The debutante protagonist invokes the aid of a hyena who impersonates her at the social gathering causing chaos and creative mayhem. Animal companions are also alter egos; food becomes both solace and instrument of deadly vengeance; cannibalism generates a necessary rebirth--all these elements are present and recur in her subsequent written work. The tone is consistently wry and helps achieve a kind of common-sense acceptance that poses the question: why would anyone think otherwise? Apart from this unsettling short story, Carrington produced several notable longer works: *Down below* (2017a), a devastating autobiographically based account of being incarcerated in an insane asylum where the protagonist is subjected to horrific chemical invasions that leave a lasting legacy and her novel *The hearing trumpet* (2005) dealing with the unexpected 'reflowering of the crone' to borrow Acker's title.[6]

That latter work was composed in either 1950 or 1960 when Carrington had moved to Mexico City, where she remained for the remainder of her long life (Suleiman 1990, p. 169). *Down Below* was written in the 1940s, not long before *The Hearing Trumpet* (if we accept the 1950 date). As Susan Suleiman points out, *The Hearing Trumpet* is to some extent a rewriting of *Down below*, as the replication of madness in *Down below* is transmuted into a controlled artistic complexity in *The Hearing Trumpet* (1990, pp. 171–172). The helpless young 'victim' protagonist of *Down below* eventually becomes the agent of her own destiny. This shift has been analysed as Carrington's reversal of the *femme enfant* worshipped by Surrealist male artists who reduced her and other women to this role (Chadwick 1985, p. 74). Both texts draw on autobiographical material and both are flanked by the complex iconography, the visual grammar, of her paintings. Particularly in *The Hearing Trumpet*, support is bestowed by female bonding along the lines that several heads are best for plotting subversion. Although it was written when Carrington was in her early 30s (Smith 2005, p. x), it concerns a group of elderly inhabitants of a care home run by a sinister doctor, who engineer their own liberation in a context that is eerily prescient, amongst other things, of the devastations of climate change. Along the way we also have transgender manifestations (an old woman revealed to be an old man in death)[7] as well as inter-species procreation where life on earth will likely be incarnated in werewolves. The home appears to be situated in Mexico (but this remains somewhat vague) and the text ends with a new Ice Age when the poles become inverted. Meanwhile, the 92-year-old protagonist Marian Leatherby basks in her designated utopia – Lapland (sic).[8]

As one would expect from the title, *The Hearing Trumpet* features sound as an important element. In her first novel, *The stone door*,[9] music is a soothing element that facilitates communication in difficult circumstances (Carrington 1977, p. 86) whereas in *The Hearing Trumpet* sound delivers hidden truths. Analysts from Marina Warner to Ali Smith have provided readings of this text and Smith's introduction conveys the insight that:

> Fundamentally, *The hearing trumpet* is a book about profound disconnection; at its centre are people unable to hear each other, or unwilling to. It's about how we hear, and how we don't, or can't, and it's about what happens when people can hear or see differently.
> (Smith 2005, p. xii)

As a long-term friend, Gloria Orenstein figures as commentator and interpreter in Acker's film but her reading of Carrington's work sometimes appears to be a little too schematic – this equals that. However, she offers illuminating links to the many mythic systems explored by Carrington including Tibetan, Mayan, and Celtic (Orenstein 1982, p. 65). She also translates the old Irish inscriptions in Carrington's painting *The Ancestor* (Orenstein 1990, p. 69). As Suleiman suggests in her 1987 study, Orenstein misses out on the humour that Carrington's work exudes. The winking nun or the old ladies who enjoy their odd feast of sardines and port as the new Ice Age descends are elements that recall the nuanced comedy of Angela Carter and Ali Smith. The text's moment of revelation is contained after all in a hot broth of oneself:

> As I drew near the fire the woman stopped stirring the pot and rose to greet me. When we faced each other I felt my heart give a convulsive leap and stop. The woman who stood before me was myself.... She nodded gravely and pointed into the soup with her long wooden spoon. "Jump in the broth, meat is scarce this season."...I never had any pretensions of a glorious death, but ending up as meat broth had never entered my calculations. ...When I was well within range she suddenly jabbed the pointed knife into my backside and with a scream of pain I leapt right into the boiling soup...A mighty rumbling followed by crashes and there I was stirring the soup in which I could see my own meat, feet up, boiling away merrily...From a speculative view I wondered which of us I was...Holding the mirror at arm's length I seemed to see a three-faced female whose eyes winked alternatively...I felt very much refreshed after the hot broth....
> (Carrington 2005, pp. 136–138)

And like all good cauldron stories (critics have noted that it is a retelling of the Grail story) the protagonist's new incarnation is a somewhat rejuvenated version of herself. Suleiman's pioneering work on Carrington links her to the burgeoning feminist revisionism of writers in the 1970s such as Monique Wittig and Hélène Cixous (Suleiman 1990, pp. 144–145). More recent publications have situated Carrington more broadly as a significant avant-garde artist (Eburne & McAra 2017).

While Carrington's work has yet to be turned into film, it is not a stretch to imagine this occurring in the future and Acker's film begins by animating some of her paintings to great effect. Barb Creed's work is located in the field of contemporary film studies and the examples she uses are from the domain of the horror film, a marginalised genre, when she wrote *The Monstrous-Feminine*. One might suggest that, generally speaking, the representation of old women on screen could also be deemed as belonging to the category of horror films since old women tend to be tied to witches and other negative manifestations of the monstrous feminine usually associated with anti-life forces. But perhaps this trend is changing. Because of current demographics there appear to be a greater range of options for representing old age and women.[10] My next examples are taken from contemporary Bulgarian films by female directors where there is an honouring of the 'granny', which appears to arise as much out of social contexts as from artistic imaginations. In communist Bulgaria, women had to work outside the home while at the same time sustaining the home itself, and this simply could not have been accomplished without the help of the granny (Ghodsee & Bernardi 2012). They also share a certain kinship with the many female figurines from prehistoric times that were found to litter the region (after all this was Thrace!). Scholars such as Marija Gimbutas (1989) have used these archaeological finds to make a case for evidence of goddess religion and have encountered dismissive and toxic criticism. Without getting into the pros and cons of that debate, there is certainly an alternative representational grammar here that can be attached to the feminine. One can look, as Creed did herself, to Kristeva and other pioneering feminists to produce possible readings of this legacy without flattening it too much into archetypes that, in the effort to universalise them, retain limited explanatory powers.

Iglika Trifonova: *Letter to America* (dir. 2001)[11]

In Trifonova's *Letter to America*, music is a generative force that resurrects the dead in all its metaphorical complexity. Dedicated to her own grandmother, this film explores (arguably somewhat sentimentally) the healing power of returning to one's rural roots from the alienation of the urban scene where people speed past life – as exemplified by Kamen's opening footage from NY. The next thing we learn, via a phone call to his friend Ivan in Sofia, is that Kamen has been hit by a car and is lying in a coma. Ivan tries unsuccessfully to gain a month-long visa to America from a scoffing US bureaucrat and states in broken English 'I really really do not want to emigrate to America' (hence the importance of 'to' rather than 'from' in the film's title). In the course of dealing with his thwarted mission, Ivan recalls that there is a song that is meant to have healing powers and begins to hum it when he first hears the news about Kamen but cannot recall it fully. As Ivan (named after the archetypal wanderer in Slavic folktales) crosses the country to find Kamen's grandmother who knows the song, he encounters a range of guides who lead him to explore other layers of Bulgarian life. In particular (but not exclusively), he meets a number of grandmothers who have all encountered tragedy but have 'gone forward' (a refrain in the film).

Each of the grannies is permitted her singularity (for example, one shows him her immaculately woven and knitted burial clothes, renewed regularly, while another does a sprightly dance after a few glasses of fiery rakia). Each of them sings a song but it is the wrong one. When Ivan begins hitchhiking to Kamen's village, his first guide is an icon restorer with an icon of St John the Baptist eerily seated on the back seat of the car. The driver, Nevena, tells him about the semi-remembered song, one that brings the dead back to life, but of which people have forgotten either the lyrics or the melody. She links it to the Orphic mysteries inevitably associated with the Thracian ur-history of Bulgaria. After she conveys this, they enter a dark tunnel and emerge into light suggesting a rebirth.

Thereafter his quest begins in earnest and Ivan is not only directed towards grannies. He encounters a truck driver sceptical of this folkloric tradition and a tractor driver looking for a mate who wants Ivan to film him for a lonely hearts TV programme. The cinematic style of the film shows a consistent pleasure in the unvarnished realities of these ordinary characters whose affective power is compellingly registered on each of their idiosyncratic faces. As part of his education Ivan watches the grannies perform a death ritual where the dead person's clothes are dipped in water and then a scythe is passed over the water to cut away death's contamination. Perhaps his most mysterious guide is a young boy who does not speak but takes him to the grave of Kamen's grandmother (the keeper of the song) and directs him to perform a mourning ritual before pointing him towards another grandmother, Rusa, who is also supposed to know the song. When Ivan first encounters the boy he has just lost his paper boat on the stream so he is lightly associated with the ferryman of the dead.

Sound is a significant aspect of the film's signifying frame – the silence of the young spirit guide and the miraculous song that is recovered in spite of a taboo. Because her own son has died, Rusa is in mourning for two years and cannot sing or even listen to music. However, she is moved by Ivan's story and Kamen is, after all, part of her village. To lessen the taboo, Rusa removes her kerchief before singing the magic tune. But in fact Ivan already knows the song and merely has to recover it. The film ends with Ivan back in Sofia, together with his now pregnant girlfriend, watching footage from NY where a recovered Kamen is participating in a Japanese tea ceremony with his friend Seiji (the one who had made the initial phone call to Ivan) and it is Seiji who sings the magic song into the camera. One might conclude that the grannies in the film function as the repositories of a robust folk wisdom that is in danger of being forgotten and when remembered, restores a fractured society that has lost its way to health.

Zornitsa Sophia: *Mila from Mars* (dir. 2004)[12]

Mila, who is fleeing from her murderously abusive partner to whom she had been trafficked out of an orphanage, lands in a crumbling and almost deserted village somewhere near the Greek border. Sporting a black eye and split lip from her latest beating and wearing fishnet stockings and short leather shorts Mila slumps on the step of one of the ruined houses. She is watched by a bevy of grannies and older men (the remaining guardians) who discuss whose child or grandchild she might be while passing around (what viewers identify later as) a toke. Eventually, in spite of warnings concerning the murderous intentions of such emissaries of modernity, one of the grannies takes Mila into her custody. Gradually it becomes clear that Mila is pregnant and the villagers set about making one of the houses habitable for her. She is led in like a bride, dressed in improvised traditional white clothes. The grannies ensure that she is properly nurtured and that she gives birth – around Christmas. The son is therefore named Christos and since the father (Alex the abuser) is absent, there are subtle suggestions of a parthenogenetic birth.[13] Throughout, flashbacks reveal Mila's life in the orphanage where Alex is a creepy benefactor who occasionally brings cakes for the deprived children – implying that while he may have lived there himself in the past he now traffics girls from there. Meanwhile, viewers have discovered (as has Mila) that Alex comes to the village once a year to buy the pot the elders have grown–illustrative of their enterprise and survival tactics in a context where there are few resources. After giving birth, as a modern girl, Mila is frustrated and bored in the village and her various acts of rebellion include writing graffiti on the walls with her menstrual blood––the word 'Maika' (mother) – for her a curse as much as a statement about her condition. The implication is that she may also be suffering from post-partum depression.

Mila also learns about the mysterious 'Teacher' who lives in a nearby tower along which he rappels by means of ingenious ropes and pulleys. The vertical dwelling contains sleeping and cooking areas as well as books that he burns for fuel. When Mila eventually moves there with her son she discovers that he has written down the 'essentials' gleaned from all his reading – the four Buddhist vows––on the walls of the tower, using the soot from the burnt books. Meanwhile, he survives by means of his herd of sheep. Haunted by fear of Alex's reprisal (he has vowed to find her wherever she is) Mila tries to persuade Teacher to kill Alex. However, she also discovers that Alex has links to Teacher whose life he saved in a recent war (presumably in the former Yugoslavia). Teacher is evidently suffering from post-traumatic stress disorder (PTSD) and trying to heal. While he and Mila form a couple to some degree they do not tell each other their names, that is, there are limits to the trust between them. Teacher eventually confronts Alex in the ruined church with Christos (Alex's son) in his arms. While we don't hear the dialogue we do see Alex pointing a gun at Teacher who stares him down. Mila has meanwhile joined the volatile mix but once again we don't hear the dialogue because the point of view has shifted to that of the old people who watch the exchange with acute anxiety. Alex eventually drives away and Mila and Assen tell each other their names and the film ends.

What is clear here in relation to the themes I have been examining is that, in terms of the monstrous feminine, Mila (significantly) gives birth within the domain of the grannies who are increasingly and demonstrably prepared to let *her* go but not the child: they are the guardians of continuing life. Towards the end of the film, Mila's room is covered in the 'Maika' graffiti although she herself is not particularly maternal in any traditional manner. For example, she leaves her infant son at the roadside and, in her frustration at being held captive in the village combined with her fear of Alex, attempts to hang herself. This is where Assen finds her and prevents the suicide. He also takes care of the child and does all the cooking, showing more maternal/nurturing characteristics than Mila does. As well the inside of the (phallic) tower has been upholstered in sheepskins so that it is transformed into a soft and welcoming space – more like an extended cradle. The faux phallic tower has a parallel former patriarchal structure in the ruined church. There the granny leader sits in its cathedra (implicitly usurping the power of the bishop) and it is where the final confrontation that frees Mila from her oppressor also takes place, ushering in a new and more equitable sociality. Christos really will be brought up by both parents as well as the idiosyncratic community. What prevails here is that no-one is defined as a victim – neither the old people stranded by versions of modernity, nor Mila, in spite of her abuse by both institutions and individuals, nor Assen the traumatised soldier. These are survivors and the implication is that there is a 'new' holy family (like Joseph, Assen is not the biological father) and that eventually they too will become the guardians of the village community.

Goddess Redux

References to the 'goddess' tend to split readers into opposing categories: those who see this concept as a deluded quest for comfort by subjects designated as victims, and the enthusiastic goddess worshippers who inhabit latter-day New Age alternative universes consisting of Goop treatments at one end and crystals and corporate mindfulness at the other. My examples of granny depictions suggest another kind of approach. Perhaps the problem lies with considering that there is a pre-existent world or religion of which the many prehistoric artefacts and figurines are the 'proof' and that many attributes of the assumed societies can be established, such as peaceful lives without conflict and a better status for women. What if instead we considered this archaeological record in terms of the reality that each age constructs its own truths (present and future) out of these data? In other words, just as Carrington and her female friends created narratives (including visual ones) that nurtured their mysterious and compelling life-as-art, we do the same now in turning to this archive: we extract what we need and use it to fuel our own curiosity about what might be attached to what, underpinned by the continuing feminist enterprise whereby we persist in trying to change the terms of engagement for women. Diverse trends, including Celtic mythology (linked or not to alchemy) and a pre-Christian world that produced the female figurines that are littered across Thrace and Anatolia, may indeed have a continuing life in the folklore of various regions including Bulgaria (formerly Thrace). And perhaps these traces contribute to a different perception of, in this instance, old women, that could be utilised as a basis for reconsidering the ways in which post-menopausal women signify within culture.

In the *Zeitgeist* we inhabit, we probably want to leave behind the interpretive certainties of Gloria Orenstein or Marija Gimbutas but should not dispose of their useful insights (in connecting the dots or trying to decode the data). This is where psychoanalysis as a tradition and the framework within which Creed and many others work demonstrates its usefulness since psychoanalysis functions outside linear time, and this has profound implications for how we consider history–– both public and private.[14] The creative frameworks provided by Carrington, Zornitsa Sophia, and Trifonova suggest new ways of considering the signifying possibilities of the crone. What undoubtedly animates both Zornitsa Sophia's and Carrington's work in particular is a revolt against authoritarian and abusive patriarchal structures. Looking for an alternative grammar of representation to articulate this rebellion means that the reimagined crone prevails. In Carrington's case, her recourse to Celtic myth, alchemy (the hidden history of chemistry that includes the reign of Big Pharma),[15] should not preclude her being seen as an important artistic conduit to the avant-garde, and this is the animating principle of recent critical reappraisals of her work. The crone is both a repository of painfully acquired knowledge and a keeper of many confluent knowledge systems, and artists are skilled at mashing up these systems to generate unexpected futures. The humour in Carrington and Zornitsa Sophia, in particular, endows their work with an endearing lightness that is missing from the earnest attempts to connect Carrington, for example, to goddess quests. Carrington operated until the first decade of the twenty-first century and the vehicle for her continuing relevance is the postmodernist playfulness her work exudes. What is sacred is that nothing is sacred.[16]

It is clear that each feminist attempt to re-vision the representation of the feminine, including post-menopausal women, is usually met with a vicious backlash. For instance, Gimbutas was reviled, as were figures such as Mary Daly, Judy Chicago, and Germaine Greer. Their scholarly reputations were trashed, enveloped in a miasma implying something fraudulent about their creativity, that there is something inherently hysterical or unhinged about their discoveries and insights (and their work is often misconstrued). But does this amount simply to a case of inter-generational matricide? Not just a case of killing the mother but the sense that women are nothing outside the maternal function – that this alone is meant to define them.[17] Women who do not espouse that function do not fare well within history. The Bulgarian grannies in the films examined are the glue that holds their crumbling communities together, nurturing each other as well as the men and children. Carrington resisted the *femme enfant* stereotype and as her art (including *The Hearing Trumpet*) shows, she animated a different and self-contained universe. She refused to be defined by others as an aberration to the rules of their representational cultural grammar – something she found confining in many different ways. Her writing and art open up other interpretive frameworks for the feminine, including her own versions of the monstrous feminine. As in the case of Creed's work, Carrington gave us new points of view on a familiar archive.

Notes

1 My thanks to Valerie Raoul and Margery Fee for comments on earlier drafts of this essay and to Emilia Slavova for introducing me to the two films. Thanks to her as well and to Kornelia Slavova for helping me to navigate the (at times) less-than-accurate subtitles to the films.
2 See Orenstein (1982, p. 65).
3 In 2010, Pallant House Gallery in Chichester mounted an exhibition entitled *Surreal Friends: Leonora Carrington, Remedios Varo, Kati Horna* that juxtaposed the work of those three artists who were also close friends and lived in Mexico City. See van Raay (2010), Kaplan (1988), p. 93ff.
4 In relation to this, Carrington has her character the Artisan say in *The stone door*: 'My womb is no larger than a grain of rice because its powers have all been used in discovery' (1977, p. 40).
5 Suleiman takes issue with Gloria Orenstein. But see as well Carrington's son Gabriel Weisz (2017, p. 132). See also Catriona McAra who makes the point that due perhaps to her dramatic biography, Carrington often functions as a character constructed through the accounts of others (McAra 2017, p. 179).
6 There is also her first novel, *The stone door* (Carrington 1977), which is out of print, although an extract is included in *The seventh horse* (Carrington 1988b). Anna Watz's (2017) essay points to its importance.
7 Madeleine Cottenet-Hage (1991) reads this episode as 'we might conclude that one's sexual identity is a matter of personal choice and should be left at that' (p. 87).
8 The Sami have rejected the term 'Lapland' as the name for their lands.
9 Published in French in 1976 but actually written in 1946 (Warner 1988, 20).
10 The recent films of Agnès Varda come to mind.
11 Iglika Trifonova. In 2001 she made her feature debut as director and screenwriter of the film *Letter to America*. The film received the Special Prize at the Golden Rose Bulgarian Feature Film Festival after the jury decided not to bestow a grand prix. *Letter to America* was the Bulgarian nomination for best foreign language film at the 73rd Academy Awards.
12 Zornitsa Sophia. Her first film *Mila from Mars* (dir. 2004) was declared 'the dreamed beginning of Bulgarian independent feature moviemaking' (in Women Film Directors in the Bulgarian Cinema, para. 2). *Variety* magazine wrote that 'the film marks the bow of a director to watch' (ibid.). It has won many awards.

13 One is reminded of Creed's point that 'the womb signifies "fullness" or "emptiness" but always it is its own point of reference' (Creed 1993, p. 27).

14 It is worth recalling here Kristeva's influential essay 'Women's time' in which she states the following: 'Some contemporary thinkers maintain that modernity is the first era in human history in which human beings have attempted to live without religion. As it stands today, is feminism not about to become a sort of religion? Or will it manage to rid itself of its belief in Woman, Her power, and Her writing and support instead the singularity of each women, her complexities, her many languages, at the cost of a single horizon, of a single perspective, of faith?' (Kristeva 1997, p. 366). In spite of reinventing herself as a Frenchwoman Kristeva started her life in Bulgaria and her writing is, and continues to be, haunted by this fact.

15 It is worth recalling that Carrington's father was the major shareholder of Imperial Chemical Industries.

16 What I am trying to convey is akin to Svetlana Boym's very useful distinction between 'restorative' and 'reflective' nostalgia: 'Restorative nostalgia stresses *nóstos* (home) and attempts a transhistorical reconstruction of the lost home. Reflective nostalgia thrives in *álgos*, the longing itself, and delays the homecoming – wistfully, ironically, desperately. These distinctions are not absolute binaries, and one can surely make a more refined mapping of the gray areas on the outskirts of imaginary homelands. Restorative nostalgia does not think of itself as nostalgia, but rather as truth and tradition. Reflective nostalgia dwells on the ambivalences of human longing and belonging and does not shy away from the contradictions of modernity. Restorative nostalgia protects the absolute truth, while reflective nostalgia calls it into doubt'. (Boym 2010, para. 10)

17 Suleiman, for example, constantly ties Carrington to the maternal.

Bibliography

Acker, A (dir.) 2014, *The Flowering of the Crone: Leonora Carrington. Another Reality*, Reel Women Media, New York.

Boym, S 2010, 'Nostalgia', *Atlas of Transformation*, viewed 1 August 2018, http://monumenttotransformation.org/atlas-of-transformation/html/n/nostalgia/nostalgia-svetlana-boym.html

Carrington, L 1947, *The giantess*, online image, viewed 5 March 2019, http://antiquesandartireland.com/wp-content/uploads/2013/08/carring.jpg

Carrington, L 1975, *Grandmother Moorhead's aromatic kitchen*, online image, viewed 5 March 2019, www.irishtimes.com/opinion/lionising-leonora-an-irishman-s-diary-about-artist-leonora-carrington-1.3037851

Carrington, L 1977, *The stone door*, Routledge & Kegan Paul, London.

Carrington, L 1988a, *The house of fear. Notes from Down below*, Virago, London.

Carrington, L 1988b, *The seventh horse and other tales*, E. P. Dutton, New York.

Carrington, L 2005, *The hearing trumpet*, Penguin Books, London.

Carrington, L 2017a, *Down below*, The New York Review of Books, New York.

Carrington, L 2017b, 'The debutante', in *The complete stories of Leonora Carrington*, Dorothyproject, St. Louis, pp. 3–7.

Chadwick, W 1985, *Women artists and the surrealist movement*, Thames and Hudson, London.

Cixous, H & Clément, C 1986, *The newly born woman*, trans. B. Wing, U. of Minnesota P, Minneapolis.

Cottenet-Hage, M 1991, 'The body subversive: corporeal imagery in Carrington, Prassinos and Mansour', in Caws, M, Kuenzli, R & Raaberg, G (eds.), *Surrealism and women*, The MIT Press, Cambridge, pp. 76–95.

Creed, B 1993, *The monstrous-feminine: Film, feminism, psychoanalysis*, Routledge, London.

Eburne, J & McAra, C (eds.) 2017, *Leonora Carrington and the international avant-garde*, Manchester UP, Manchester.

Ghodsee, K & Bernardi, L 2012, 'Starting a family at your parents' house: multigenerational households and below replacement fertility in urban Bulgaria', *Journal of Comparative Family Studies*, vol. 43, no. 3, pp. 439–459.

Gimbutas, M 1989, *The language of the goddess*, Harper & Row, San Francisco.

Kaplan, J 1988, *Unexpected journeys. The art and life of Remedios Varo*, Virago, London.

Kristeva, J 1997, 'Women's time', in Oliver K (ed.), *The Portable Kristeva*, Colombia UP, New York, pp. 349–368.

McAra, C 2017, 'A nonagenarian virago: quoting "Carrington" in contemporary practice', in Eburne, J & McAra, C (eds.), *Leonora Carrington and the international avant-garde*, Manchester UP, Manchester, pp. 177–197.

Orenstein, G 1982, 'Reclaiming the Great Mother: a feminist journey to madness and back in search of a goddess heritage', *Symposium*, vol. XXXVI, no. 1, pp. 45–70.

Orenstein, G 1990, *The reflowering of the goddess*, Pergamon Press, New York.

Purkiss, D 1996, *The witch in history: early modern and twentieth-century representations*, Routledge, London & New York.

Smith, A 2005, 'Introduction', in Carrington, L (ed.), *The hearing trumpet*, Penguin Books, London, pp. v–xv.

Sophia, Z (dir.) 2004, *Mila from Mars*, motion picture, Kirov Consult, Bulgaria.

Suleiman, S 1990, *Subversive intent: gender, politics, and the avant-garde*, Harvard UP, Cambridge, pp. 169–178.

Trifonova, I (dir.) 2001, *Letter to America*, motion picture, Phanta Vision Film International B.V., Bulgaria.

van Raay, S 2010, 'Surreal friends; Leonora Carrington, Remedios Varo and Kati Horna', in van Raay, S, Moorhead, J & Arcq (eds.), *Surreal friends: Leonora Carrington, Remedios Varo and Kati Horna*, Lund Humphries, Surrey, pp. 8–29.

Warner, M 1988, 'Introduction', in Carrington, L (ed.), *The house of fear. Notes from down below*, Virago, London, pp. 1–21.

Watz, A 2017, '"A language buried at the back of time": *The stone door* and post-structuralist feminism', in Eburne, J & McAra, C (eds.), *Leonora Carrington and the international avant-garde*, Manchester UP, Manchester, pp. 90–104.

Weisz, G 2017, 'Shadow children: Leonora as storyteller', in Eburne, J & McAra, C (eds.), *Leonora Carrington and the international avant-garde*, Manchester UP, Manchester, pp. 126–140.

Women Film Directors in the Bulgarian Cinema, viewed 5 March 2019, http://jeni-bg-kino.com/en/zornica_sofia.php

10 The 'Monstrous-Feminine'

Dementia, Psychoanalysis, and Mother-Daughter Relations in Dana Walrath's *Aliceheimer's*

E. Ann Kaplan

In her groundbreaking volume, Barbara Creed (1993) reworks psychoanalytic theories to show how dominant culture has constructed a feminine that is 'monstrous' – a monstrosity evident in horror film after horror film. Relying especially on Julia Kristeva's (1982) concept of abjection, Creed demonstrates how women have been relegated to the margins of culture, abjected, cast aside, and thereby rendered 'monstrous'. Creed's interest in how women's biology, sexuality/sexual difference, and especially their reproductive functions create a crisis for men and their masculinity which results in their inventing what Creed calls 'a monstrous feminine'.

In this project I show how pervasive images unconsciously continue to render women 'monstrous' only now in relation to age. Older women have long been abjected: As Creed reminds us,

> The place of the abject is "the place where meaning collapses," the place where "I" am not. The abject threatens life; it must be "radically excluded" (Kristeva 1982, p. 2) from the place of the living subject, propelled away from the body and deposited on the other side of an imaginary border which separates the self from that which threatens the self.
>
> (Creed, p. 9)

Older women are abjected because threatening for economic, political, and social reasons. Their abjection takes the form of being made invisible, rendered ridiculous in off-colour jokes, or pushed to the margins, even to the other side of the border, because no longer fitting the youthful, slender, sexual being men fantasise and desire, no longer, then, *bearing meaning.* Older women have also long been linked to the image of the wicked witch, who, with her long pointed nose seems to have co-opted the penis for evil ends. In Creed's (1993, pp. 76–77) words, in psychoanalytic theory 'woman as witch is positioned as the oral sadistic mother and the phallic woman…'. Creed further adds that the words 'irrational, scheming, evil… are used to define the witch,' who is also associated with a range of abject things from puss to cannibalism.

Anxiety about ageing – especially as regards older women – has increased exponentially in the Millennium for several reasons: First, simple demographics. In most advanced nations, people are living longer, putting pressure, not only on healthcare systems, but also on economics, politics, transportation, education; second, while dementia is far from being inevitable as people age, incidence is increasing. Alzheimer's disease – the debilitating illness – is on the increase, especially among women. Five million people, most of them women, currently have dementia in the US, and this is expected to grow to 17 million in 2050. The economic and social consequences of so many women with dementia is heightening an ageism always already in place. Finally, people living longer lives, often healthy ones, can seem threatening to upcoming generations seeking to replace older people in the workforce. If such people keep on working, age panic can set in (See Kaplan/Chivers 2018).

With this larger framework, in this chapter I want to turn the tables on the construction of older women as monstrous much as Creed does in revealing the seemingly hidden power underlying the diverse kinds of monstrous feminine she explores in the Horror Film – a power that creators of these female monsters apparently deny, or perhaps, unconsciously take some pleasure in. The most obvious threat offered by women with dementia (AD for short) is their apparent loss of a 'self,' their no longer having a recognisable *subjectivity*. The pervasive view, especially within neuroscience discourse is that once a person loses her memory, she no longer can be a subject.[1] She is no longer the autonomous, self-directing, independent individual that neo-liberal capitalism requires. Western culture eschews dependency as a weakness. The reality of not being in control is terrifying in this context. Thus, people with dementia create what I call 'age panic'.

Let me briefly indicate how this kind of 'monstrous feminine' is evident in the images of dementia widely circulated in the media. My selection is mainly from journalism between 2014 and 2015, when the panic about dementia was reaching its height. The AD figure as 'absent' dominated reports. For example, a *New York Times* report (November 2014), 'Facing the Challenges of Keeping an Aging Nation on its Feet,' included a somber photo of a fragile grey-haired woman, bent over and struggling to move with the help of a walker. Another *New York Times* report in April 2015 was titled 'In Race for Medicare Dollars, Nursing Home Care May Lag,' and it showed an image of a frail elderly lady sitting in a cluttered room with a lost expression on her face. The story discussed the neglect and injuries AD people suffer in many poorly funded facilities. In November 2015, a report, 'As Cognition Slips, Financial Skills Are Often the First to Go,' showed a rare frail elderly man (usually, women are imaged) with a blank face, staring straight ahead, while his depressed female relative looked on. Significantly, the article discussed the difficulties for AD subjects to keep atop of their finances, given that the US and individual States do not allocate much funding for long-term care facilities.[2] A 2018 *New York Times* article, 'Continuing Care Homes Need a Financial Checkup,' discussed the enormous upfront fees demanded for Continuing Care Retirement Centers (CCRC's) and people's fears that the home may go bankrupt, as some have done. In Europe, by contrast, at least until recently, long-term care has been seen as a human right.[3] In all the images noted, it's as if the person is not there in any shape or form as a viable subject. Blank looks predominate.

Things are changing rapidly, partly in response to intervention by certain outlier neuroscientists, some younger gerontologists and by the coming together of scholars from these disciplines and many in the humanities in the growing international field of Age Studies. But this ageist 'monstrous feminine' has not gone away.[4]

For the rest of this chapter, I want to counter the pervasive negative image of women with dementia, using Creed's Kristevan mother-daughter psychoanalytic formulations, together with some of Melanie Klein's concepts, in relation to a powerful graphic memoir, Dana Walrath's *Aliceheimer's: Alzheimer's Through the Looking Gla*ss (2013). The ageing protagonist in the text is far from 'monstrous' when viewed through a very different lens than that of popular media's repeated abject stereotypes of women with dementia. I'll suggest some of the psychoanalytic mechanisms undergirding this fear of loss of 'self,' and then turn to analyse mother-daughter relations as these are dramatically changed because of the mother's dementia. Psychic patterns and images, far different than the 'monstrous feminine' of AD subjects in popular culture, are revealed in the process.

This then becomes a study of a text that counters the demented monstrous feminine, and that offers new perspectives. It also becomes a study in how a mother's dementia impacts the prior psychoanalytic relationship of mother and daughter. That this narrative is written by a daughter confronting her mother's gradual succumbing to dementia only adds to the psychoanalytic interest of the project. How does Walrath react to the changes in her mother? How does the daughter avoid situating her mother as 'monstrous,' given Kleinian theories of early rage towards the breast and cultural frames the daughter lives within? What underlying psychoanalytic issues are expressed or inferred in each case? What is it about mother-daughter relations, viewed psychoanalytically, that makes the changes in the mother so very difficult for the daughter to handle? What strategies does Walrath discover to deal with changes in both herself and her mother? How is the pervasive dementia 'monstrous feminine' countered by the text, showing that new realities create new and altered psychic situations?

As we know from the reworking of Freud's theories in the 1950s and 1960s (especially by Melanie Klein, Lacan, Deleuze, and Guattari, and centrally, Julia Kristeva), Western culture relies on fantasies of a unified self, denying the unconscious severely split self of psychoanalytic theory. Such a fantasy of subjects as unproblematically 'whole' sets extreme emphasis on being in control – something patriarchy insists on. In classical Freudian theory, the child only separates from the mother with difficulty, largely through identification with the Father enforced by culture.

Creed's interpretation of Kristeva's mother-child theories clarified issues for me, and inspired my reading of Walrath's memoir. Especially helpful is Creed's (1993, p. 13) reading of Kristeva's concept of what she calls 'maternal authority,' versus the familiar 'paternal law'. The child early on has contact with this maternal authority through the mother's role in toilet training and in mapping out areas of the body for the child in the processes of feeding and cleaning her, separating the 'clean' from the 'dirty' body. This is different from the paternal law within which language is acquired, along with a vast number of cultural and social performances where guilt, embarrassment, and shame come into play (Creed 1993, p. 13). As the child tries to break away, struggling to become a separate subject, the mother becomes the 'abject'. Creed shows how in many horror films the maternal figure is constructed by Patriarchy as the 'monstrous feminine' in the sense of preventing the child from taking her proper place in relation to the Symbolic. But the child partly longs to remain locked 'in a blissful relationship' with the mother, and is 'terrified of separation'. So the child easily succumbs to the comforting pleasure of the dyadic relationship, while simultaneously resenting the mother for apparently holding her back (Creed 1993, p. 12).

Lacan calls this sphere, where mother and child perhaps long to remain, the Imaginary (Lacan 1949/1977). Building on Freud, Lacan argues that the mother and child first reside in this sphere, but culture insists the mother release the child into the Symbolic – a situation which inevitably causes extreme ambivalence towards the mother, even in some cases, passive aggression. The child is caught between conflicting desires: psychically yearning for symbiosis, while patriarchal culture pushes for separation.

For Patriarchy, there are also conflicting processes. While the image of the saintly mother, holding and caring for her child, may be comforting in patriarchy, there is always looming her opposite, namely the 'Maternal Authority,' controlling, powerful and dangerous, a threat to male dominance, a violation of paternal law. She is linked to the figure Creed discusses, namely woman, not *castrated*, but *castrating*. And this mother can be intimidating for the child.

If new family structures are now in place as a result of the Women's Liberation Movement and developments within psychoanalytic practice and theory, the Father is still crucial as an authority, if to a lesser degree than before. Indeed, with more maternal authority allowed to the mother, a daughter's ambivalence might be increased. So a major question is what happens when the mother, as this authority, suddenly relinquishes her position because of oncoming dementia? How does the daughter respond to her mother no longer being in control? How does she respond to the boundary issues suddenly changing as the mother becomes dependent on her daughter, instead of the reverse? I will try to show that, in a sense, once the mother has dementia, positions *are* reversed, but long-held psychic patterns *remain*. Where the mother in Kristeva's reading yearns to keep the child down with her in the imaginary but is forced to release her into the Symbolic, where the mother herself inevitably resides, now the mother cannot help but retreat from the Symbolic, back, we could say to the imaginary. This raises interesting psychoanalytic questions, including exploring how far that 'monstrous feminine' lurks around the margins of the narrative as the protagonists are forced to play reversed roles.

Dana Walrath's (2013) engaging Memoir, *Aliceheimer's: Alzheimer's Through the Looking Glass*, belongs in a relatively new graphic-medical genre about AD. As I have argued elsewhere, *Aliceheimer's* expands perspectives of the AD subject towards a more complex view than is generally found in at least Western culture (Kaplan/Chivers 2018). In her introductory essay, Walrath speaks in her professional, somewhat distanced voice, as is appropriate. She tells us she is approaching her mother's dementia through the lens of her training in medical anthropology, and she insists that 'the biomedical story of dementia and how we approach aging globally' is in desperate need of revision (Walrath, p. 4). She discusses how medical anthropologists, like herself, 'locate sickness and health in three interconnected bodies...' which Walrath names 'the political, the social and the physical' (p. 4). In *Aliceheimer's*, Walrath shows her mother creating a new subjectivity as her dementia advances, as against becoming the blank 'absent' subject of popular media noted earlier, or even returning to a stereotypical normative self as in some AD narratives. In a sentence that could almost come from Kristeva writing on abjection, Walrath (p. 5) notes that 'Stigma, silence and social death surround rejected ways of being and echo through the hallways of hospitals'. She claims however that comics can 'rewrite the dominant narrative' (p. 5).

But much more is ongoing in the drawings and text of the memoir itself, as Walrath herself realises without trying to tease out hidden meanings, as I will try to do. For my purposes, it's significant that Walrath's interest in AD emerged from direct experience with her mother's illness. The complex view partly arises because Walrath attempts as best she can to show events as Alice experiences them, which is partly aided by the author's chosen graphic form. Complexity is achieved through the integrated combination of narrative and drawings. As Walrath (p. 3) notes, talking about her form, a graphic image is able to slow things down, and to capture 'the complexity of life and death, sickness and health' (p. 3). She indicates that the drawings embody the subconscious, and the text the conscious, and that moving back and forth between the visual and the verbal 'lets us tap into our collective memory' (p. 3). Walrath implies that in so doing, her text comes closer to revealing her mother's inner experience than can words alone.[5] Walrath's narrative (usually on the page opposite the drawings) situates what the drawings reveal; the combination allows the reader to access some of Walrath's own emotions and inter-personal issues vis-à-vis her mother. Thus is set up a sort of duality that runs throughout the text of on the one hand, Walrath's consciousness about events, and on the other, unconscious tensions from the past that stealthily emerge. These reveal complex psychic conflicts following what Walrath presents as an almost idyllic early year or two.

Starting with the lens of Kristevan psychoanalytic mother-daughter theories, especially as interpreted by Barbara Creed, what does Walrath tell us about her relationship with her mother before Alice started to show signs of dementia? What unconscious aspects emerge in the drawings or between image and text? Significantly, as one opens the book, one finds an image of a mother and child in a forest landscape, with the label 'Alice and Dana Camping 1960'. The mother is smiling, and her body arches protectively over the contented child, who looks directly at the camera. The inserting of the image with blurred outlines, not a frame as such, on the lower right hand corner of a totally white page, suggests an almost dreamlike or ghostly quality, which as we'll see, is also conveyed in the largely pallid palette Walrath uses for most of the drawings. The photo presents an image of intimacy and harmony, suggestive of Lacan's imaginary. Yet almost immediately, in her introduction detailing how her project came about, we learn that later on Walrath (p. 1) saw herself 'as the daughter who got on her (that is, her mother's ed.) nerves. The feeling was mutual'. It was this 'unfinished business,' as Walrath calls it (a desire for Kleinian reparation, perhaps, as her words below suggest), that motivated Dana to invite her mother to live with her as her Alzheimer's progressed. 'I wanted to create a bond with my mother, to redo the past, and to fill the hole inside of me. In the middle of dementia, somehow, my mother wanted to do the same' (Walrath, p. 1).

The process does seem very much that which Melanie Klein theorised in the 1930s regarding the urge for reparation to ease guilt for unconscious aggressivity towards the mother as the child struggles to become a subject. Klein argues that a crucial period in the child's development is the change from seeing the mother as only a partial object-relation 'to the relation to a complete object' (Klein 1935/1975, p. 264). Klein continues to note that 'Not until the object is loved *as a whole* (ibid.) can the loss be felt as a whole'. Part of this process involves making reparation to the object. The ego, Klein (1935/1975, p. 265) continues, 'feels impelled...to make restitution for all the sadistic attacks that it has launched on that object'.

Soon, in the section 'Disappearing Alice,' Walrath (p. 11) tells us that Alice, 'a proud, hardworking career woman,' had often 'wished aloud' that she had gone to medical school instead of becoming a biology teacher. Walrath then observes, 'The years of her pushing me in this direction and away from creative work made sense at last'. This is significant in its inference of prior tension between mother and daughter: Walrath would have preferred studying the arts, but Alice insisted on her going to medical school. We find, then, the child struggling to separate from the mother, and the mother not letting go. Alice projects her own desires onto her daughter, thereby showing that she is unconsciously unable also to fully separate. The early symbiotic relationship has not quite been mastered on either side.

Significant in this section are comments that implicate the level of the Symbolic as it pertains to Alice's new condition: Walrath notes that Alice's 'internal governor' (basically, the Paternal Law) was disappearing, so that parts of Alice's self, previously hidden, could now emerge. Alice is finally able to appreciate her daughter's artistic creativity evident in objects around the house, marking an important change in their relationship – a coming to terms not possible before Alice began to change with her illness. Alice no longer projects her desires onto her daughter.

The drawing opposite the text on this page is frightening, almost a kind of 'monstrous feminine' somewhat out of place: I wondered why Walrath chose this image to accompany a narrative which, on the surface, suggests reconciliation between mother and daughter. The heading for the drawing is 'Alice is Disappearing; Soon There will be None'. The cut-up *Alice in Wonderland* pages that form the shape of Alice's body do not show any head! Indeed the 'heading' takes the place of Alice's head. In addition, the furry framing of Alice's cut out body renders her not quite human. Was there unconscious aggression here, remaining from the days of tension mentioned earlier? Was Alice in her new way of being unconsciously 'monstrous' to Walrath?

In the next related text entitled 'None is Hard to Draw', Walrath seems to repair the possible prior aggression, including guilt, towards her mother. For she has painstakingly drawn an elaborate page of marks in her mother's honour, to the tune of 28, 126. The text also suggests reparation, with Walrath expressing how she exhausted her young mother struggling in a period of wartime scarcity. Her mother also seems to desire healing, for when Walrath (p. 13) returns home to visit her dying father, Alice hugs her and thanks her for her help: 'And you used to be so annoying,' she adds. Walrath, as often, ends the page with the note, 'Aliceheimer's,' indicating that these changes are due to the condition.

But more may be going on: Perhaps the next two pages, which situate the two drawings side-by-side, aim to reconcile Walrath's ambivalence about her mother, on the one hand, and her trauma at seeing her mother 'disappear'. Does the focus on her mother 'disappearing' reflect a complicated unconscious wish in play? Since consciously Walrath will go on to show how very much *there* her mother still is!

The following page suggests the Kleinian relationship between aggression and reparation, since it repeats both the disturbing 'Alice is Disappearing' drawing *and* the restitution page of 28, 126 marks. Taken together, these pages resonate with some aspects of Kristeva's insights into the role of art as catharsis and psychic healing, enabling a move away from abjection. In *Black Sun,* for example, Kristeva (1989, p. 24) talked about the cathartic possibilities of literature: '...the literary (and religious) representation possesses a real and imaginary effectiveness that comes closer to catharsis than to elaboration; it is a therapeutic device used in all societies throughout the ages...'. Meanwhile, in *Powers of Horror,* Kristeva (1982, p. 200) discussed the power of language in literature to 'reveal an intense, passionate attitude through which the speaking subject displays his desire and calls upon the reader to embrace it, beyond words, through the archaic configuration of melody...'. What she says here applies also to Walrath's techniques in *Aliceheimer's* with the rhythm and flow of her images providing affects from extreme sadness (and abjection) (as in the drawing discussed above) to exuberant joy (catharsis) (when her mother hallucinates her husband up in a tree) paralleling the melody intonation in speech can provide.

In addition, in an interview dealing with an exhibition, *Rites of Passage: Art for the End of the Century* at the Tate Gallery a few years ago, Kristeva (1995, p. 26) noted the weakening and banalisation of signs, 'which means,' she says, 'that we are subject to psychosomatic reactions'.[6] Artists use the body as a sign, but 'it is always subverted, transformed, an object at the frontier of subject and object, of word and flesh' (p. 26), basically abjected, as in some of Walrath's images.

In the section, 'Missing Pieces,' we learn about another issue from Walrath's childhood, namely her mother's 'distorted affinity to all things blond' (Walrath, p. 17) – something Walrath couldn't understand at the time. An Armenian immigrant, Alice was (according to Walrath) 'beautiful, with thick, curly black hair, olive skin and big dark eyes' (17). Knowledgeable about Lamarckian inheritance theories, Alice would try to push her nose upwards in the hopes of changing her body to US norms. Walrath was supposed to drop everything Armenian in order to fit in. 'Hiding,' she says, 'had always been Alice's friend,' the 'missing pieces' kept out of sight. The drawing again insists on 'missing pieces,' showing Alice's face with only one eye, or her head without any facial features. While sympathetic now to her mother's plight, clearly as a child Walrath resented having to hide her Armenian inheritance. With Alzheimer's 'blond values begin to disappear,' and her mother dresses 'like an Armenian princess' (Walrath, p. 17). The 'missing pieces' are being revealed.

Here Kristeva's notion of art opening out to catharsis from abjection may again be helpful. In creating her mother's body out of cut-up text, especially in the first half of the graphic memoir, Walrath creates a subjectivity for her mother that does not rely on memory or what many call 'patriarchal' time. Her mother's textual body has its own kind of being, something many do not attribute to people with Alzheimer's. Images convey ambivalence and fear, since sometimes they are disturbing (Alice's face may miss an eye or other detail, for example), and often fragmented.

But as we'll see the catharsis emerges in her mother's sheer joy at imagining her husband up in the trees. Walrath adds colour – bright reds and green – to convey this joy. In the following sections, 'Flight,' 'Alice Ungrounded', and 'Aliceheimer's,' Walrath attempts to give us access to this joy happening to her mother. The drawings express even more than can the words accompanying them, something of changes involved with Alzheimer's. One drawing shows her mother in the process of using her new 'special powers' to 'take off'; another draws Alice half up in the air, with the text below reading 'She's still here. She's just losing her memory, the part that kept her grounded'. In these sections, we learn that Alice tried to keep the 'double dose of authority and confidence' she had when Walrath was a child (the Kristevan 'Maternal Authority'). This voice enables her to carry on, even if, as we learned already, in fact it had no actual power behind it anymore. The description of playing scrabble with Alice, when she made up words, offers a glimpse again into past conflict between mother and daughter. When Walrath (p. 19) notes, 'Challenge her? Never' (19), we assume that in the past she did challenge her mother, with the predictable resulting conflict. Reading to Alice now enables them to find common ground.

As the condition continues, it seems Walrath begins to accommodate to the inevitable reversal of mother as the abjected, and herself the child struggling to be free. Now Alice is released from the Symbolic, living in a kind of Imaginary of her own making, while Walrath assumes the position of reason and the law, gradually coming to terms with, and beginning to understand, the radical changes in Alice.

These changes are marked by Walrath changing the ghostly palette that has dominated the text so far, now adding splurges of colour, as noted. This suggests a vitality and energy lacking in earlier sections. In a wonderful section, just called 'Up,' Walrath first conveys, and then interprets, some of Alice's hallucinations. One is that 'Alice often sees my father high in the branches of one of our maple trees'. Walrath (p. 27) wonders what this means, and finally decides that, after years of tumultuous marriage, Alice's vision reveals 'longing – longing for him, longing to make amends'. And 'There he is, up in the branches, waiting for her'.

The drawing opposite has two big panels: in one, Walrath and her mother stand together, Walrath with her arm around her mother, watching Dave (Father, husband) dancing up in a tree. The other shows her mother with her hand on her breast – the gesture a gifted therapist, Martha Whitney, taught Alice to make when it was dark and she couldn't see Dave up in the tree! One senses here Walrath's new tenderness towards her mother, a love that enables her to see from within Alice's new mind how Alice now sees the world. Obviously, with the changes in Alice, so her daughter, Dana Walrath, is gradually able to let go of hostility, ambivalence, and aggression from inevitable childhood conflicts, and come to love her 'new' mother. But not all at once: there are more steps they have to go through.

An example of Walrath's ability to follow her mother's new mental processes is when, enjoying meat for dinner, Alice asks her daughter where she got the meat, stating, 'Isn't there rationing'? Walrath immediately understands her mother to be mentally back in the Second World War, when indeed there was rationing. As always, Walrath does not try to bring her mother back to the present; she is simply glad to see that her mother's comment made sense given a certain context. What may seem like arbitrary fantasies or hallucinations Walrath rather sees follow a certain logic. Alice's brain, in other words, still works, but it's working *differently*. Walrath comments that instead of sticking with science and biomedicine, which define visions as symptoms to be eradicated, she and her husband rather used 'other branches of science,' validating Alice's special power, from their point of view, to accommodate simultaneous realities in accordance with relativity theory.

As the memoir continues, Walrath turns to her very early life with her mother, as if unconsciously drawn to explore the realm of the imaginary when she and her mother were in a harmony depicted in the photo at the book's opening. It's as if, because now her mother is no longer a controlling, somewhat aggressive presence, a space has been opened up for Walrath to look back at their relationship more objectively. And Walrath actually returns to the moment of her birth. The section 'Umbilicus' starts with a drawing on the left-hand side, of a man (her father? Or, given the strap with a light on it over the man's head, the doctor?) holding up baby, saying 'It's a girl child'. On the right-hand side, the narrative starts with a reflection that is a bit startling because, like that photo, so intimate: 'I was never close to my mother, not counting those first nine months and the six months that followed when she breastfed me, unlike most mothers in the scientific 1960s' (Walrath, p. 39). Her mother no longer threatening provides room finally for Walrath to explore how she felt about her mother, and how she now feels. Walrath describes the pleasant home Alice created for her, but what was missing was intimacy: 'But no, we were never close (that is after her first year, ed.) until Alzheimer's'. Further, Walrath explains that she didn't invite her mother to live with her (once Alice was sent to the lockdown Alzheimer's unit at the facility) because wanting to repay her mother or something like that. Rather, 'it was our unfinished business of finding a good "close,"' she says.

And indeed Alzheimer's does allow Walrath's mother to behave quite differently to her daughter, even if Alice does not really know what she's saying. It's as if Alice's split off self is now able to speak: For example, Alice tells Walrath (in the course of a memory about her own childhood), 'You know, you must have been a cute little kid. I wish I had known you then'. This suggests that unconsciously Alice had appreciated her daughter more than she could consciously acknowledge or indicate at the time (unconscious competition? Envy of opportunities her daughter had which Alice hadn't?)

In the last sections of the graphic novel, it seems Walrath earns more warm words from her mother, just because (ironically) her mother does not consciously know that the woman taking care of her is her daughter. So it's a sort of bitter irony for Walrath, although it seems also rewarding because the emotion Alice expresses is genuine. For example, in the section 'Because You Are My Mother,' Alice asks her daughter, 'Dana, why are you so good to me?' Walrath answers 'Because you are my mother,' a concept Alice has a hard time accepting. Having been reminded about her husband and Walrath's siblings, Alice says 'I wasn't very good to you. I'm sorry'. A remarkable moment of lucidity allows Alice to reach back in time and finally finish that 'unfinished business' that Walrath says is the reason she brought Alice into her home. Alice asks to be forgiven, and Walrath accepts her wish. When Alice wants to know why Walrath is forgiving, Walrath tells her 'it's because you did the best you could'.

This shows how far Walrath herself has come in moving from unconscious hostility and aggression towards the 'Maternal Authority' of her childhood to empathy for that 'authority' (p. 43) now that Alzheimer's had ironically opened up space for difficult and conflicting feelings to emerge. Walrath sees herself as able to 'redo the past,' reworking her prior fantasy of yanking her mother's hair while brushing it, or getting annoyed at the knots and 'chopping all her hair off'. This last phrase shows just how angry Walrath had been at her mother, and how much now her feelings have changed. Walrath tells us she wants to listen to her mother and help her through her mental difficulties. The moment of lucidity, of course, passes as it must with AD, when her mother says 'Running a hotel must be very hard'!

As the narrative comes to an end, we learn even more about Walrath's childhood and family difficulties of two distinct kinds. One was that evidently Walrath had looks closer to her white American father, while her siblings were dark skinned with black hair. Neighbours queried

Walrath as to where she came from, obviously making her feel very awkward. The second was her brother being disabled – something that Alice experienced as shameful, especially when other parents refused play dates with her son. Somehow, Walrath was to make things right, but was also to blame when her brother had angry outbursts. Walrath, being light-skinned, was to show Alice deserved her 'wonderland,' namely her neat American suburban home and life.

It's easy to see why Walrath would have built up a resentment towards her mother that could not be confronted and that smouldered all these years until Alice's condition. Now things can be said because Alzheimer's allows for moving beyond social codes and conventions that inhibit frank speaking. One snapshot reveals the merging of roles between mother and daughter – a merging that, if confusing, allows frank talk. Alice's hands are hurting from IV's put in them while Alice was ill in hospital. Walrath takes her hands and kisses them where it hurts. Alice thanks her and asks 'Are you my mother?' Walrath replies: 'I am your daughter,' although her motherly attention justifies the question. When Alice says that it's nice that Walrath is her daughter, Walrath (p. 55) says: 'It is nice. At last'.

Another snapshot reveals still more about Walrath's childhood and Alice's inability to nurture her properly. Walrath is reminded of an incident when Alice confuses memories of her having periods with her current Alzhheimer's induced incontinence. Tending to her mother's resulting messes, Walrath is reminded of how her mother was unable to talk to Walrath about anything to do with the body, resulting in Walrath having no preparation for when her periods began. Alice gave her the most curt of instructions, and Walrath (p. 57) says: 'I double bagged and smoldered. The rage only surfaced when facts born from the filmstrip (shown in school, ed.) didn't pan out. No. Bleeding doesn't stop when you go swimming, that is, if you are from the Hair Belt'.

Walrath finally spends some time recounting details about her mother's life and family in Armenia, where Walrath went to track down older family members and do some family archival research. It seems her project is part of a reparation process, involving coming to terms with her genetic and historical background.

At the very end of the memoir, in a section 'Who Are You?,' Walrath has some important insights about relationships and social roles inspired by her experience with her mother's Alzheimer's. As Walrath puts it, 'Identity is the public side of self. Daughter, mother, anthropologist, wife – each of these prescribes a series of social behaviors that go with the role'. But Walrath learns that in fact what's important, more so than social roles, 'is recognition of intention and behavior…'. Alice's constant questioning of Walrath as to her role (is Walrath her mother, her sister?) leads Walrath to say that somewhere Alice knew Walrath was her daughter, and this, in turn, says Walrath (p. 69), '…helped me know my deepest self'. 'Alice,' Walrath says, 'remained with me even when we weren't on Skype, because now, thanks to Alice, I recognize myself'.

This is a very profound result of Walrath's experience caring for her mother. It seems that in the process of writing about this time Walrath was in fact working through a lot of unconscious rage which could now become conscious. Meanwhile, in her own way, Alice too is able to work through her unconscious guilt at how she failed Walrath as a mother, and how she was unable to properly nurture her. Because of Alzheimer's, Alice is able to articulate as if to a stranger how she failed her daughter, and to ask for forgiveness. Both mother and daughter seek reparation and reconciliation (à la Melanie Klein) as Alice's life is coming to an end. The very last sequence of exchanges between the two over Skype might well be showing the two back enjoying a kind of rare harmony found in a kind of fantasy (Lacanian) imaginary visualised in the opening photograph.

Notes

1 There is by now a substantial sub-field in Age Studies with humanists dealing specifically with dementia and Alzheimer's in literature, film, the Arts. The work of Anne Davis Basting (2009) is exemplary both in terms of theory and practice, writing, and performance. See her ground-breaking monograph, *Forget Memory,* See also bibliography in Kaplan/Chivers (2018), a forthcoming collaborative essay where the many authors working in this area are detailed.

2 In some States, Medicare may be used, but it's mainly left to the families of AD subjects to find and fund their care, being ground down to poverty before being eligible for Medicare dollars See Peter Finch, 'Continuing Care Homes Need a Financial Checkup'. *New York Times,* Sunday Review, Sunday March 1, 2018, p. 7.

3 For information regarding vastly different provisions for elderly care in European nations still retaining elements of prior State Welfare programmes, see a series of essays in *Aging in European Societies* (2013), edited by Constantinos Phellas.

4 For more on continuing abjection of AD subjects and on arts and humanities theories and practices for alternatives to prevailing dementia discourses, see E. Ann Kaplan/Sally Chivers (2018), 'Alzheimer's, Age Panic, Neuroscience: Media Discourses of Dementia and Care'. Forthcoming in *The Oxford Encyclopedia for Research in Communication.*

5 Much has been written in recent years about unique opportunities offered by the comic form. Art Spiegelman's (1986) graphic memoir *Maus* about the Holocaust first generated attention to what the form could achieve, above and beyond the long-standing popular comics prevalent across the globe. One might say that *Maus* ushered in a new era for the comic form, hitherto seen as an art form below 'literature'. Increasingly, in the intervening years, artists have gravitated to the form, re-inventing in each case new approaches and different results, as for example in Alison Bechtel's (2006) *Fun Home* or Marjane Satrapi's (2003) *Persepolis.* For more on the virtues of the comic form and details of its history, see Hillary Chute (2010, 2017).

6 I want to thank Nicholas Chare for letting me know about this interview, and further yet, providing a copy.

References

Basting, A. D. (2009) *Forget Memory: Creating Better Lives for People with Dementia*. Baltimore: John's Hopkins University Press.

Bechdel, A. (2006) *Fun Home: A Family Tragicomic*. New York: Houghton Mifflin.

Chute, H. (2010) *Graphic Women: Life Narrative and Contemporary Comics*. New York: Columbia University Press.

Chute, H. (2017) *Why Comics? From Underground to Everywhere*. New York: Harper.

Creed, B. (1993) *The Monstrous-Feminine: Film, Feminism, Psychoanalysis*. London and New York: Routledge.

Kaplan, E. A. & S. Chivers (2018). 'Alzheimer's, Age Panic, Neuroscience: Media Discourses of Dementia and Care.' in the *Oxford Research Encyclopedia of Communication* [Online resource]. http://oxfordre.com/communication/view/10.1093/acrefore/9780190228613.001.0001/acrefore-9780190228613-e-765.

Klein, M. (1975) *Love, Guilt and Reparation and Other Works 1921–1945*, Vol. 1. of *The Writings of Melanie Klein*. Ed. R. E. Money-Kyrle. London: Hogarth Press and The Institute of Psychoanalysis.

Kristeva, J. (1982). *Powers of Horror: An Essay on Abjection*. Translated from the French by L. S. Roudiez. New York: Columbia University Press.

Kristeva, J. (1989) *Black Sun: Depression and Melancholia*. Translated from the French by L. S. Roudiez. New York: Columbia University Press.

Kristeva, J. (1995). 'Of Word and Flesh: An Interview with Julia Kristeva by Charles Penwarden.' In S. Morgan and F. Morris (eds.), *Rites of Passage: Art for the End of the Century*. London: Tate Gallery Publications, pp. 21–27.

Lacan, J. (1949/1977). 'The Mirror Stage as Formative of the Function of the I as Revealed in Psychoanalytic Experience.' In J. Lacan (ed.), *Ecrits: A Selection*. Translated from the French by Alan Sheridan. New York and London: W.W. Norton & Co, pp. 1–7.

Satrapi, M. (2003) *Persepolis: The Story of a Childhood*. New York: Pantheon.

Spigelman, A. (1986) *Maus I: A Survivor's Tale, My Father Bleeds History*. New York: Pantheon.

Walrath, D. (2013) *Aliceheimer's: Alzheimer's Through the Looking Glass*. Yerevan: Harvest Publishers.

Part IV

Introduction

Rethinking the Monstrous-Feminine through a Transnational Frame

Nicholas Chare, Jeanette Hoorn, and Audrey Yue

Most of the films discussed in *The Monstrous-Feminine* derive from American and European cinema. In this final section, four chapters consider the monstrous-feminine as it manifests in cultural productions from other geographical contexts. The sections open with Brett Farmer's 'Polluted Water', which examines abjection in Thai cinema in relation to the films of Poj Arnon. Arnon is a major force in the Thai film industry but one whose corpus is often viewed ambivalently. Farmer reads this ambivalence as, in part, a symptom of class-based snobbery. In Thailand's taste economy, admitting to admiring Arnon's oeuvre risks being perceived as evidence of a lack of cultural refinement. The intensity of repulsion directed towards Arnon, however, leads Farmer to argue that turning to class to explain his negative critical reception is insufficient. Arnon's films, Farmer explains, are identified as *nam nao*, as 'polluted water', dangerously impure and therefore unfit for common consumption. Arnon makes pictures that are abject.

Farmer carefully unpacks the make-up of this abjection, finding this boundary-troubling manifests across genre, form, and content. The two major topoi of abjection in Arnon's films are female ghosts and queers. Foregrounding the need to address issues of cultural specificity, Farmer builds on Katarzyna Ancuta's (2017) and Rachel Harrison's (2017) critically reflexive employment of Barbara Creed's conception of the monstrous-feminine in the context of Thai culture to explore how patriarchal anxieties in Thailand manifest by way of efforts to control the unruly, abject feminine. Many of Arnon's female characters can be read as embodying this abject. Farmer gives the example of Dao (Mai Charoenpura) in *Tai Hong* [Still] (Dirs. Poj Arnon, Chatchai Katenut, Tanwarin Sukkhapsit & Manussa Vorasingha, Thailand, 2010), whose character is middle-aged sex worker. In shots at the beginning of the film, Farmer describes her as embodying 'the ageing female grotesque'. Age intersects with gender and class to produce a vision of abject femininity. This vision, however, based on surface appearances and the preconceptions they encourage, is subsequently replaced, subverted, when Dao is shown to be 'a sassy working-class wisecracker' who endears herself to the audience through her world-weary wit. Dao reappears in the final story of the quartet forming *Tai Hong*, a nonsensical horror story which Farmer suggests 'with its cavalcade of abject sexual and social marginals – prostitutes, queers, ageing women – [...] is classic Poj Arnon'.

This practice of placing the socially marginalised at the centre of the action also characterises Arnon's signature work, his Ho Taeo Taek series of films which centres upon a group of *kathoey* who run a haunted boarding house. Farmer traces the etymology of *kathoey* and also draws attention to its shifting usage and contemporary complexity. *Kathoey* signals being '[b]etwixt and between masculinity and femininity', therefore embodying a capacity for border-crossing. In the Ho Taeo Taek series, *kathoey* function as an interface between 'the living and the dead, the monstrous and the human'. The *kathoey* in the films possess agency and are rebellious and transgressive. Farmer contrasts their depiction with those of other *kathoey* in contemporary Thai cinema which frequently operate in the service of national fantasies of unity and social reconciliation. In Farmer's persuasive sociopolitical reading, Arnon's *kathoeys* function as a reminder of the real social tensions that continue to characterise Thai society. The disqualification of Princess Ubolratana from running as a candidate in the 2019 Thai general election gave recent international exposure to these ongoing social tensions. Ubolratana's candidacy was intended to reconcile the rival political factions of the exiled Shinawatras and their rural powerbase and the urban middle class who are opposed to them. Arnon's films, as Farmer discusses, have been censured for threatening 'national morality'. His queer ribaldry clearly perceived as a challenge to moral propriety as a source of social cohesion and compliance.

Alongside his sociopolitical readings of Arnon's films, Farmer also compellingly argues that their popular appeal lies not so much in their formulaic storyline but in their 'ritualised structures of feeling'. The intense affect registered by audiences viewing these horror-comedies is central to their popularity. Like essays such as Cowie's and Pisters' in this volume, Farmer is therefore attuned to the importance of attending to sub-narrative dimensions within films. Understanding Arnon's films is not simply a case of following their storylines but also of appreciating their affective dimensions.

Valerie Wee's chapter, 'The Monstrous-Feminine in the Millenial Japanese Horror Film', also extends the insights afforded by the monstrous-feminine beyond Western cinema. Additionally, Wee's analyses parallel Farmer's in their attention to how horror films register social change. She reads millennial Japanese horror films as expressing anxieties arising from a weakening in Japan of traditional patriarchal values. Wee begins with an historical overview of the figure of the *onryō* [vengeful ghost], a common feature in recent Japanese horror cinema appearing in films such as *Ringu* [Ring] (Dir. Hideo Nakata, Japan, 1998), *Hongurai Mizu* [Dark Water] (Dir. Hideo Nakata, Japan, 2002) and *Ju-on* [The Grudge] (Dir. Takashi Shimizu, Japan, 2002). Inspired by *The Monstrous-Feminine* (Creed 1993), she reads the *onryō* as an abject figure. For Wee, traditional tales featuring the *onryō*, in which women who have been murdered by the men responsible for protecting and caring for them return from the dead to exert violent revenge, cannot be read as affirming women's autonomy as they end with the revengeful spirit returning to the supernatural realm from whence they came. In this sense, traditional patriarchal society is left untouched, unchanged. The role of the *onryō*i is simply to warn men to fulfil their prescribed duties towards women (Wee 2011). These wrathful wraiths do not challenge the status quo.

Wee then situates the *onryō* within the sociopolitical situation of Japan at the end of the twentieth century, convincingly demonstrating ways in which the figure of the vengeful female spirit has been revised to respond to societal change. She outlines how traditional feminine roles revolving around motherhood and caring are being increasingly challenged despite the persistence of traditional gender hierarchies. Wee describes the growing emergence of sexually liberated young women unwilling to conform to traditional expectations of chasteness and submissiveness. The *onryō* in millennial Japanese horror cinema can be read as a response to these trends. In films such as *Ringu* and *Hongurai Mizu*, for instance, the vengeful spirits are not adult women as was common in traditional tales of *onryō* but pre-teenage girls. The age differential has come into being as concerns have risen in Japanese society about the rise of 'selfish personal indulgence' in *shojo*, young females. The ghosts in *Ringu* and *Hongurai Mizu*, Sadako and Mitsuko, are excessive, with their rage and zeal for revenge insatiable, refusing to be bounded by convention. Wee reads this unappeasable dimension to their characters as registering anxieties about conspicuous consumption and self-indulgence in Japanese girls.

Building on her sensitive analysis of abjection in *Ju-on* in *Japanese Horror Films and their American Remakes* (Wee 2014), Wee also traces how the ghost in that film, Kayako, can be read as extending the *onryō* tradition. Kayako is a woman rather than a girl but she possesses similarities with Sadako and Mitsuko in that she supports fears of the feminine as 'essentially unfixable, indeterminate, and unknowable'. The three films of *Ringu*, *Hongurai Mizu*, and *Ju-on* each demonises the maternal even if their envisioning of the monstrous-feminine as it is incarnated in *onryō* is qualitatively different from traditional representations of the spirit. They all also explore the collapse of the traditional family though many of their female characters. For Wee, therefore, the films contribute to the demonisation of a new generation of young women unwilling to conform to traditional norms of comportment and seeking intellectual, social, and sexual independence. After a period of decline, the Japanese film industry is resurgent and more cinemas are being built to meet consumer demand (Yamamura 2008). Viewing films at the cinema is a leisure activity. As Laura Spielvogel (2003) has discussed, in Japan both the home and the workplace can be sources of pressure and responsibility. In this context, leisure spaces such as the cinema potentially provide a valuable opportunity for women to relax and escape social norms. As Wee demonstrates, however, the ideological underpinnings of contemporary Japanese horror films work to reaffirm those very norms.

The penultimate essay in this section also examines the monstrous-feminine in the context of non-Anglophone cinema, in this case from Slovenia. There is a strong personal dimension to Polona Petek's chapter 'Women in the Way?' as Petek was taught by Creed who also went on to supervise her doctoral thesis. Creed's *The Monstrous-Feminine* was a touchstone for Petek's subsequent thinking in relation to Slovenian cinema, a film industry in which women were, for a long time, highly marginalised. It was while Petek was studying at the University of Melbourne that the first Slovenian feature-length fiction film directed by a woman was released, *Varuh meje* [Guardian of the Frontier] (Dir. Maja Weiss, Slovenia/Germany, 2002). A decade later, Petek begin to study in depth the position of women in Slovenian cinema.

The Monstrous-Feminine has been important for Petek as it offers rich ways in which to theorise marginality and reflect on efforts to exploit marginal status for positive political ends. One of Petek's case studies in this context has been the director Maja Weiss whose film *Varuh meje* was a revelation when Petek came across it listed as a feature at the 2003 Melbourne Queer Film Festival. Weiss' films frequently include borders and boundaries (physical, emotional, figurative, and literal) as a theme. The border also informs another of Petek's case studies, the films of Sonja Prosenc. Petek reads Prosenc's *Zgodovina ljubenzi* [History of Love] (Dir. Sonja Prosenc, Slovenia, 2018) as a work where the narrative is less important than the emotions it enables the director to stage. This is reminiscent of Farmer's emphasis in the first chapter of this section on the importance of feeling in Arnon's films. Petek's sensitive analysis of *Zgodovina ljubenzi* emphasises the significance of the repeated visual references to water in the film. Petek also notes its sophisticated use of sound. Given the importance of the border as a theme in the films of Prosenc and Weiss, *The Monstrous-Feminine*, with its many insights into boundary-crossings and anxieties about border-dissolutions is an invaluable resource. Petek also turns for inspiration to the work of Henk van Houtum on borders, the ordering of space and the claiming of place.

The final essay in this section and the volume, is Jeanette Hoorn's 'In-Your-Face' which adopts a transnational approach to the monstrous-feminine exploring how it manifests in examples of modern and contemporary art from Australia, Mexico, and the US. Like the three preceding essays, Hoorn's complex exploration of the role of the abject in Australian Indigenous artist Destiny Deacon's works and also those of the multi-cultural Mexican painter Frida Kahlo demonstrate the value of Creed's ideas for cross-cultural analysis. Hoorn deftly outlines the value of the monstrous-feminine for analysing a range of artistic media and movements including bio-art and art exploring animal-human relations. Her primary focus, however, is on how representations of the abject female body relate to issues of male power and colonialism.

Hoorn begins by analysing Kahlo's works as art produced from a liminal position. The limen is, as Stephen Greenblatt (1995, p. 29) notes, 'the threshold or margin, the place that is no-place'. By identifying Kahlo as a painter of the margins, the marginalised, Hoorn, like Petek in the preceding essay, emphasises the value of the monstrous-feminine as a way of conceptualising social ostracism and means to contest and resist it. Some of Kahlo's paintings provide an uncompromising portrayal of parturition. Hoorn reads these as breaking with a sanitised rhetoric of birth that suppresses its bloody, painful reality. Hoorn then moves to a consideration of the American feminist artist Judy Chicago, specifically her much celebrated installation *The Dinner Party* (1979) and the controversies it initially generated. In her subsequent discussion of Cindy Sherman's photography, Hoorn examines how Laura Mulvey (1996) drew inspiration from Creed's *The Monstrous-Feminine* for her own interpretations of Sherman's work. Mulvey discusses Creed's influence on this research in her interview for this volume. Remaining in a North American context, Hoorn then considers Carolee Schneemann's performance works and her portfolio of photographs *Eye Body*. Some of the photographs in *Eye Body* could easily pass as stills from a horror film. Taken cumulatively, the analyses of the works by Schneemann, Sherman, Chicago, and Kahlo in their varied media, painting, performance, photography, and installation demonstrate the extent to which the monstrous-feminine can serve as an important explanatory framework for modern and contemporary art.

Hoorn concludes with an in-depth reading of Deacon's art. Deacon is principally known for her photographic works which draw attention to the racism and structural violence that are a legacy of settler colonialism. She has always been attuned to the role of language as an oppressive force as her use of word play and neologisms attests to. Hoorn's subtle and perceptive reading of Deacon's artworks builds out from a consideration of them as reflections on liminality. For Hoorn, Deacon's engagement with abjection is understated and nuanced in contrast with some of the more visceral takes that can be found in contemporary art. Hoorn's essay, like those of Farmer, Petek, and Wee, powerfully demonstrates the kinds of insights the monstrous-feminine can provide outside of the context of Anglophone horror cinema in which it was initially conceived.

References

Ancuta, K. (2017) 'Beyond the Vampire: Revamping Thai Monsters for the Urban Age,' *eTropics: Electronic Journal of Studies in the Tropics* 16(1), pp. 31–45.

Creed, B. (1993) *The Monstrous-Feminine: Film, Feminism, Psychoanalysis*. London: Routledge.

Greenblatt, S. (1995) 'Liminal States and Transformations,' in S. Morgan and F. Morris (eds.), *Rites of Passage: Art for the End of the Century*. London: Tate Gallery Publications, pp. 28–30.

Harrison, R. (2017) 'Dystopia as Liberation: Disturbing Femininities in Contemporary Thailand,' *Feminist Review*, 116(1), pp. 64–83.

Mulvey, L. (1996) *Fetishism and Curiosity*. London: BFI.

Spielvogel, L. (2003) *Working Out in Japan: Shaping the Female Body in Tokyo Fitness Clubs*. Durham: Duke University Press.

Wee, V. (2011) 'Patriarchy and the Horror of the Monstrous Feminine,' *Feminist Media Studies* 11(2), pp. 151–165.

Wee, V. (2014) *Japanese Horror Films and Their American Remakes*. New York: Routledge.

Yamamura, E. (2008) 'Socio-economic Effects of Increased Cinema Attendance: The Case of Japan,' *The Journal of Socio-Economics* 37, pp. 2546–2555.

11 Polluted Water

Demotic Thai Cinema and Queer Abjection in the Films of Poj Arnon

Brett Farmer

In 2015, Poj Arnon,[1] one of Thailand's most successful contemporary film-makers, celebrated his 20th anniversary as a feature film director. In the two decades since his breakout directorial debut with the 1995 hit comedy, *Sati Taek Sud Khua Lok/Crazy*, Arnon directed close to 30 other motion pictures and executive-produced a dozen more. It is a prodigious output made all the more impressive by the fact that the majority of these films were solid box office performers with several ranking among the highest-grossing domestic releases of recent times (Nainapat 2017). Given this extraordinary track-record, it shouldn't surprise that Arnon's anniversary milestone garnered considerable attention in both the print and online Thai media. What might prove less expected is that, for the most part, the tenor of the coverage was distinctly icy – even derisive. The respected film magazine, *Bioscope*, provides a characteristic example. Devoting a multi-page retrospective to 'Poj Arnon ... 20 Years,' complete with photographic highlights and specially commissioned portraits, the tributary guise of the lavish spread was quickly undercut by the accompanying commentary which starts:

> Love him or loathe him, you can't have escaped the cinematic vision of Poj Arnon in some form. His name is never out of the film industry and, reviewed on the basis of numbers alone, there's no denying he has worked regularly and continuously. Of all our current generation of filmmakers, it must be said that he alone is the person who makes Thai movies, one of the few who can survive making real old-style movies.
>
> (Pimnam 2016, p. 45)

Damning with faint praise – and, even then, through gritted-teeth – the thinly veiled condescension evidenced here indicates the ambivalent position Poj Arnon has come to assume in contemporary Thai film cultures. His brash and often vulgar brand of populist film-making plays well with substantial segments of the domestic Thai audience, but among others, notably the middle-classes and cultural elites, he is, to quote the headline of another media profile, 'a man maligned' (Pajee 2017, p. 12) branded as everything from 'Thailand's reigning cinematic snakeoil salesman'

(Wise Kwai 2014, para. 2) to its 'infamous master of schlock' (Winston 2016, p. 7). Detractors of Arnon's films, writes Kong Rithdee, 'never get tired of ridiculing, disparaging and raising eyebrows (or something else) at what they see as pre-packaged nonsense that corrupts the integrity of Thai cinema in the director's prolific output' (Rithdee 2012, p. 4).

As the moralising rhetoric of ridicule and raised-eyebrows might suggest, a good deal of the disdain for Arnon's brand of populist film-making is an effect of class-based taste economies, pure and simple. Scratch the surface of even the most benign aesthetic judgement, faithful readers of Bourdieu (1984, pp. 2–6) will know, and one will inevitably find a correlative social judgement working to index and affirm taxonomies of status and rank. It's a process of taste-based social distinction that assumes a particularly intense cast in Thailand, a deeply status-oriented country where complex codes of hierarchical relationality govern nearly every aspect of social and cultural interaction (Mulder 2000, pp. 43–55). Thailand has, moreover, undergone tumultuous processes of economic growth and social modernisation in recent times that has seen the rise to ascendancy of vast new urban middle-classes who explicitly stake, and often fiercely guard, their precarious claims to legitimacy in the valorised taste economies of spectacular cultural consumption and commodity lifestyles (Phongpaichit and Baker 2016; Vorng 2017).

Cinema has been a significant part of this latter-day history of expanded social distinction in Thailand. Prior to the economic boom of the late-twentieth century, Thai movies were a largely déclassé affair, consisting of quickly produced, low-budget products geared to socially devalued markets of teenagers, urban labourers, and Thailand's massive agrarian sector – 'fit only for low-class people and rural nobodies' as one observer of the time put it (Hamilton 1994, p. 151). In addressing these popular audiences, Thai films cultivated a strategically sensationalist style of attractional cinema rooted in misprized traditions of rural folk culture and demotic carnivalesque. Widely described through the culinary idiom of *khrob tuk rot* or 'bursting with all flavours' (Fouquet 1989; Herrera 2015), vernacular Thai movies mixed disparate elements, styles, and genres into a multiform ensemble that offered optimal points of appeal to the heterogeneous reading formations of the popular classes but bore scant resemblance to the well-wrought ideals of international film aesthetics, thus further reinforcing the domestic industry's reputation for unrefined boorishness. In the 1990s, however, Thai cinema experienced a marked reversal of fortunes when a raft of factors stemming from the era's economic boom and the increased internationalisation of capital and cultural flows led to an exponential improvement in the range, style and cultural cachet of local film-making (Harrison 2006; Lewis 2003). Sporting vastly improved production values and international-style 'quality aesthetics' and screened in the gleaming new multiplexes of Thailand's roaring consumerist infrastructure, the renovated products of the so-called 'new

Thai cinema' surged in popularity and status, becoming part of the era's 'upwardly mobile, bourgeois culture of "globalized" consumption' (Ingawanij 2006, p. 149).

Within this context, older models of vernacular Thai film didn't disappear, but, freighted with further negative attributes of archaic anachronism, they became ever more marginal and devalued. It's here that we can begin to contextualise the widespread disdain for a film-maker like Poj Arnon who, to repeat the telling description from *Bioscope* above, remains one of the few who continues to 'make Thai movies ... real old-style movies' (Pimnam 2016, p. 45). A self-avowed populist––'I make movies for the masses,' he asserts, 'the lower and middle market ... movies that are fun and easy to understand' (in Petvirojchai 2017, p. 23)––Arnon is the latter-day heir to the fast-and-furious traditions of demotic Thai film, complete with *ad hoc* production practices and patchwork *khrob tuk rot* textuality. With little formal education and no film training, he churns out movies at lightning speed, typically without a script and improvising as he proceeds. 'I'm not a person who studies theory, I just do it', he declares with characteristic chutzpah (Pimnam 2016, p. 45). It is a utilitarian, quick-and-dirty approach to film-making as provisional trade that, not surprisingly, sits uncomfortably with the bourgeois quality ideals and 'world-class' aspirations of the 'new Thai cinema'. Detractors 'may say [my films] are tasteless', the director declares, but 'I have the audience on my side. I make films for my fans' (Rithdee 2009, p. 1).

On its own, however, a class-based taste analysis isn't quite sufficient to account for the full weight of revulsion – or, for that matter, fascination – elicited by the cinema of Poj Arnon. As the director himself points out, he is hardly the only Thai film-maker to churn out populist fare, so 'I have to wonder what I did ... that they come down so heavily on my films' (Pajee 2017, 12). To answer that requires, perhaps, a deeper probe. One of the Thai language terms used most frequently to denote the demotic style of films made by Poj Arnon – as indeed other 'lowbrow' media entertainments – is *nam nao* or 'polluted water' (Eaosriwongs 1980; Fouquet 2003). Typically translated into English via the much weaker cognate of 'trash', *nam nao* is charged with a deep frisson of cultural anxiety that 'evokes the look and smell of stagnant water and rotting garbage ... of decay and refuse,' of a 'social pollution that need[s] to be expelled or quarantined' (Farmer 2015, p. 215). It is, in other words, a potent expression of abjection.

Julia Kristeva famously defines abjection as that which 'disturbs identity, system, order [... and] does not respect borders, positions, rules. The in-between, the ambiguous, the composite' (1982, p. 4). In her primarily psychoanalytic purview, abjection is linked to processes of identity constitution as the developing subject – or in the case of collective identities, the developing social group – comes into being through processes of differentiation and expulsion, drawing borders around self and other, subject and object. The abject, she writes, is 'what is jettisoned from the symbolic system ... the logic of prohibition ... of excluding filth ... establishing the "self and clean" [*corps propre*] of each social group if not of each subject' (Kristeva 1982, pp. 64–65). To the extent that abjection remains the grounds of subjective production, what is deemed abject and unclean is never entirely ejected, never completely erased. It broods over the very borders it defines, ever poised to revolt, to return, to pollute, setting in motion a perpetual *pas-de-deux* of attraction and revulsion. 'We may call it a border', Kristeva writes, but 'abjection is above all ambiguity ... a composite of judgment and affect, of condemnation and yearning, of signs and drives' (1982, pp. 9–10).

It is a theoretical image that corresponds suggestively both to the semiotic valences of *nam nao*––with its metaphoric condensation of borderless fluidity and profane contamination – and to the outrageous mongrelism of demotic Thai cinema. In the case of Poj Arnon, his films present a giddy web of abject border-crossings that fuel much of the anxiety at play in the love-him-or-loathe-him, dread-and-desire extremes of his polarised reception. Aesthetically, they continue the pronounced textual eclecticism of *khrob tuk rot* – with moments of comedy, romance, pathos, fear, action, and music rubbing cheek by jowl with little sense of logic or cohesion – while upping the attractional ante with a rash of more contemporary cultural flourishes and allusions. The result is something of a sensorial assault that, depending on perspective, can be exhilarating or disorienting. 'The movie has romance and family drama parts throughout, with a bit of everything squeezed in,' huffs one disapproving reviewer of Poj's 2018 film *Toot Too Ku Chart*, 'The result is a sense of "too muchness" (*kwam-lon-ti-woe-wang*) in the film. There's no control, whatever happens happens' (23Scenes 2018, para. 5). Faced with the aesthetic lawlessness of Arnon's mongrel films, readers primed for meaning, order, and control experience the anxious *non-sense* and *dis-order* of the abject – 'the place', as Kristeva asserts, 'where meaning collapses' (2).

It is part of the reason commentators almost universally struggle to denominate, let alone evaluate, his films and routinely fall back on either a *sui generis* exceptionalism – where a 'Poj Arnon film/*nang Poj Arnon*' acts as a taxonomic register unto itself (Petvirojchai 2017, p. 21) – or resort to strings of awkward hyphenates[2]:

> The bottom line is: [Poj Arnon] has been accused of making bad films. Stupid films. Of producing Trash ... Of promoting crimes against artistic integrity by giving birth to the cine-hybrid that can only be witnessed in Thai cinema: the homosexualised horror-comedy, featuring gays and ghosts and gags, inwardly multiplied among one another into a species that's garish, vulgar and, hell, fun.
> (Rithdee 2009, p. 1)

The turbid mix of weighted metaphors here – trash and criminality, birth and hybridity, death and perversion – indicates that abjection in the films of Poj Arnon isn't limited to the scandalous impurities of its mongrel aesthetics but saturates every level: form and content, strategy and statement, discourse and narrative. And taking the alliterative allusion to 'gays and ghosts and gags' as a cue, there are two topoi of abjection that loom particularly large in Poj's films: female ghosts and queers.

In terms of the former, the female ghost or *phi* – a category that in the Thai language includes not just spectres but animistic spirits, deities, and demons – is a longstanding staple of Thai cinema across multiple forms (Fuhrmann 2016; Knee 2005). It is also a classic figure of cinematic abjection. In her influential elaboration of Kristevan theory for feminist studies of horror cinema, Barbara Creed (1993) identifies female ghosts as a privileged expression of what she terms 'the monstrous-feminine': 'what it is about woman that is shocking, terrifying, horrific, abject' (1). As Creed argues, female corporealities and other manifestations of the feminine operate as a powerful source of abjection in phallocentric imaginaries, playing out primal fantasies of incorporation and separation from the maternal body and the violent secondary elaborations of patriarchal misogyny. With its spectacular catalogue of monstrous female archetypes – 'archaic mother, monstrous womb, vampire, possessed monster, *femme castatrice*, witch, castrating mother' (Creed 1993, pp. 151–152) – horror cinema functions as 'a form of modern defilement rite [that] attempts to separate out the symbolic order from all that threatens its stability, particularly the mother and all that her universe signifies' (Creed 1993, p. 14).

It is a provocative account that has generated widespread critical interest and enquiry, even in cultural contexts far removed from Creed's principal focus on Hollywood film (Dumas 2018; Lee 2015; Ng 2014). Rachel Harrison, in exploring the monstrous-feminine as a lens for reading 'disturbing femininities in contemporary Thailand' (2017, p. 64), wisely cautions against an erasure of cultural specificities, noting that 'Creed's Eurocentric focus' and adoption of 'theoretical positions derived from ... Judaeo-Christian philosophical thought' don't always translate automatically into the Thai context (p. 72). Nevertheless, as 'a way of understanding how woman is made monstrous ... and a threat to the moral, spiritual, and social status quo', theories of the monstrous-feminine, Harrison avers, remain 'highly relevant to Thai cultural studies and to instances of its cinematic horror genre'(ibid.), where 'female spirits and ghosts' (ibid.) abound. Katarzyna Ancuta similarly argues that 'Creed's model of the monstrous feminine can be criticized ... for promoting cultural conceptualisations of gender that may be incompatible with Southeast Asian realities' (2017, p. 35), but it resonates powerfully with Thai patriarchal anxieties around sexual difference and psychosocial measures 'to exercise control over [female] sexuality' through cultural spectacles of demonisation and abjection (ibid.).

Importantly, both Harrison and Ancuta extend the hermeneutic ambit of the Thai monstrous-feminine to encompass inter-related modes of sexual and social difference such as class, ethnicity and region. Thailand's 'skewed gender and socio-economic hierarchies which favour men over women, rich over poor, and Bangkok over the rest of the country' (p. 36), writes Ancuta, imbue its cinematic iterations of female monstrosity with multiple modes of abjection deemed threatening to the authority of not just masculinities but 'the public image of a country focused on the urban middle classes' (ibid.). In a similar vein, Harrison suggests that Thai cinematic images of the monstrous-feminine condense and speak to a range of anxieties and struggles between opposing sexual, social and spatial realms:

> the rational, enlightened and conservative-nationalist masculine thrust, perceived as being 'modern' and represented by Siam's political and cultural elite at the centre, and the unrestrained, supernatural expressions of the feminine as sexualised body, aligned with the supposedly pre-modern 'irrationality' of 'the natural world' at the periphery.
>
> (Harrison 2017, p. 75)

It is an argument that chimes evocatively with the cinematic articulations of feminine monstrosity in the work of Poj Arnon which is, as we have seen, centrally coded as scandalous 'other' to Thailand's hegemonic bourgeois subject positions and sensibilities. Instructively, the multiple monstrous spectres that haunt Arnon's films are typically drawn from the twilight world of social subalterns: premodern revenants, provincials, urban workers, and sexual outsiders.[3]

Consider, by way of example, *Tai Hong/Still* (2010), an omnibus quartet of interlinked ghost stories which was conceived, produced, and (partially) directed by Arnon. Taking its name from *phi tai hong* or 'ghosts of bad death', the classic vengeful spirits of Thai folklore, *Tai Hong* weaves together four separate tales – each helmed by a different director – based loosely around a series of real-life murders and tragedies ripped from the headlines of recent Thai news. Though it is a somewhat more sober affair than most entries in the Poj Arnon oeuvre – due, no doubt, to the tempering contributions of the other three film-makers – *Tai Hong* still exhibits the maverick film-maker's trademark textual transgression and thematic focus on social and sexual misfits.

A prologue sequence, directed by Arnon, introduces the central characters who will subsequently feature in the constituent tales by way of a framing device where they cross paths in the lead-up to a New Year's Party at Santaka nightclub. This diegetic location is an obvious riff on Santika Club, a Bangkok entertainment venue that tragically burned down during New Year's celebrations in 2009, killing 66 partygoers, and that forms the basis for the first of the film's four tabloid-driven ghost stories ('Fire' 2009).[4] Chief among the characters introduced in this opening sequence is Dao, an ageing exotic dancer, played with tough brillo by celebrated Thai singer and veteran TV-film actor, Mai Charoenpura. Apart from the star casting, Dao's textual centrality is underscored by the fact she is afforded the very first shot in the film: a studied close-up of her mouth, lips moist and slightly parted, as she meticulously paints them with a run of blood red gloss, accompanied by the ominous strains of an atonal musical score. The marked combination here of sexualised femininity and uncanniness is further accented as we watch Dao – intercut in parallel montage with shots of the other characters – progressively make up her face in a series of fragmentary close-ups. At one point, she stops abruptly and, in a weighted moment of literal abjection, plucks out a nasal hair with her fingers, momentarily staring at the detached and abjectified body part with unsettling dispassion before resuming her ritual of cosmetic sexual enhancement. The fact that Dao is evidently coded as a sex worker, a literal painted lady, and one moreover who is past the flush of youth – Mai Charoenpura was 41 at the time of filming – further enshrouds her character with additional registers of illicit sex and the ageing female grotesque.

Yet, having introduced Dao through a classic horror tropology of abjectified female sexuality, the film sets about subverting or at least problematising its signifying effects. Setting off to her job in a cheap and forlornly empty gentlemen's club, Dao gives it her all in an increasingly desperate pole dance, accompanied by a pronounced musical shift on the soundtrack to a hackneyed disco-beat backing track. A quartet of young men enter the bar, take one look at the slightly long-in-the-tooth woman gyrating like a mad thing on the stage, and promptly leave. Engrossed in her athletic performance, Dao continues for several beats, all forced toothy smiles and backside wiggles, when, suddenly realising her potential clients have fled, she stops mid-twerk, drops the act, and mutters to herself in coarse argot, 'Where the fuck did they go ... all the other girls went to Dubai, I should have gone too. I'm outta here!' Played with sharp self-deprecating irony, the sudden switch from the enigmatic, threatening seductress of the opening shots to a sassy working-class wisecracker recodes Dao as an endearingly comic – and very human – presence, suggesting that whatever guise of monstrous femininity she may assume is a knowing performance. It is an interplay between monster and human, mask and self, deception and truth that the film keeps in abeyance through the fourth and final story of the omnibus quartet where Dao returns as a protagonist.

Titled 'Khuen Khru/Haunting Motel', the final story, which is entirely directed by Arnon, signals a marked change in the film's style and tenor. Where the preceding stories are all presented with relative naturalism designed for optimal chills, 'Kheun Khru' is geared for horror-comic excess.

It is also the only one of the four entries to use a female-dominant narrational economy with Dao serving as primary focalising agent throughout. As it opens, we see Dao saunter with feigned nonchalance to the end of a line of very young streetwalkers. She sports a prominent surgical mask in an ostensible attempt to conceal her age, while literalising the interplay of mask and role established in the prologue. After a bit of humorous business with failed client negotiations, Dao is approached by a pair of bumbling young men on a motorcycle, Thua (Rutchanon Sookprakorb) and Dam (Kachapa Tancharoen). The fact that their names combine to form a colloquial Thai expression for anal sex is a none-too-subtle index of the queer dynamics at play in the set-up where the outrageously gay Dam is urging his reluctant straight friend Thua to engage Dao's services for a threesome. Engineering a deal, the three set off rather ungracefully on the motorbike to one of Bangkok's many curtained drive-in 'love motels'. There they encounter a crazed cat-stroking 'Gold-Toothed Aunty' (Wasana Chalakorn) who manages the motel and tells the hapless trio that the room they have rented is haunted by a *phi tai hong*. Cue the scene for a delirious sequence of spoofed Thai horror conventions, shifting identities and sexual farce that sees all four of the characters in the motel assume and then relinquish the roles of seducer and seduced, haunter and haunted, killer and victim, living and dead. At one point, Dao is identified as the terrifying spectre, slithering across the floor with the classic menacing moves of the long-haired female ghost of Thai and other Asian cinemas, only to have it redefined in the next instant as a lapse of perception. In the end, Dao is actually revealed to be the only figure in the tale who *isn't* a ghost via a flashback sequence where we see Dam, crossdressed in skirt and wig, trying to seduce a protesting Thua in the motel room. In a fit of homophobic panic, Thua kills Dam, only to have the Gold-Toothed Aunty enter the room and kill Thua, but not before he, in turn, uses his last breath to kill the Gold-Toothed Aunty. The net effect is patently nonsensical and logically inconsistent, but lots of disorienting fun and, with its cavalcade of abject social and sexual marginals – prostitutes, queers, ageing women – it is classic Poj Arnon.

Without doubt, Arnon's penchant for abject social and sexual dissidence finds it fullest expression in the hugely successful Ho Taeo Taek series of queer comic horror films, widely regarded by most commentators, including the director himself, as his signature work (Petvirojchai 2017, p. 20). With a crude play-on-word title that defies translation but equates roughly to 'the dormitory hotel of chaotic sissies', Ho Taeo Taek focusses on a trio of ageing flamboyant *kathoey* – a Thai gender/sexual category of transfemininity – who run a haunted boarding house for young men in provincial Thailand. Launched in 2007, the first *Ho Taeo Taek* (Arnon) proved such a winner at the Thai box office that it generated not only a series of direct sequels – six to date and counting – but an emulative mini-cycle of *kathoey*-themed horror-comedies.[5] Each Ho Taeo Taek film works to a programmatic formula: the *kathoey* protagonists encounter some manner of supernatural haunting, and their efforts to exorcise the malevolent spectres furnish the pretext for 90+ minutes of 'wacky homo-gags, succulent expletives and flippant horror' (Rithdee 2009, p. 1).

The formulaic recursiveness of the series suggests that the pleasure of these films is rooted not so much in story or even meaning, as in ritualised structures of feeling, the intense affective and psychical energies afforded by their sensationalist spectacles of wanton unruliness. It's not without significance that the series is grounded in a hybridised register of horror-comedy: two genre forms known for their ritual repetitions and 'lowbrow' status as what Linda Williams terms 'body genres', so-called because they 'privilege the sensational' and play out reactive effects on the body of the viewer (1991, p. 4).[6] Moreover, both genres are, as we have seen with horror, constitutively invested in spectacles of abjection linked, more often than not, to the body. Whether in terms of their iconography of befouled objects – corpses, ghouls, freaks, blood, excrement – or their comic rhetoric of filth – toilet jokes, sexual innuendo, profanities – the Ho Taeo Taek series revels in the obscene detritus of corporeal, erotic, and social abjection. Refusing injunctions against the monstrous Other, the films bring the occluded spectres of abjection from the margins to the centre, creating a surreal and potentially subversive realm of riotous possibility not unlike a Bakthtinian carnivalesque, 'a world inside out' where 'rank, privileges, norms, and prohibitions' are suspended and hierarchies inverted 'from top to bottom' (Bakhtin 1984, p. 11).[7]

That the Ho Taeo Taek series positions transgendered *kathoey* at the heart of this topsy-turvy derangement accentuates the sexual and, arguably, political dimensions of its destabilising operations. Popularly translated as 'ladyboy', but also known in Thai as 'second kind of woman/*sao braphet song*', *kathoey* is a liminal category with long roots dating back to pre-modern Siamese cosmologies and their ternary systems of gender/sexual organisation (Morris 1994). In recent times, the category has been subject to multiple revisions and modernisations – opening up into 'an array of *kathoey* varieties ... in the domains of sex (hermaphroditism), gender (cross-dressing, transsexualism) and sexuality (homosexuality)' (Jackson 2000, p. 411) – but it is certainly not quit of its interstitial status nor, indeed, of its archaic associations with pre-modern traditions (Käng 2014). Betwixt and between masculinity and femininity, the past and the present, *kathoey* signify a resonant and highly visible register of trans-categorical displacement or what Marjorie Garber calls 'category crisis' (1992, p. 16): 'a failure of definitional distinction, a borderline that becomes permeable, that permits border-crossings from one (apparently distinct) category to another' (ibid.). It is part of the reason *kathoey* figure so prominently in Thai folk cultures as spirit mediums where, as Rosalind Morris argues, 'the *kathoey* becomes the displaced synonym ... for a space (a spacing) through which alterity, and thus death, passes' (2000, p. 134).

The radical capacity of the *kathoey* for border-crossing and liminal displacement is vital to the semiotics of the Ho Taeo Taek series where the *kathoey* protagonists are positioned across multiple, intersecting categories of difference. Apart from the obvious aspect of their sexual intermediacy, *kathoey* function in the films as a literal interface between the living and the dead, the monstrous and the human. They are the ones who confront the haunting entities and who ultimately serve to pacify them at film's end, frequently after more 'conventional' figures of institutional authority – Buddhist monks, Brahmin priests, male shamans, and ghostbusters – have failed. Indeed, one of the *kathoey* protagonists, Pancake, played by beloved comic Kohtee Aramboy, is herself a ghost, killed in the first episode and returned as a spectral force who aids her sisters' engagements with the other side. In keeping with these ghostly dimensions, the *kathoey* characters also denote a blurred temporality, mixing iconographic signifiers – costume, props, settings – from vastly different eras to the point where it becomes impossible to place them and the films historically. Are they in the past, the present, or somewhere in-between?

The *kathoey* of Ho Taeo Taek assume an equally ambivalent social status. Though *kathoey* in Thailand seldom face the kind of violent transphobic ostracism suffered by trans- and genderqueer-identified people in many other societies, they are still subject to stigmatisation in what Peter Jackson calls 'the tolerant yet unaccepting character of Thai discourses about non-normative sexuality and gender' (1999, p. 230). *Kathoey* are figures of ambivalent fascination in contemporary Thai culture and the degree to which they are tolerated is almost always indexed to socially conservative scripts of classed Thainess. The most tolerated, even admired, *kathoey* are those who 'exhibit a high standard of feminine beauty' and 'adopt the reserved, polite manners and speech of a genteel Thai man or woman', Jackson contends, while the most stigmatised *kathoey* are 'those considered loud-mouthed, aggressive or lewd, qualities widely regarded as low-class' (ibid.). No prizes for guessing where the Ho Taeo Taek crew sit on this spectrum. Indeed, a good deal of the films' scandalous comedy arises from the slippage between the protagonists' outward assumption of a demure classed Thai femininity and their sudden eruptive vulgarity of speech and comportment as they curse, shriek, spit, fart, and, in a particularly Thai social taboo, use their feet to humiliate each other and their opponents. Moreover, while their spectacular consumerist style and professional ambitions as small business operators suggest an aspirational bourgeois habitus, there is never any doubt about their precarious subaltern status in the rigid hierarchies of the Thai class system. In the series' third instalment, *Ho Taeo Taek Waek Chi Mi* (Arnon dir. 2011), the women make a 'step up' the social ladder when they are contracted to run the dormitory at an elite boarding school for boys, but in their initial meeting with the college's headmistress – Khun Waeosawat Miruluem, a wildly over-the-top parody of a Thai high-society matron played to camp excess by Apaporn Nakornsawan – they are reminded in no uncertain terms of their subordinate position: 'just remember you are here as dormitory caretakers only, you are *not* teachers!'

These compounded codings of sexual, social, and discursive alterity render the *kathoey* characters of Ho Taeo Taek what might be termed 'revolting subjects' in both senses: as disgusting and obscene but also transgressive and rebellious. They are abjectified figures of disgust but they assume a determinative agency as active subjects, driving the narrative and serving as vehicles of audience identification. Here it is instructive to compare the *kathoey* of Ho Taeo Taek with the long line of other *kathoey*-themed comedies that have emerged in Thai cinema in recent years. Dubbed 'the *kathoey* wave' (Schoonover and Galt 2016, p. 200), these films exploded in the wake of *Satri Lek/Iron Ladies* (2000), Yongyoot Thongkongtoon's hugely successful feel-good underdog sports comedy about a real-life *kathoey* volleyball team from Lampang who battled the odds to become national champions.[8] Notable for a structural centralisation of *kathoey* characters from the discursive periphery of comic relief or paternalistic pity to the limelight of active protagonism, these films have been widely read as restorative nationalist fantasies that work to reimagine 'Thai national identity and its renewed positioning in a global cultural field' (Schoonover and Galt 2016, p. 206). In their emblematic status as social outliers fighting to achieve a place within the national community, the *kathoey* protagonists of these films function as therapeutic agents of national conciliation, bringing the wayward heterogeneity of Thai social and sexual difference into symbolic harmony and restoring order in the dominant cultural narrative of 'Thainess' (*kwam-pen-thai*). As Serhat Ünaldi notes, 'this post-2000 wave of ... Thai *kathoey* movies is progressive to the extent that it grants *kathoeys* [sic] more agency [b]ut this agency is seldom used to challenge underlying power structures, being exercised to become a good member of Thai society' (2011, p. 68).

One would be hard pressed, however, to claim the 'revolting' *kathoey* of Ho Taew Taek as 'good members of Thai society'. Far from it. They are, if anything, social iconoclasts, upending notions of sacralised Thainess and highlighting the cleavages of class, region, gender/sexuality, and ethnicity that, as David Streckfuss notes, have been 'long papered over and held together by incessant calls for unity and a century-old construction of an ossified national identity' (2011, p. 313). Acting in flagrant contravention of middle-class Thai ideals of social and corporeal comportment, speaking loudly and defiantly in the vilified base tongues of *pasa talat* (marketplace Thai) and regional/subcultural dialects, and lampooning the orthodox gatekeepers of hegemonic Thainess (social, religious, and governmental elites), the *kathoey* of Ho Taew Taek are brazen recalcitrants of sociopolitical dissidence, abject 'others' excluded from the dominant narratives of Thai nationhood who, quite simply, refuse to know, let alone stay in, their place.

That this performance of 'revolting Thainess' should occur against the historical backdrop of one of the most violent and sustained periods of social and political instability in Thailand's history – what has been described as 'a slow-burn civil war' between 'hierarchical and egalitarian conceptions of the Thai nation' (Ferrara 2015, p. 264) – lends added import to the spectacle, while at the same time suggesting yet another level of contention in the culture of violent polarisation around the cinema of Poj Arnon. More than one commentator has, in fact, joined these speculative dots. 'The scathing reception that invariably greets Poj's every new film,' writes Kong Rithdee, 'speaks of the gap, or the tension, between old and new, urban and rural, the masses and the rest, perhaps not unlike the messy politics we've found ourselves in' (2009, p. 1). It is instructive, therefore, that the Ministry of Culture, the state agency charged with monitoring and policing 'appropriate' expressions of cultural Thainess, should have made one of its most explicit interventions against a Poj Arnon film during the period of heightened political anxiety that followed the bloody state crackdown on pro-democracy protesters in central Bangkok in mid-2010. Amidst a systemic purge of any and every kind of sociopolitical dissent – which, not incidentally, often took the rhetorical cast of a cleansing of polluting forces (Montesano, Chachavalpongpun and Chongvilaivan 2012, pp. 122–123) – the Ministry of Culture ordered Arnon to change both the title and the poster art of his third instalment in the Ho Taew Taek series, citing unspecified 'threats to national morality' (Wasana 2010, para. 2). Though it amounted to little more than a symbolic gesture of disciplinary control, it evidences the genuine disquiet felt by state hegemons in the face of Arnon's 'revolting *kathoey*'. In the end, the minor changes were made and the film came out to the inevitable bad reviews and just as inevitable strong box office. The obnoxious *kathoey* and other irreverent subalterns that populate the carnivalesque demotic cinema of Poj Arnon might be subject to measures of repression but, like the abject, they are bound to return.

Notes

1 This chapter uses the Royal Thai General System of Transcription (RTGS) to render Thai names unless, as is the case here, a divergent form is already in common use. Unless otherwise noted, all translations from the Thai are the author's.

2 It's also why Arnon's films seldom get an international release as they are all but unintelligible outside domestic Thai frames of reference and sensibility. In a rare non-Thai review of an Arnon film, US critic Peter Nelhaus recounts his bewildered reaction watching, *Ho Taeo Taek /Haunting Me* during a 2007 visit to Bangkok:

> Imagine the stupidest Thai horror-comedy combined with outtakes from *Wigstock*. That pretty much describes *Haunting Me* ... I would have hoped to be even slightly amused. Obviously there is a culture gap as

> I was surrounded by an audience that couldn't stop laughing... The film is my introduction to Poj Arnon, a guy who admittedly knows how to please Thai filmgoers.
>
> (Nelhaus 2007)

3 In one of the few appreciative critical assessments of Arnon's oeuvre, Prepanod Nainapat (2017) argues that a concern with social subalterns or minority groups (*khon klum noi*) is a defining theme of his work, singling out the frequency of queer characters in his films and the young protagonist with Down syndrome in *Oe Rue/Beautiful Wonderful Perfect* (2005): 'The work of Poj [Arnon] opens a space for minorities as people who persevere against difficulties no matter how many times' (para. 16).

4 The practice of mobilising true-life news stories, often grisly and of recent occurrence, as the basis for otherwise fictional films is a common feature of Thai horror that can seem unethical, even exploitative, to the outside observer. In part it is designed to increase a film's topicality and, therefore, marketability – something Poj Arnon does to a notoriously naked degree in many of his films, not just horror – but it also speaks to the distinctive cultural status of horror in the Thai popular imaginary. Belief in the supernatural and spirit world remains an integral, if diversely articulated, aspect of contemporary Thai cosmologies. As such, there isn't the same epistemological division between real/unreal, truth/fiction – or, by extension, the same requirement for suspension of disbelief – that typically frames horror in Western contexts. For a further discussion of these matters, see Ancuta (2016).

5 Notable entries here include: *Koi Thoe Ke/Ghost Station* (Sippapak dir. 2007); *Phi Ta Wan Kap Achan Ta Po/The Ghost and Master Boh* (Pothineth dir. 2008); *Phi Tum Tim* (Narintr dir. 2009); *Nam Phi Mong Sayongkhwan/H2-Oh!* (Cheamcharoenporn dir. 2010); and *Phi Kathoei/Drag Ghost* (Saengsoi dir. 2011).

6 Williams brackets comedy out from her original model, suggesting it lacks the same degree of bodily mimicry between image and spectator that characterises her paradigmatic examples of horror, melodrama, and pornography. Other critics, however, mount a convincing case for including comedy films as a 'body genre', the success of which is directly 'measured by bodily response' and 'the excessive sensation and emotion they produce' (Martin 2006, 190).

7 In an insightful reading of an earlier Arnon *kathoey* film, *Phlon Na Ya / Spicy Beauty Queen of Bangkok* (dir. 2004), Atit Pongpanit (2011) draws parallels to a close corollary of the carnivalesque, the 'theatre of the absurd'. Like the absurd, Pongpanit argues, the films of Poj effect an 'abandonment of the straitjacket of logic, social norms and conventions' and 'a sense of enjoyment which results from this new sense of freedom' (198).

8 Examples here include: *Phrang Chomphu/Saving Private Tootsie* (Liasirikun dir. 2002); *Satri Lek 2/Iron Ladies 2* (Thongkongtoon dir. 2003); *Wai Bum Cheer Krahuem Lok/Cheerleader Queens* (Arnon dir. 2003); and *Beautiful Boxer* (Uekrongtham dir. 2003).

References

23Scenes 2018, 'Movie review: *Toot Too Ku Chat*', *Pantip*, viewed 1 March 2019, www.pantip.com/topic/37724863

Ancuta, K 2016 'The smiling dead; or: on the empirical impossibility of Thai zombies', in D Fischer-Hornung & M Mueller (eds.), *Vampires and zombies: transcultural migrations and transnational interpretations*, University Press of Mississippi, Jackson, pp. 21–42.

Ancuta, K 2017, 'Beyond the vampire: revamping Thai monsters for the urban age', *eTropics: Electronic Journal of Studies in the Tropics*, vol. 16, no. 1, pp. 31–45.

Arnon, P (dir.) 1995, *Sati Taek Sud Khua Lok*, motion picture, Five Star Productions, Bangkok.

Arnon, P (dir.) 2003, *Wai Bum Cheer Krahuem Lok*, motion picture, Five Star Productions, Bangkok.

Arnon, P (dir.) 2004, *Plon Na Ya*, motion picture, Five Star Productions, Bangkok.

Arnon, P (dir.) 2007, *Ho Taeo Taek*, motion picture, Five Star Productions, Bangkok.

Arnon, P (dir.) 2011, *Ho Taeo Taek Waek Chi Mi*, motion picture, Five Star Productions, Bangkok.

Arnon, P, Katenut, C, Sukkhapisit, T, & Vorasingha, M (dir.) 2010 *Tai Hong*, motion picture, Phra Nakorn Film, Bangkok.

Bakhtin, M 1984, *Rabelais and his world*, trans. H Iswolsky, Indiana University Press, Bloomington.

Bourdieu, P 1984, *Distinction: a social critique of the judgement of taste*, Routledge, London.

Cheamcharoenporn, O (2010), *Nam Phi Mong Sayongkhwan*, motion picture, M-Thirtynine Talk, Thailand.

Creed, B 1993, *The monstrous-feminine: film, feminism, psychoanalysis*, Routledge, London.

Dumas, R 2018, *The monstrous-feminine in contemporary Japanese popular culture*, Palgrave Macmillan, Cham.

Eaosriwongs, N 1980, 'Kwamlamluek khong namnao khong nang thai', *Sinlapa Watthanatham*, vol. 1, no. 10, pp. 44–53.

Farmer, B 2015, 'Battling angels and golden orange blossoms: Thai television and/as the popular public sphere', in J Tay & G Turner (eds.), *Television histories in Asia; issues and contexts*, Routledge, London, pp.74–91.

Ferrara, F 2015, *The political development of modern Thailand,* Cambridge University Press, Cambridge.

'Fire in Bangkok nightclub kills scores of New Year's Eve revellers' 2009, *The Guardian*, 1 January, viewed 1 March 2019, www.theguardian.com/world/2009/jan/01/bangkok-nightclub-fire-deaths

Fouquet, G 1989, 'Of genres and savours in Thai film', *Cinemaya*, vol. 6, pp. 4–9.

Fouquet, G 2003, 'Présentation: profondeurs insoupçonnées (et remugles?) des 'eaux croupies' du cinéma thaïlandais', *Aséanie*, vol. 12, pp. 143–156.

Fuhrmann, A 2016, *Ghostly desires: queer sexuality and vernacular Buddhism in contemporary Thai cinema*, Duke University Press, Durham.

Garber, M 1992, *Vested interests: cross-dressing and cultural anxiety*, Penguin, Harmondsworth.

Hamilton, A 1994, 'Cinema and nation: dilemmas of representation in Thailand', in W Dissanayake (ed.), *Colonialism and nationalism in Asian cinema*, Indiana University Press, Bloomington, pp. 141–161.

Harrison, R 2006, 'Amazing Thai film. the rise and rise of Thai cinema on the international screen', *Asian Affairs*, vol. 36, no. 3, pp. 321–338.

Harrison, R 2017, 'Dystopia as liberation: disturbing femininities in contemporary Thailand', *Feminist Review*, vol. 116, no. 1, pp. 64–83.

Herrera, A 2015, 'Thai 16mm cinema: the rise of a popular cinematic culture in Thailand from 1945 to 1970', *Rian Thai: International Journal of Thai Studies*, vol. 8, pp. 27–62.

Ingawanij, MA 2006, 'Un-Thai *Sakon*: the scandal of teen cinema', *South East Asia Research*, vol. 14, no. 2, pp. 147–177.

Jackson, P 1999, 'Tolerant but unaccepting: the myth of a Thai "gay paradise"', in P Jackson & N Cook (eds.), *Genders and sexualities in modern Thailand*, Silkworm Books, Chiang Mai, pp. 226–242.

Jackson, P 2000, 'An explosion of Thai identities: global queering and re-imagining queer theory', *Culture, Health and Sexuality*, vol. 2, no. 4, pp. 405–424.

Käng, D 2014, 'Conceptualizing Thai genderscapes: transformation and continuity in the Thai sex/gender system', in P Liamputtong (ed.), *Contemporary socio-cultural and political perspectives in Thailand*, Springer, Dordrecht, pp. 409–429.

Knee, A 2005, 'Thailand haunted: the power of the past in the contemporary Thai horror film', in S Schneider & T Williams (eds.), *Horror international.* Wayne University Press, Detroit, pp. 141–159.

Kristeva, J 1982, *Powers of horror: an essay on abjection*, trans. L Roudiez, Columbia University Press, New York.

Lee, H 2015, 'Transformations of the monstrous feminine in the new Asian female ghost films', *Diogenes*, vol. 62, no. 1, pp. 100–114.

Lewis, G 2003, 'The Thai movie revival and Thai national identity', *Continuum: Journal of Media and Cultural Studies*, vol. 17, no. 1, pp. 69–78.

Liasirikun, K (dir.) 2002, *Phrang Chomphu*, motion picture, Thailand.

Martin, N 2006, 'Never laugh at a man with his pants down: the affective dynamics of comedy and porn', in P Lehman (ed.), *Pornography: film and culture*, Rutgers University Press, New Brunswick, pp. 189–205.

Montesano, M, Chachavalpongpun, P, & Chongvilaivan, A 2012, *Bangkok May 2010: perspectives on a divided Thailand*, Institute of Southeast Asian Studies, Singapore.

Morris, R 1994, 'Three sexes and four sexualities: redressing the discourses on gender and sexuality in contemporary Thailand', *Positions*, vol. 2, no. 1, pp. 15–43.

Morris, R 2000, *In the place of origins: modernity and its mediums in northern Thailand*, Duke University Press, Durham.

Mulder, N 2000, *Inside Thai society: religion, everyday life, change*, Silkworm Books, Chiang Mai.

Nainapat, P 2017, 'Poj-Universe: Samruat jakkrawan nang kong Poj Arnon', *The Matter*, viewed 1 March 2019, https://thematter.co/rave/to-infinity-and-beyond-in-pot-anon-universe/22769

Narintr, S (dir.) 2009, *Phi Tum Tim*, DVD, Happy Home Entertainment, Thailand.

Nelhaus, P 2007, '"Haunting me": tubby Thai tranny terror', *ScreenAnarchy*, viewed 1 March 2019, https://screenanarchy.com/2007/03/haunting-me-tubby-thai-tranny-terror.html

Ng, A 2014, 'Sisterhood of terror: the monstrous feminine of Southeast Asian horror cinema', in H Benshoff (ed.), *A companion to the horror film*, John Wiley and Sons, Malden, pp. 442–459.

Pajee, P 2017, 'A Man Maligned', *The Nation*. 18 April, p. 12.

Petvirojchai, S 2017, 'Interview Poj Arnon, oops I did it again', *Hollywood Reporter Thailand*, vol. 25, pp. 18–23.

Phongpaichit, P & Baker C 2016, 'Introduction: inequality and oligarchy', in P Phongpaichit & C Baker (eds.), *Unequal Thailand: aspects of income, wealth and power*, NUS Press, Singapore, pp. 1–31.

Pimnam, C 2016. 'Poj Arnon: saep saep woe baeb phloe phloe ko', *Bioscope: South Asian Screen Studies Journal*, vol. 146, pp. 44–55.

Pongpanit, A 2011, The bitter–sweet portrayals of expressing and maintaining 'non-normative' genders and sexualities in Thai mainstream cinema from 1980 to 2010, Doctoral Thesis, University of London SOAS, London.

Pothineth, W (dir.) 2008, *Phi Ta Wan Kap Achan Ta Po*, motion picture, Pranakorn Films, Thailand.

Rithdee, K 2009, 'Populist and proud of it', *Bangkok Post*, 13 November, Real Time Section: p. 1.

Rithdee, K 2012, 'Poj Arnon and love during the flood', *Bangkok Post*, 5 March, Real Time Section: p. 4.

Saengsoi, K (dir.) 2011, *Phi Kathoei*, motion picture, Thailand.

Schoonover, K & Galt, R 2016, *Queer cinema in the world*, Duke University Press, Durham.

Sippapak, Y (dir.) 2007, *Koi Thoe Ke*, motion picture, Sahamongkol Film International, Bangkok.

Streckfuss, D 2011, *Truth on trial in Thailand: defamation, treason, and lèse-majesté*, Routledge, London and New York.

Thongkongtoon, Y (dir.) 2000, *Satri Lek*, motion picture, Tai Entertainment, Bangkok.

Thongkongtoon, Y (dir.) 2003, *Satri Lek 2*, motion picture, Tai Entertainment, Bangkok.

Uekrongtham, E (dir.) 2003, *Beautiful Boxer*, motion picture, GMM Pictures, Bangkok.

Ünaldi, S 2011, 'Back in the spotlight: the cinematic regime of representation of *kathoeys* and gay men in Thailand', in P Jackson (ed.), *Queer Bangkok: 21st century markets, media, and rights*, Hong Kong University Press, Hong Kong, pp. 59–80.

Vorng, S 2017, *A meeting of masks: status, power and hierarchy in Bangkok*, NIAS Press, Copenhagen.

Wasana 2010, 'Poj talaeng yuen yan tam wa "chi mi" mai tam pasa wibat', *MovieMThai.com*, viewed 1 March 2019, https://movie.mthai.com/movie-news/81836.html

Williams, L 1991, 'Film bodies: gender, genre and excess', *Film Quarterly*, vol. 44, no. 4, pp. 2–13.

Winston, C 2016, 'Poj lines up another romp for his monks of mirth', *The Nation*, 17 March, p. 7.

Wise Kwai 2014. 'Review: Mor 6/5 Pak Ma Tha Mae Nak', *Wise Kwai's Thai Film Journal*, web log post, May 11, viewed 1 March 2019, http://thaifilmjournal.blogspot.com/2014/05/review-mor-65-pak-ma-tha-mae-nak.html

12 The Monstrous-Feminine in the Millennial Japanese Horror Film

Problematic M(O)thers and Their Monstrous Children in *Ringu*, *Honogurai mizo no soko kara* and, *Ju-On*

Valerie Wee

> All human societies have a conception of the monstrous-feminine, of what it is about woman that is shocking, terrifying, horrific, abject.
>
> Barbara Creed, The Monstrous Feminine, 1.

The alignment of horror with the feminine has long prompted the assertion that horror texts reveal patriarchy's enduring fear of the female, a claim insightfully explored by Barbara Creed in her seminal book, *The Monstrous-Feminine*. Published in 1993, Creed examined American and British horror cinema's obsession with representations depicting the female propensity for terrifying deviance, violence, and destruction. As Creed argues, women and the feminine exist in horror films as persistent and disturbing threats to society's dominant patriarchal structures, values, and beliefs. In marking the 25th anniversary of Creed's influential study of the monstrous-feminine in Western horror film, this chapter extends Creed's observations beyond Western cinema and examines their relevance to Japanese horror films with a particular focus on the millennial J-Horror tradition that rose to prominence with the release of *Ringu* (Nakata dir. 1998), *Honogurai Mizu no Soko Kara* (Nakata dir. 2002, henceforth *Honogurai Mizu*), and *Ju-on: The Grudge* (Shimizu dir. 2002, henceforth *Ju-on*). These three films, which revolve around ambiguous maternal figures and their monstrous children, drew global attention to Japanese cinematic horror.

In examining the horror film, Creed focussed on the genre's mediation of the abject and abjection, highlighting three prevailing tendencies: (1) the genre's propensity for images of abjection; (2) the notion of the border as a means of identifying the abject; and (3) horror film's overreliance on abjecting the maternal figure (1993, pp. 10–11). Unsurprisingly, these three elements dominate millennial J-horror.

Japanese horror films have a long history of addressing the concerns and anxieties resulting from social and cultural changes within the nation, in particular, shifts that have undermined or destabilised traditional gender roles and identities (Balmain 2008; Wee 2014). The millennial J-horror films examined here express fears rooted in social changes that were undermining long-held patriarchal values and behaviours in modern Japan. The horror in *Ringu*, *Honogurai Mizu*, and *Ju-On* is explicitly aligned with maternal actions and (ir)responsibilities that reference larger socio-cultural shifts in gender behaviour, reflecting the growing gender tensions in contemporary Japan.

This study begins with a brief historical overview of the *onryō*, a vengeful female ghost, as a figure of the uncanny, the abject, and the monstrous, before advancing to consider Japan's socio-cultural and political environment at the end of the twentieth Century. These discussions provide the backdrop against which I then interrogate millennial J-horror's representations of femininity and the female through the lens of Barbara Creed's psychoanalytic framework of the monstrous feminine. Notably, while Creed offers significant insights into cinematic female monsters such as the archaic mother, the castrating mother, the possessed monster, the vampire, and the witch, she does not engage with the figure of the female ghost. By examining J-horror's representations and revisions of the traditional *onryō*, I hope to add to the existing discussions of female monstrosity, while also considering how the complexity and ambiguity of these films' treatments of the female, the maternal and the (m)Other align with the anxieties that dominated Japan in the millennial era.

Japanese *Kaidan*: A Brief Historical Overview of the *Onryō*

Kaidan are supernatural myths and folktales that date back to the Edo period (1603–1867). These stories typically feature monsters, demons, and ghosts (Hearn 1971). A sub-category of these pre-modern *kaidan* focusses on women who are betrayed and murdered by their husbands and/or samurai masters. The dead women then return as terrifying *onryō* to wreak vengeance on their murderers, and in some instances, on the society that allowed their mistreatment.[1]

In *Tokaido Yotsuya Kaidan/Ghost Story of Yotsuya*, Iemon, a samurai, poisons his devoted wife, Oiwa, so that he can marry another woman of higher status. Oiwa's ghost returns to haunt her faithless husband, causing him to murder various people, including his new wife and father-in-law. Oiwa's ghost is appeased only after Iemon is killed. In *Kaidan Bancho Sarayashiki/The Story of Okiku*, a maid, Okiku, is murdered by Tessan Aoyama, her samurai master, who throws her body down a well. Okiku's ghost haunts Aoyama, finally driving him mad. Another Japanese fable, *Kuroneko/The Black Cat* features a woman and her daughter-in-law who are robbed, raped, and murdered by samurai. The women then return as vengeful demon cats that kill any samurai they encounter.[2]

In *The Monstrous-Feminine*, Creed examines the 'woman as monster', aligning the monstrous-feminine with the abject. Creed builds on Julia Kristeva's assertion that the abject is that which ignores 'borders, positions, rules', and 'disturbs identity, system, order' with impunity (Kristeva 1982, p. 4). *Onryō* clearly epitomise the abject; they terrify and destabilise because they transcend the boundary between life and death, between human and demon/monster. *Onryō* are also free from patriarchally imposed limits on female power, agency and independence, and are allowed to exact their terrifying vengeance on the men who betrayed them.

Japanese horror cinema's depictions of the traditional *onryō* conform to Creed's assertion that 'the horror film abounds in images of abjection, foremost of which is the corpse, whole and mutilated, followed by an array of bodily waste such as blood, vomit, saliva, sweat, tears, and putrefying flesh' (1993, p. 10). Nabuo Nakagawa's 1959 cinematic version of *Tokaido Yotsuya Kaidan* offers lurid images of the poisoned Oiwa's putrid, disfigured face. And after Oiwa's death, her corpse, which was unceremoniously thrown into a river to rot, is later seen surfacing in a mucilaginous pool of blood-red gore. *Kuroneko*'s raped and murdered mother, Yone, and her daughter-in-law, Shigei, are abject in their ability to transform between human and demon cat form, an ability that clearly disrupts natural order. Kaneto Shindo's 1968 film version included close-up shots of the women in human form, but in stylised kabuki-like make-up that represented their feline Otherness, lapping up milk from bowls. Yone and Shigei clearly embody 'were-creatures, whose bodies signify a collapse of the boundaries between human and animal' (Creed 1993, p. 10).

These *kaidan* reveal the underlying values and dominant ideologies that historically organised the Japanese worldview. In Japan, social harmony and stability was (and remains) of crucial importance, and these beliefs were grounded in Confucian teachings that stressed idealised notions of order, and personal and social responsibility. As Yoko Sugihara notes, 'the Confucian ethical system emphasizes a harmonious society in which a hierarchical structure is maintained … which assumes … men's dominance over women and children' (2002). For the Japanese, this highly patriarchal view was not historically deemed oppressive. Rather, the view was that 'there were certain benefits for women under this system. In theory at least, the extreme dependence of women upon their menfolk meant that *the [men] had the obligation to ensure [women's] well-being and protection*' (Kanematsu 1993, p. 58; emphasis mine). These *kaidan*, therefore, explored the consequences when men cast-off their responsibilities and murdered the women they were obligated to protect, causing these women to return as *onryō*.

One might be inclined to see the *onryō* as a terrifying and destructive supernatural female force threatening patriarchy and masculinity. Yet a careful examination of these folktales reveals the opposite. While the appearance of an *onryō* was indication that individual men had betrayed their patriarchal duties, it is vital to recognise that the validity of the patriarchal system itself is never in fact questioned in traditional *kaidan*. Rather, the *onryō* served a crucial function in destroying the flawed individuals threatening the security of the patriarchal structure so that traditional social order could be re-established. While clearly terrifying and malevolent, the *onryō* should in fact be viewed as serving a crucial role in punishing and destroying those masculine elements within society who had abandoned their prescribed duties, and in doing so, ultimately threatened the order, stability, and harmony so prized in Japanese society.[3] Such an interpretation aligned with Confucian teachings that state: 'if a ruler, a subject, a father...do [sic] not fulfill their duties, they abuse their titles...this is the beginning of the collapse of ritual/propriety..., and is one of the causes [of] social disorder and political chaos' (Yao 2000, p. 35). In such situations, Confucian teaching prescribes that it is in fact necessary for subordinates to rise up against these irresponsible figures of authority, as only then can order and balance be reestablished.

This perspective is clearly dramatised in the historical *onryō*-centred *kaidan*, which adhered to a typical pattern. While alive, the women represent the idealised Japanese female – Oiwa, Okiku, Yone, and Shigei are innocent, submissive, and obedient; they defer to dominant patriarchal power and are explicitly depicted as content with their subordinate and domestic positions in life. It is only *after* they have been betrayed and murdered that they return as terrifying, destructive, beings. No longer human and no longer admired, they are feared for possessing the supernatural power to destroy men. As Samuel Leiter notes of the traditional *kaidan* narrative,

> one of the chief ways in which women who have been trampled on become empowered is to turn into vengeful spirits after they have died. The entire world of selfish, unfaithful husbands and lovers must take cover when one of these women comes back from the other world to seek revenge on those who have wronged her.
>
> (2002, p. 225)

Onryō, therefore, embody the two distinct female tropes that Creed identified within the horror film; they are initially 'woman as victims of the (mainly male) monster', before becoming 'woman-as-monster' (Creed 1993, p. 1). Once these women have effected their vengeance and their anger has been appeased by the destruction of the men who betrayed them, however, these monstrous females then return to their supernatural realms, leaving the larger patriarchal society reinstated and intact. As Creed notes, 'the horror film attempts to bring about a confrontation with the abject (the corpse, bodily wastes, the monstrous-feminine) in order finally to eject the abject and redraw the boundaries between the human and the non-human' (Creed 1993, p. 14).

Thus, while these classic *kaidan*'s depictions of the empowered female as a destructive, terrifying, and vengeful wraith play into a typical patriarchally inflected fear of the feminine – as Fumiko Enchi observes, 'Just as there is an archetype of woman as the object of man's eternal love, so there must be an archetype of her as the object of his eternal fear, representing, perhaps, the shadow of his own evil actions' (1983, p. 57) – the figure of the *onryō* in fact exists to reinforce Japan's patriarchal structures, in so far as she serves to warn men against neglecting their duties or betraying their roles. Should this warning not be heeded, her actions ensure the reinstatement of the proper hierarchical patriarchal system.

The vengeful *onryō* reemerges as a critical figure in millennial J-horror. *Ringu*, *Honogurai Mizu*, and *Ju-on* all feature memorable versions of betrayed females who return as terrifying female ghosts intent on haunting the living.

Millennial J-Horror: *Ringu*, *Honogurai mizu*, and *Ju-On*

In *Ringu*, Reiko, a divorced single mother, works as a reporter. While investigating several mysterious deaths linked to a videotape, Reiko and her son, Yoichi, inadvertently become the tape's next victims. She and her ex-husband, Ryuji, try to uncover the tape's origins in the hope of saving both mother and son. Their investigation reveals that the tape is haunted by a young girl, Sadako, who was brutally murdered by her father. Seven days after the tape is viewed, Sadako's terrifying form appears to claim the viewer's life.

The theme of a hapless mother trying to protect her child from a malevolent pre-teen wraith also shapes the plot of *Honogurai Mizu*, in which another divorced single mother, Yoshimi Matsubara, is trying to raise her daughter, Ikuko, in a small urban tenement. Psychologically fragile and struggling to cope with her job, Yoshimi inadvertently neglects Ikuko, who gradually comes under the sway of another child whose presence she senses around the apartment building. After a series of mysterious and creepy events, it is revealed that this child, Mitsuko, had been neglected and ignored by her own parents. Left to fend for herself, she drowned after falling into the building's roof-top water tank. Mitsuko's ghost is determined to find another mother to give her the attention she craves, and she chooses Yoshimi as her intended surrogate.

Ju-On, like *Ringu* and *Honogurai Mizu*, revolve around a failed marriage and familial betrayal. The film opens with a violent murder that includes jarring shots of torn family photographs, a man's bloody hands, and a close-up of a woman's dead face. This act of violence against the female taints the house in which this murder occurs so that the site is cursed by malevolent forces. Those who enter the haunted house meet various disturbing ends after encountering the ghosts of the murdered woman, Kayako, and her son, Toshio.

As these brief plot synopses show, the *onryō* is a crucial figure in millennial J-horror. Like their pre-modern *onryō* sisters, Sadako,

Mitsuko, and Kayako are female victims betrayed and destroyed by the patriarchal systems they inhabited, and in the case of Sadako and Kayako, by specific patriarchs. However, these millennial J-horror films have revised the *onryō* in ways that reference the dominant anxieties of the modern age, reflecting the specific challenges that were plaguing Japanese society at the time.

Patriarchal Anxieties in the New Millennium

Ringu, *Honogurai Mizu*, and *Ju-On* reveal a growing patriarchal anxiety that is best understood against the backdrop of gender-rooted conflicts which arose in the final decade of the twentieth century, developments that have steadily undermined the conventional gender roles and relationships that once formed the stable foundations of traditional Japanese life.

Ever since the *Meiji* and *Taisho* periods (1868–1926), two feminine ideals have dominated Japanese culture: the idea of *bosei honno,* which defined motherhood and child rearing as an innate and immutable female inclination, and the ideal of *ryosai kenbo*, essentially the paradigm of the 'good wife, wise mother'. As McKinlay observes,

> In Japanese society, the notion of motherhood has traditionally served as a powerful and pervasive symbolic function which transcends the pragmatic aspects of the role. To become a mother is not simply to give birth, but to achieve *ichininmae*, to become a real woman.
>
> (2011, para. 1)

This view persists even in the twenty-first century, for 'as recently as 2000 ... Japanese women are still assessed on their motherhood roles, and most particularly their skills in nurturing and educating children, regardless of other roles they may have – such as participants in the paid workforce' (McKinlay 2011, para. 4). Well into the 1990s, even after the passage of the Equal Employment Opportunity Law in 1986, discrimination continued to be informally practised both institutionally and in the workplace, where women were largely relegated to lowly clerical positions, which they were promptly expected to leave when they married (Morley 1999, pp. 72–73, p. 78). Much of modern Japanese culture and society remains committed to traditional hierarchies in which the male/masculine remain superior to the female/feminine, where the female submits to the male, and where the public constituted the 'male' domain while the 'feminine' is relegated to the domestic.

By the late 1990s, however, Japan was beginning to witness a growing number of young women rejecting conservative values, roles, and behaviours that previously circumscribed female potential and contained the perceived 'hazards' posed by female independence and agency. A growing number of media reports detailed the emergence of a generation of sexually liberated young women who deliberately abandoned traditional notions of the chaste and submissive Japanese female and instead actively pursued sexual independence and (potentially controversial forms of) empowerment. These included 'wealthy and leisured young Japanese women who travel[led] to exotic locales to pursue... sexual liaisons' with foreign men (Kelsky 1996, p. 173) and Japanese schoolgirls (particularly *kogyaru*) who engaged in *enjo kosai* ('subsidized companionship'), an activity that evoked notions of teenage prostitution wherein young girls received an allowance or gifts to 'date' (and have sex with) adult men (Leheny 2006, p. 16; Miller 2004, p. 239). Japanese women were also rejecting traditional notions of marriage that emphasised submissiveness and domesticity, instead embracing (Western) notions of romantic love, greater personal and professional freedom, and demanding a more equitable division of labour – expectations that were motivating women to delay marriage until they could find husbands who shared these attitudes (Tipton 2002, p. 230).

Far from endorsing or celebrating the apparent advances that Japanese women were experiencing in the period, contemporary Japanese films largely offered conservative critiques of how female empowerment and independence were dangerous and destructive to both tradition and patriarchy. In 1996, Susan Napier observed that 'women seem to have become increasingly other, unreachable, even demonic' in contemporary Japanese cinema and fantasy literature (1996, p. 56). In the final years of the twentieth century, contemporary Japanese horror films resurrected the figure of the vengeful *onryō*, reimagining her in ways that reflected contemporary socio-cultural anxieties.

The following examination of these millennial versions of the monstrous-feminine further builds on Creed's framework of horror and the abject to better understand the underlying anxieties that shaped the modern versions of the J-horror *onryō*. As I will show, the *onryō* has been reinterpreted in new and interesting ways.

J-Horror: The *Onryō*, Abjection, and the Border

According to Creed, the abject 'threatens life, [and] must be radically excluded from the place of the living subject, propelled away from the body and deposited on the other side of an imaginary border which separates the self from that which threatens the self' (Creed 1993, p. 65). Encapsulated in this assertion are the notions of abjection as a threat, the crucial need to establish the border between what is 'us' and the abject 'not-us'/dangerous to us, and the importance of reinstating and maintaining that clear distinction. The treatment of the *onryō* in traditional *kaidan* largely adhered to this.

J-horror's modern depictions of the abject *onryō* borrow from established *kaidan* traditions in many ways. Like their predecessors, Sadako, Mitsuko, and Kayako are dead females who refuse to respect the border between life and death, who escape their graves and return to haunt and threaten the living. All three make their appearances in sequences characterised by notable moments of horror, where feminine abjection and monstrosity are deliberately associated with corruption, bodily deformities, and putrefaction.

In *Ringu,* our first sight of the dead Sadako centres on her decaying corpse, which, like her predecessor Okiku, had been left to rot in a well. In attempting to appease Sadako's vengeful spirit, Reiko descends into the watery pit to reclaim Sadako's body for proper burial. The scene is rooted in the abject. There is a terrifying instance in which Sadako's rotting corpse appears to be attacking Reiko as the former flails around in the water, before she gains her balance and is seen cradling Sadako's body. Where water is traditionally associated with cleanliness, purity, and by extension, life, the scene instead associates the well water with putrefaction, contamination, and death.

These instances of Sadako's abjection are intensified only a few scenes later. Having retrieved Sadako's body, Reiko and Ryuji, Reiko's ex-husband, assume that all is well, effectively setting up perhaps the singularly most infamous sequence in *Ringu* in which Ryuji returns home to notice that his television has switched itself on. As he watches, the contorted figure of the dead Sadako is seen crawling out of the well towards the television screen and then out of the screen into the physical realm. Sadako's emergence from the television is coded for terror – she is visually disturbing, possessing the long, dank hair, and swollen, deformed face historically associated with the classic depictions of *onryō* found in Japanese woodcut prints, cinema, and on television. Furthermore, the sight of Sadako emerging from the two-dimensional screen image and taking malevolent three-dimensional form is terrifying in its incoherence. It is essentially the moment of abjection where meaning collapses, for Sadako's appearance effectively overturns the rules of reality and dismantles established natural order as it foregrounds her uncanny ability to cross the suddenly permeable border/boundary between the natural and supernatural world, between the television image/screen and the physical world, between image and materiality, between death and the living. On her destructive and malevolent quest for vengeance, Sadako shows that she is the abject that is not constrained by any limits or boundaries.

While the horror and abjection that Sadako represents echoes that of her *onryō* predecessors, unlike the traditional *onryō*, Sadako's monstrosity is further heightened by the fact that she prevails despite Reiko's many efforts to assuage the former's anger. Despite Reiko's success in solving the mystery of Sadako's death and seeking out her body for proper ritual burial, Sadako's anger remains unassuaged, indicating that the traditional rules of the *kaidan* no longer hold; this *onryō* will not return to her side of the border, she will not be repudiated, appeased, or contained. Reiko's quest to save her son, to reinstate a safe world for patriarchy, fails. As the film concludes on Reiko's phone call to her father to ask him to sacrifice himself to Sadako to save Yoichi, it becomes apparent that Sadako's threat against patriarchy endures. Unlike her predecessors, therefore, Sadako refuses to be 'ejected'; she thwarts any attempts to 'redraw the boundaries between human and non-human' (Creed 1993, p. 14).

Honogurai Mizu similarly equates horror with the abject and the feminine. In the film's climactic sequence, after Yoshimi has a vision that reveals the circumstances of Mitsuko's death – the child's accidental drowning in the apartment's roof-top water tank – the water tank begins to bulge, gushing out water. There is a cross-cut to Ikuko drawing a bath in their apartment. As the bathtub begins to fill with filthy water, Ikuko tries to turn off the taps only to be attacked by a pair of rotting arms bursting out of the water, a shot that echoes Sadako's corpse in the well, and the classic horror images of Oiwa and Okiku rotting in their watery graves. Like her predecessors, Mitsuko's rotting body clearly evokes notions of impurity and decay, marking her as the abject.

This scene culminates in one of the film's most powerfully disturbing moments. Rushing back to their apartment to save Ikuko as the walls and corridors are drenched in water, Yoshimi sees an unconscious child in the bathroom, picks her up, and rushes into the elevator, only to see Ikuko stagger out into the hallway unharmed. Yoshimi realises that the child she is holding is the corporeal form of Mitsuko, who clasps Yoshimi's neck while calling her mother. At that point of realisation, the lift doors close on Yoshimi. When the doors re-open, the lift is empty.

The terror and incoherence of this sequence lies in the disintegration of the vital boundary that distinguishes the living Ikuko from the dead Mitsuko, the difference between Yoshimi's innocent daughter and a malevolent supernatural ghost. In this scene, the human Self and the monstrous Other are indistinguishable. When the difference cannot be seen, there is no means to identify, avoid, or escape from the dangerous abject.

While Mitsuko and Yoshimi's disappearance might appear to signal the reestablishment of the vital border that separates the subject from the abject, the safe from the dangerous, the living from the dead, this moment of relief is short-lived. In the film's final coda, a teenage Ikuko returns to the old, abandoned tenement years later. Yet she finds the apartment where she and her mother used to live, clean and seemingly still occupied by her mother. When Ikuko asks if she can stay with her mother, a brief glimpse of Mitsuko is seen in the shot, standing behind Ikuko, even as Yoshimi denies Ikuko's request. Ikuko, sensing Mitsuko's presence, turns to look behind her, but sees nothing. As Ikuko turns back to her mother, she finds herself alone in the apartment. While *Honogurai Mizu* concludes with Ikuko exiting the apartment, leaving her mother's ghost with Mitsuko, the final shot also suggests that the supernatural remains at large in the physical world. Clearly, Mistuko and the dead Yoshimi continue to haunt the old apartment building. They have not been banished or confined to the other side of the border, separate from the living; the boundary between the natural and supernatural realms remains porous.

Although *Ringu* and *Honogurai Mizu*'s treatment of Sadako and Mitsuko clearly reference elements of earlier *onryō*, they deviate from tradition in one notable aspect – their youth. Unlike Oiwa, Okiku, Yone, and Shige, who are adult women, Sadako and Mitsuko are younger pre-teen girls.

The emergence of the young (often adolescent) female ghost hints at Japanese society's growing anxieties regarding the young Japanese female, culturally labelled *shojo*. The term – literally meaning 'little female' – traditionally refers to a girl aged 7–18, who is 'socially unanchored, free of responsibility and self-absorbed – the opposite of the ideal Japanese adult' (Orbaugh 2003, pp. 258–259). Originating in the *Meiji* period, *shojo* were initially depicted as 'innocent girls who were sedate, smiling, and unassuming' (Ogi 2001, p. 172). However, the term *shojo* took on more problematic and negative inflections in the 1990s, when it evolved from describing young girls engaging in innocent, unrestrained consumption, and self-involved enjoyment, and took on connotations of selfish personal indulgence, an apparent thoughtless disregard for others, and a rejection of established social mores. As Tomoko Aoyama notes, contemporary Japanese society tends to view *shojo* as 'free and arrogant' (2005, p. 53). According to Fran Lloyd, rising economic independence and sexual freedom resulted in changing perceptions of Japanese teenage girls: 'presented by the media as bodies to be consumed, they were also seen as consuming bodies who congregated in Tokyo's fashionable shopping centers awaiting opportunities to acquire the latest luxury goods' (2001, p. 78). By the 1990s, the term had 'become a shorthand for a certain kind of liminal identity' (Napier 2001, p. 118); *shojo* were viewed as existing on the boundary between adulthood and childhood, power and powerlessness, awareness and innocence. This liminality echoes the abject's refusal to respect borders. *Ringu* and *Honogurai Mizu* appear to foreground this alignment between the *shojo*'s 'in-between' status and her propensity for abjection.

This evolving perception of the *shojo* also coincided with the advent of other negatively inflected (stereo-)types of female adolescence. The *kogyaru* (or *kogal*) emerged as another problematic young female figure. The *kogyaru* is commonly viewed as 'impertinent, vulgar or indecent, egocentric, lacking manners, absurd or lacking in common sense' (Miller 2004, p. 238) in media depictions and public perceptions; she is often deemed transgressive, decadent, self-indulgent, hedonistic, materialistic and prone to excessive consumption (Miller 2004, p. 241). As Balmain notes, 'in a similar manner to the moral panics that accompanied other sub-cultural movements ... the Japanese and foreign media in the 1990s constructed the *kogal* lifestyle and language in terms of deviant behavior' (2008, p. 123). Both the *shojo* and the *kogyaru* are associated with notions of (negative) independence, freedom, self-absorption and selfishness; they are deemed adolescent females who feel entitled to consume and destroy heedlessly.

Ringu and *Honogurai Mizu* offer exaggerated representations of the demanding, greedy, increasingly deviant attitudes associated with the *shojo* and *kogyaru* in their depictions of Sadako and Mitsuko, reflecting contemporary Japanese horror's growing tendency to locate the terrifying, disruptive, supernatural forces within the figures of young girls.[4] Unlike their processors, all of whom were either defeated or withdrew from the physical realm after attaining their revenge, Sadako and Mitsuko resist exorcism or appeasement. As mentioned earlier, Sadako's threat endures even after her body was reclaimed and ritually buried, and Mitsuko continues to hold Yoshimi hostage to her demand for maternal attention. Their insatiable desires, their insidious haunting of their victims, and the impossibility of containing their threat and abjection all hint at contemporary Japanese society's growing fears regarding the rise of a new generation of females increasingly outside patriarchal control and containment. J-horror therefore continues the genre's enduring practice of associating horror and monstrosity with the feminine, while also extending patriarchal fear of the feminine onto the figure of the female adolescent.

Ringu and *Honogurai Mizu*'s treatment of the *onryō* figure further deviates from tradition by emphasising Sadako's and Mitsuko's ambiguity. Where Oiwa, Okiku, Yone, and Shige all begin as victims and transform into monstrous villains upon their betrayals and murders, Sadako and Mitsuko are *simultaneously* victims and monstrous villains. This is particularly clear with Sadako, whose monstrous ability to kill people at will even as a living child is made apparent long before she is murdered by her father. While little is known about Mitsuko while she was alive, her demand for maternal attention as 'payment' for her unfortunate accidental drowning, alongside her continued malevolence towards Ikuko even years after Yoshimi's death, casts her as both victim and irrational monster. In both cases, these *onryō* are inherently ambiguous and abject because they inhabit a space where the border between villain and victim cannot be established.

Contemporary J-horror's increasing ambivalence towards the *onryō* is also found in *Ju-On*, where the ghosts of a wife, Kayako, and her young son, Toshio, haunt the home in which they were murdered. *Ju-On*'s cycle of supernatural violence begins with (what we later learn is) Kayako's brutal murder[5]; the film's ambiguous monstrous-feminine, she is another female who is both victim and (possible) villain.

Kayako and her son Toshio bear the visual markers of the supernatural and abject; there are numerous shots of both mother and son looking unnaturally pale with blue lips and vacant eyes. Kayako possesses the long, lank black hair that characterises the *onryō*. In one horrific scene, Kayako's deformed, broken body creeps down the stairs towards Rika, a young woman who has entered the haunted house. In her appearances, Kayako is marked as abject Other, monstrous, and threatening. Like Sadako and Mitsuko, Kayako references her historical predecessors. She is the *onryō* of a murdered wife, haunting a cursed family home. Her encounters with the living are terrifying and lethal.

While Kayako is easily placed within the *onryō* tradition, however, like Sadako and Mitsuko, Kayako's abject Otherness is tinged with the ambiguous and irresolvable. Throughout *Ju-On*, Kayako's motivations, intentions, and actual actions are intentionally left unclear and incoherent, for while she appears to be implicated in the demise of several people who have come in contact with the haunted home, the film deliberately obscures her actual role in their deaths. In one disturbing sequence, we see an unidentifiable dark shadow menacing a guard sent to investigate some mysterious noises coming from a restroom. Later investigations of the security tapes show the guard being consumed by the dark shadow while Kayako stands apart, gazing directly into the camera. Later, when Kayako is seen creeping up on and grabbing hold of Hitomi, whose brother Katsuya had moved into the haunted house, the scene that immediately follows simply shows that both Kayako and Hitomi have disappeared. In these various instances, Kayako is implicated in the supernatural events, but it is deliberately left unclear if Kayako is controlling the shadow that kills the guard, if she is a passive supernatural witness to the guard's demise, or if she in fact kills Hitomi. This ambiguity is reinforced in a later sequence in which Kayako approaches but does not harm Rika, moments before Rika is attacked and murdered by Takeo, Kayako's husband and murderer. Thus, while Kayako is clearly haunting the various victims in *Ju-On*, she remains a largely mysterious and ambiguous force, as she is never seen actually killing the victims.

In fact, *Ju-On* utilises heightened ambiguity and incoherence to intensify horror and anxiety. The film deliberately dispenses with a clear, linear narrative, and instead presents the events in the film in fragmented, disordered vignettes with obscure causal or temporal connections. This sense of disorder and instability, anathema to a culture that reveres order and harmony, is reinforced by several scenes of feminine abjection that are deliberately constructed to confound and confuse. In one scene, when Rika is in the haunted house, she looks in a mirror only to see an image of Kayako trying to break out of her (Rika's) body. Rika raises her hands to cover her eyes in horror, only to see what appears to be Kayako's hands covering her eyes. The moment is grounded in a loss of bodily integrity and ambiguous identity, provoking deep anxiety and uncertainty for it dissolves any reliable boundary between Self and Other, raising the idea that just as it is impossible to distinguish Rika from Kayako, it is impossible to distinguish villain from victim. In fact, it is not even possible to conclusively identify Kayako as the villain. Notably, *Ju-On* refuses to offer any explicit explanation for Kayako's murder, further reinforcing her ambiguity.[6] *Ju-On* intensifies the fear that Woman and the feminine are essentially unfixable, indeterminate, and unknowable.

Ringu, *Honogurai Mizu*, and *Ju-On* depict the harrowing consequences that ensue when traditional values and behaviours are abandoned evoking a heightened state of anxiety – one reflective of the fear, insecurity and increasing paranoia experienced by Japanese patriarchy, which was witnessing its previously unassailable power and authoritative position being steadily undermined by a growing generation of youth and, in particular, young women, who actively reject the established norms of conservative tradition.

J-Horror, Abjection, and the Maternal

Yet even as millennial J-horror introduced a new type of monstrous femininity, it nonetheless continued to adhere to the popular horror tradition of demonising the maternal, for *Ringu*, *Honogurai Mizu*, and *Ju-On*, with their emphasis on divorced, irresponsible, and/or ineffectual mothers, offer largely negative depictions of adult femininity that explicitly deviate from the traditional Japanese ideals of *bosei honno* and *ryosai kenbo*.[7]

In *Ringu*, Shizuko, Sadako's psychic mother, appears only briefly. Asked to participate in a press event to demonstrate her psychic gift, Shizuko is denounced as a fraud despite offering proof of her abilities. Conforming to the idealised notion of the submissive and docile Japanese female, Shizuko remains silent and endures the taunts of the press. Moments later, when a male journalist falls down dead with a terrified expression on his face, a horrified Shizuko exclaims, 'Sadako, you did that!', publicly condemning her daughter who was presumably acting in defence of her mother. Shizuko's behaviour in this brief scene positions her as a woman who has fully entered into a patriarchally organised symbolic order serving the law (and the interests) of the father.

This view of Shizuko is, however, undermined by later revelations. While investigating Sadako's past, Reiko visits a village where Shizuko once lived. An old man who remembers Shizuko suggests that Sadako's father 'wasn't human', mentioning that Shizuko spent long hours by the sea, and commenting that Shizuko conceived Sadako with a sea demon. While the film does not overtly confirm this claim in any way, this revelation effectively aligns Shizuko with the abject, introducing the implication that like her daughter, Shizuko also scorned the boundary between human and non-human, between the land and the sea, between the natural and the supernatural. This one revelation further suggests that far from being the chaste female and submissive wife, Shizuko herself flouted patriarchal and natural laws, and in doing so, brought the monstrous Sadako into existence. These narrative developments hint at the heightened masculine anxieties structuring the film's narrative, aligning J-horror's concerns with those that Creed already identified in Western horror films: 'popular images ... which represent woman as monstrous also define her primarily in relation to her sexuality, specifically the abject nature of her maternal and reproductive functions' (1993, p. 151). As Creed notes, such representations 'reinforce the phallocentric notion that female sexuality is abject', while also '[challenging] the view that femininity ... constitutes passivity'; rather, the opposite is true, woman terrifies because she is castrating (ibid.). In possibly conceiving a child with a demon (which might explain Sadako's powers), Shizuko served as the conduit by which a supernatural threat is born, a threat that refuses to recognise male patriarchal power, and who kills at will. These revelations clearly align both mother and daughter with terrifying acts of deviance and associate them with a destructive supernatural feminine power.

Ringu's ambivalence towards mothers extends to Reiko, *Ringu*'s heroine, who is also presented as a woman who rejects Japan's dominant patriarchal structures and ideologies. Reiko is a divorced mother pursuing a career as a journalist, two qualities that distinguish her from the idealised, domestically confined, traditional Japanese woman. Notably, the film also explicitly links Reiko to dangerous and destructive supernatural forces. Reiko's journalistic curiosity drives her to investigate reports of fatalities linked to a mysterious videotape. She is the one who seeks out, finds, and brings the malevolent tape into her own home, ultimately endangering herself and her son, Yoichi. In subsequently seeking help from her ex-husband, Reiko damns him to a terrifying and deadly encounter with the supernatural. Furthermore, after her plan to appease Sadako's destructive spirit fails, she turns to her father and asks that he sacrifice himself to Sadako to save Yoichi.[8] Reiko, as daughter, wife, and mother, brings danger and potential destruction to her father, ex-husband, and son.

Honogurai Mizu, with its narrative focus on wives and mothers who divorce their husbands only to struggle to raise their daughters, also directly engages with the *ryosai kenbo* ('good wife, wise mother') ideal. In the film, women remain tethered to the maternal identity, even as anxieties about the collapse of the traditional family are explicitly linked to maternal failure resulting in neglected and endangered children. These circumstances shape the relationships between Yoshimi and her mother, Yoshimi and Ikuko, and Mitsuko and her mother. These intersecting stories, with their shared elements and resonating echoes of tensions and betrayals between mothers and daughters place increasing stress on the mother-child bond.

The film's conservative stance is clearly reflected in an early scene that contrasts a stereotypically neurotic and superstitious Yoshimi with her (overly-)rational, facts and detail-oriented ex-husband, Kunio. His subsequent revelation that she has suffered an emotional breakdown foregrounds Yoshimi's mental and psychological fragility. In emphasising Yoshimi's frail, neurotic state, the film casts her decision to leave her husband in highly problematic terms, especially as this decision ultimately places her and her daughter, Ikuko, in the path of a dangerously threatening supernatural force. From a conservative, patriarchal Japanese perspective, Yoshimi appears thoughtless and irresponsible, particularly where Ikuko's well-being is concerned. In rejecting the socially approved role of good wife and wise mother within a marriage, and a domestic existence that promises security, social position, and respectability, Yoshimi has placed herself and her daughter outside patriarchal society's safe and protected norms. Mother and daughter are not only socially exiled to a rundown apartment after the divorce, they find themselves plunged into an increasingly disturbing, confined, and threatening space haunted by an *onryō.*

The film's depiction of the mother-child bond also deliberately undermines the traditional ideal of *bosei honno*. Rather than representing the idealised mother-child connection, the film undermines and problematises the traditional ideal of motherhood via three different portrayals of women/mothers in modern Japan, women who either through circumstance or choice, must raise their daughters alone without a husband/father's presence.

The film's opening sequence offers a flashback to Yoshimi as a child waiting in vain for her mother to pick her up after school. When a teacher tells Yoshimi, 'No one's come for you', Yoshimi's sense of abandonment and loneliness is explicitly emphasised. A cut to the present shows the adult Yoshimi looking out a window, setting the stage for the subsequent revelation that her relationship with Ikuko mirrors the one she had with her own mother.

This opening prologue, of a neglected child and an absent mother, raises the film's key fascination with maternal failures, in which these shortcomings inevitably lead to supernatural mayhem, for the young female ghost, Mitsuko, who stalks Ikuko and Yoshimi, died as a result of maternal neglect and irresponsibility when she was left alone to accidentally drown in the apartment's water tank. *Honogurai Mizu*'s plot weaves together the fates of three daughters, Yoshimi, Ikuko, and Mitsuko, who find themselves entwined in a supernatural battle for maternal attention, atonement, and survival after suffering from maternal indifference and neglect.

In *Ju-On*, Kayako's and her son's murder at the hands of her enraged husband raises the spectre of her failure as good wife and wise mother. Her subsequent appearances, haunting her home and stalking those who enter the space equates her with the malevolent, threatening, and mysterious female Other that contains echoes of Creed's archaic mother, 'everything associated with the archaic mother belongs to (a) the idea of an empty, forgotten house, that first mansion or dwelling place, and (b) the image of that last resting place, the grave, Mother Earth' (1995, p. 148), even as the film ambiguously hints at her trapped powerlessness. Kayako's appearances throughout the film explicitly align her with death and, in the final scene, with the grave, for *Ju-On* concludes with a shot of a female body wrapped in a plastic sheet in the house's attic. The corpse's eyes open as the camera zooms into a close-up, and the uncanny croaking sound associated with Kayako is heard. This shot encapsulates Kayako's very ambiguous nature. As a broken body sealed in plastic and abandoned in the house by her murderous husband, she is the epitome of the victim, yet her life-in death, signalled by her opening her eyes and her croaking, mark her as the terrifying uncanny, abject. There is also the lingering uncertainty of whether this body is Kayako's, or Takeo's latest female victim, Rika, since the plastic sheet blurs the victim's face. All these contribute to the film's heightened opacity and ambivalence towards the female/maternal monster-victim, an attitude that permeates millennial *kaidan*. Clearly, *Ju-On* consciously problematises its depiction of Kayako – while she is clearly Takeo's victim, her actions as wife, mother, and *onryō* are deliberately left ambiguous and obscure.

The notion of maternal failure resulting in the death of a young child who then returns for vengeance has emerged as a popular trope in millennial J-horror.[9] In *Ringu*, *Honogurai Mizu*, and *Ju-On*, the mothers are not directly responsible for the children's deaths (Mitsuko drowns in an accident; Sadako and Toshio are murdered by their fathers), yet these fatal events nevertheless inevitably reflect on the failed mothers for '[there is a] pervasive belief in Japanese society that a child's actions reflect directly upon the mother, even when the mother is no longer directly responsible for or involved in the child's life' (McKinlay, para. 26). From a Japanese perspective, these mothers' failure to nurture, protect, and raise their children to conform to social expectations and acceptable behaviours makes them responsible for their offspring' deviance and monstrosity.

In fact, contemporary Japanese horror films overwhelmingly depict the mother-child relationship in dark, ambiguous, and highly disturbing terms: Shizuko utters the accusation that presumably dooms Sadako, Reiko brings the cursed video into their home and exposes her son to its malevolence, and the scene of Reiko cradling the rotting remains of Sadako's body is disturbingly gruesome; the image of Yoshimi cradling a child is fraught with horror as the child is not her daughter but a vengeful spirit; *Ju-On* features a malevolent mother-and-son pair of ghosts haunting their cursed family home where they were murdered. While clear links are drawn between monstrous children and their mothers, these depictions deviate from Creed's claim that '...the monstrous child is ultimately depicted as a creation of the psychotic, dominating mother' (Creed 1993, p. 79). In J-horror, these monstrous children are more often the products of ineffective, irresponsible or negligent mothers.

Conclusion

Ringu, *Honogurai Mizu*, and *Ju-On* all explore the collapse of the traditional family. Sadako is betrayed by her mother and murdered by her (step-?)father, while the divorced Reiko's focus on her career exposes her son, Yoichi, to Sadako's malevolence; Mitsuko and Ikuko must cope with maternal negligence and abandonment; Toshio is an innocent victim of his father's murderous and jealous rage. In these contemporary Japanese horror films, the traditional *onryō* narrative has been adapted to reflect an almost hysterical anxiety about adolescent menace and malevolence that originates from familial/parental failures and betrayals. They reveal deep social anxieties about the adolescents coming of age in modern Japan. These films appeared to be responding to a moral panic caused by a spate of reports detailing shocking and disturbingly violent crimes committed by Japanese children in the 1990s and early 2000s (Arai 2006; Faiola 2004; Kakuchi 2013; Kawakami 1999), a fear that spawned the term *kodomo ga hen da*, 'the child is turning strange' (Arai 2006, p. 222), or 'the strange-changed child' (Lury 2010, p. 29).[10] While expressing the nation's growing anxieties about an emerging generation of Japanese youth in crises, these horror films continue to ground their representations of horror and monstrosity around the feminine and the maternal.

Creed avers that 'the horror film attempts to bring about the confrontation with the abject (the corpse, bodily wastes, the monstrous-feminine) in order finally to eject the abject and redraw the boundaries between the human and non-human' (1993, p. 14). This trajectory once structured the traditional *kaidan*. As I have argued, the abject figure of the historical *onryō* served a crucial function. Her appearance signalled social dysfunction and potential crisis. Her role was to destroy that which was undermining and tainting the community, clearing the way so that the patriarchal order could be reestablished and order restored, a process that ensured that all the traditional boundaries (between dominant masculinity and submissive femininity, between the natural and supernatural, between safety and danger) would eventually be reinstated. The *onryō*, therefore, was 'the abject [that] must ... be tolerated, for that which threatens to destroy life also helps to define life' (Creed 1993, p. 9). In contemporary J-horror, however, the return to the normal and the redrawing of the necessary boundaries remains elusive; *Ringu*, *Hongurai Mizu*, and *Ju-On* all conclude on profoundly ambiguous and ambivalent notes, the abject is not effectively ejected, and once clear boundaries remain blurred and indistinct.

In evaluating the monstrous female, Creed notes, 'the presence of the monstrous-feminine in the popular horror film speaks to us more about male fears than about female desire or female subjectivity' (Creed 1993, p. 7). Millennial J-horror reinforces a system in which dominant patriarchal concerns continue to demonise a new generation of young women who are increasingly ignoring, if not actively rejecting, the traditional and socially approved roles of wife, mother, and domestic homemaker, preferring to remain single, embracing financial and sexual freedom, while actively engaging in conspicuous material consumption. These versions of the unruly Japanese female appear to be finding greater representation on screen, where the female and the feminine are quite often relegated to the supernatural, the horrific and the terrifying. The depictions of female Otherness and deviance, and the alignment of these qualities with the unnatural in Japanese horror overtly reference the on-going and publicly recognised gender anxieties that find expression and debate in Japanese public discourses. It would appear that the vengeful and angry *onryō* at the centre of contemporary Japanese horror films may, in fact, have just cause for their antagonism.

Notes

1 Notably, Japanese male ghosts or *yurei* do also appear in Japanese folk tales, but they are seldom motivated by revenge, unlike their female counterparts who are traditionally angry, vengeance driven, and often malevolent (Screech 2006). Far from displaying the violent and destructive tendencies, and terrifying demeanours characteristic of female *yūrei*, male *yūrei* are often, in stark contrast, calm, quiet, contemplative, and largely unthreatening.

2 All three folktales have received the cinematic treatment, with the most notable versions dating to the 1950s and 1960s. *Kaidan bancho sarayashiki* (*Ghost Story of Broken Dishes at Bancho Mansion*, Juichi Kono, 1957), *Tokaido Yotsuya Kaidan* (Nabuo Nakagawa 1959), and *Yaba no naka no kuroneko* (*The Black Cat,* Kaneto Shindo 1968) used the Edo Gothic setting, which is characterised by flux, insecurity, and anxiety linked to the decline and eventual disappearance of the *samurai* and the shift to modernity, to articulate fears about the erosion of tradition and the undermining of gender roles in the face of externally imposed change during and after the Japanese Occupation.

3 It is, in fact, possible to view these men as instances of the abject for they chose to ignore their 'positions' and the social 'rules' that define proper patriarchal behaviour, and by their actions, they disturb (masculine) 'identity, system, order' (Creed 1993, p. 4).

4 While the figure of the *kogyaru* is essentially a teen identity, it appears that the inner character traits associated with the figure are increasingly being mapped on younger pre-teen females in Japanese horror films.

5 While Kayako's murder is depicted on screen, Toshio's is not.

6 While *Ju-On: The Grudge*, deliberately withholds the reason for Kayako's murder, two telemovies, *Ju-On: The Curse 1* and 2, which preceded Shimizu's film, reveal that Takeo suspected Kayako of an extramarital

affair. In ignoring her marriage vows, Kayako is '[t]he [monstrous] female subject ... who refuses to take up her proper place in the symbolic order'; Kayako represents 'abjection ... constructed as a rebellion of filthy, lustful, carnal, female flesh' (Creed 1993, p. 38). Kayako's death at her husband's hands can thus be interpreted as patriarchy's attempts to punish and contain her. As Creed notes, 'patriarchal ideology works to curb the power of the mother, and by extension all women, by controlling woman's desire through a series of repressive practices which deny her autonomy over her body' (1993, p. 162).

7 Significantly, a national population survey revealed that between 1975 and 1990, there was an approximate 50% increase in single-mother families in Japan, with a majority of these families the result of divorce; furthermore, over 70% of divorces in Japan were initiated by women (Peng 1996, para. 4, para. 9).

8 In *Ringu*, the original victim can save themselves by make someone else watch the video, thereby passing on Sadako's deadly curse. Reiko, in letting Ryuji watch the tape, unknowingly saved herself and doomed him.

9 *Chakushin Ari* (Takashi Miike 2003) is another J-horror film that deals with similar themes.

10 Jessica Balanzategui offers an in-depth consideration of contemporary Japan's youth and child-focussed anxieties in her examination of the uncanny ghost children depicted in J-horror (2018, pp. 175–178).

References

Aoyama, T 2005, 'Transgendering *shõjo shõsetsu*', in M McLelland and R Dasgupta (eds.), *Gender, transgenders and sexualities in Japan*. Routledge, London, pp. 49–64.

Arai, A 2006, 'The wild child in 1990s Japan', in T Yoda and H Harootunian (eds.), *Japan after Japan: social and cultural life from the recessionary 1990s to the present*. Duke University Press, Durham, pp. 216–238.

Balanzategui, J 2018, *The uncanny child in transnational cinema: ghosts of futurity at the turn of the twenty-first century*, Amsterdam University Press, Amsterdam.

Balmain, C 2008, *Introduction to Japanese horror film*. Edinburgh University Press, Edinburgh.

Creed, B 1993, *The monstrous-feminine: film, feminism, psychoanalysis*, Routledge, London.

Creed, B 1995, 'Horror and the carnivalesque: the body monstrous', in L Devereaux and R Hillman (eds.), *Fields of vision: essays in film studies, visual anthropology and photography*, University of California Press, Berkeley, pp. 127–159.

Enchi, F 1983, *Masks*, trans. J Carpenter, Random House, New York.

Faiola, A 2004, 'Youth violence has Japan struggling for answers', *The Washington Post*, 9 August, viewed 30 September 2014, www.washingtonpost.com/wp-dyn/articles/A50678-2004Aug8.html?noredirect=on

Hearn, L 1971, *In ghostly Japan: spooky stories with the folklore, superstitions and traditions of old Japan*. Tuttle Publishing, Vermont.

Kaidan bancho sayarashiki (*Ghost Story of Broken Dishes at Bancho Mansion*). Dir. Juichi Kono. Toei, 1957.

Kakuchi, S 2003, 'Youth murder shocks Japan', *Asia Times*, 15 July, viewed 25 October 2013, www.atimes.com/atimes/Japan/EG15Dh02.html
Kanematsu, E 1993, *Women in society: Japan*. Times Book International, Singapore.
Kaneto, S (dir.) 1968, *Yabu no Naka no Kuroneko* (*The Black Cat*), motion picture, Toho, Japan.
Kawakami, R 1999, *Gakkō Hōkai* (*School Collapse*], Bungei Shunju, Japan.
Kelsky, K 1996, 'Flirting with the foreign: interracial sex in Japan's "international" age', in R Wilson and W Dissanayake (eds.), *Global/local: cultural production and the transnational imaginary*, Duke University Press, Durham, pp. 173–192.
Kristeva, J 1982, *Powers of horror: an essay in abjection*. Trans. Leon S. Roudiez, Columbia University Press, New York.
Leheny, D 2006, *Think global, fear local: sex violence and anxiety in contemporary Japan*, Cornell University Press, New York.
Leiter, S 2002, 'From gay to gei: the onnagata and the creation of kabuki's female characters', in S Leiter (ed.), *A kabuki reader: history and performance*, Routledge, London, pp. 211–229.
Lloyd, F 2001, 'Strategic interventions in contemporary Japanese art', in F Lloyd, (ed.), *Consuming bodies: sex and contemporary Japanese art*, Reaktion Books, London, pp. 69–108.
Lury, K 2010, *The child in film: tears, fears and fairytales*. I. B. Tauris, London.
McKinlay, M 2011, 'Unstable mothers: redefining motherhood in contemporary Japan', *Intersections: Gender, History and Culture in the Asian Context*, vol. 7, web, viewed 20 February 2019, http://intersections.anu.edu.au/issue7/mckinlay.html
Miller, L 2004, 'Those naughty teenage girls: Japanese kogals, slang, and media assessments', *Journal of Linguistic Anthropology*, vol. 14, no. 2, pp. 225–247.
Morley, P 1999, *The mountain is moving: Japanese women's lives*, University of British Columbia Press, Vancouver.
Nakagawa, N 1959, *Tokaido Yotsuya Kaidan* (*Ghost Story of Yotsuya)*, motion picture, Shintoho, Japan.
Nakata, H (dir.) 1998, *Ringu* (*Ring*), motion picture, Basara Pictures, Japan.
Nakata, H (dir.) 2002, *Honogurai Mizu no Soko Kara* (*Dark Water*), motion picture, Nikkatsu, Japan.
Napier, S 1996, *The fantastic in modern Japanese literature: the subversion of modernity*, Routledge, London.
Napier, S 2001, *Anime from* Akira *to* Princess Mononoke*: experiencing contemporary Japanese animation*, Palgrave, London.
Ōgi, F 2001, 'Gender insubordination in Japanese comics (manga) for girls', in J Lent (ed.), *Illustrating Asia: comics, humour magazines, and picture books*, University of Hawai'i Press, Honolulu, pp. 171–186.
Orbaugh, S 2003, 'Busty battlin' babes: the evolution of the *shōjo* in 1990s visual culture', in J Morrow, N Bryston, and M Graybill (eds.), *Gender and power in the Japanese visual field*, University of Hawai'i Press, Honolulu, pp. 201–265.
Peng, I 1996, 'Single-mother families in Japan: a conspicuous silence', *NIRA Review*, viewed 21 January 2011, www.nira.or.jp/past/publ/review/96spring/peng.html

Screech, T 1994, 'Japanese ghosts', *Haunted Times*, viewed 5 July 2006, www.hauntedtimes.com/japanese-ghosts/

Shimizu, T (dir.) 2002, *Ju-On: The Grudge*, motion picture, Nikkatsu, Japan.

Sugihara, Y 2002, 'Gender role development in Japanese culture: diminishing gender role differences in a contemporary society', *Sex Roles: A Journal of Research*, vol. 47, no. 9–10, pp. 443–452.

Tipton, E 2002, *Modern Japan: a social and political history*, Routledge, London.

Wee, V 2014, *Japanese horror films and their American remakes*. Routledge, London.

Yao, X 2000, *An introduction to Confucianism*, Cambridge University Press, New York.

13 Women in the Way? Re-reading *The Monstrous-Feminine* in Contemporary Slovenian Cinema

Polona Petek

Introduction

In 2018, the Slovenian Film Council – following the Council of Europe's recommendations and emulating the Eurimages' strategies for gender equality in European film industries[1] – commissioned researcher and film producer Nika Gričar to conduct a survey on gender equality in Slovenian film culture (Gričar 2018). The results covering the past quarter-century (the period since 1995, the year the Slovenian Film Fund, the Centre's forerunner, was established) were alarming. At the Academy of Theatre, Radio, Film and Television (AGRFT), approximately a third of students in the Film Directing programme in the Department of Film and Television are women and also approximately a third of active Slovenian film directors are women. Yet, the share of women directors backed financially by the Slovenian Film Centre in the past decade amounts to a meagre 9%. By now, only 13 fiction feature-length films have been made by eight women directors in Slovenia[2] – a dismal number compared to more than 500 titles attributed to Slovenian film-makers since 1948, the year of the release of the first Slovenian sound feature-length film (Štefančič 2005, 2016).[3]

Still, this year seems to be a watershed for women in Slovenian cinema. I write this just days after the closure of the 21st Slovenian Film Festival, the annual national showcase, whose competition programme this year featured four feature-length, one medium-length and seven short/student films directed by women.[4] Director Urša Menart was the first-ever woman to receive the Best Feature Film award for *My Last Year As a Loser* (2018).[5] She was also the first-ever woman to receive the Best Screenplay award.[6] In addition to these achievements and accolades, it is also worth mentioning that the current director of the Slovenian Film Festival is a woman (Jelka Stergel); the current director of the Slovenian Film Centre is a woman (Nataša Bučar); and I myself have just been invited on board the national Film Realisation Programme Commission, the expert body that decides which film projects are to be financially backed by the Slovenian Film Centre and which not – that is to say, the central body of the (financial) decision-making part of Slovenian film culture, in which women have thus far been most meagrely represented (Gričar 2018, p. 2).

What a different world Slovenia was 20 years ago when I decided to pursue film studies overseas! Its film production, newly established as a national cinema following the declaration of Slovenian independence in 1991, was in what seemed like a permanent state of searching: searching for funding, searching for a workable and affordable infrastructure, searching for audiences[7] and, last but not least, searching for its new pioneers, including the first woman to direct a feature film. Namely, despite the long-standing tradition of film in Slovenia, [8] 97 years passed before the first fiction feature-length film was directed by a woman in Slovenia.[9] This was *The Guardian of the Frontier*, directed by Maja Weiss, which premiered in 2002. Film scholarship in Slovenia was in an equally peculiar state. The tradition of writing about film in Slovenia is strong and long-standing.[10] Yet, in contrast to the prolific field of film journalism, Slovenian film scholarship in the late 1990s was to a large extent synonymous with a single name – Slovenia's prime scholarly export, Slavoj Žižek, who had by then published several of his academic bestsellers, including *The sublime object of ideology* (1989), *Enjoy your symptom!* (1992a), and *Everything you always wanted to know about Lacan (but were afraid to ask Hitchcock)* (1992b). There were no university programmes for studying film scholarship, only individual undergraduate courses such as *Sociology of Cinema* taught in the Department of Sociology at the Faculty of Arts in Ljubljana.[11]

No university programmes, no school of film theory (apart from the Ljubljana Lacanian School surrounding Žižek), and marginalised women film-makers. This was the climate in which I, a comparative literature graduate, decided to go overseas to pursue my interest in cinema, its history and theory. It was not a carefully planned or even calculated career decision, but rather one of those instinctive moves that only a very enthusiastic young person is capable of, a rite of passage of sorts, a leap into the unknown, for I could hardly have gone further away from what was then my home, with no friends or family to lean on.

Melbourne

Fortune favours the bold, says an old Latin proverb, which certainly proved true in my decision to move to Australia and enrol in the Cinema Studies Master of Arts programme at the University of Melbourne. It was there, in an absorbing course called 'Film, Modernity, and the Avant-Garde', that I first encountered Barbara Creed, an inspiring scholar and a most generous teacher, who guided me steadily into the world of film scholarship. It was not my conscious decision to spend my time at Melbourne getting equipped for a feminist analysis of Slovenian cinema, and I feel grateful that this was not the case, for this initial lack of determination allowed me to explore many forking paths of film history and theory. But then a decisive coincidence occurred.

It was March 2003, the beginning of a new semester at the university. I was already a confirmed PhD student supervised by Barbara Creed and also tutoring and giving occasional lectures in her courses on 'Feminist Film Theory', 'Surrealism and Cinema' and 'Film Noir'. Her book, *The monstrous-feminine: film, feminism, psychoanalysis*, was my bedside reading, so to speak, for – despite the application of its conceptual framework to horror[12], hardly my first preference when it comes to genre film-making – it proved a most useful source of ideas for how to approach and interpret feminist, surrealist, and *noir* representations of women on screen. But March in Melbourne is not just the beginning of a new school year; it is also the month of the biggest and oldest queer film festival in Australia, established in 1991 and officially called the Melbourne Queer Film Festival since 2003. In March 2003, I was leafing through the festival brochure when I noticed a Slovenian film listed in the programme. It was Maja Weiss' *Guardian of the Frontier*, hailed not only as the first Slovenian queer film but also the first-ever Slovenian fiction feature-length film directed by a woman.

This was a bizarre moment: a moment of pride and respect for a film-maker 'from home' who had made the first Slovenian queer film so soon, only a decade after the term exploded onto the global cinematic stage; but it was also a moment of shock for having realised that it was the beginning of the twenty-first century, yet, this was only the first Slovenian film directed by a woman. Up until that moment my interest in Slovenian cinema had been slight, certainly not comprehensive, and I must have repressed the fact that women were so conspicuously absent from Slovenian cinematic limelight. But this was a potent moment and it was Barbara Creed's book that made it such. Namely, it would have been a humbling, shameful moment if it was not for *The monstrous-feminine*, the book's core message, which made me realise in that moment that marginalised, victimised positions are symptomatic of those who create them, not those who assume them, or, more accurately, are forced into them. No doubt, this idea could have come from many other sources, feminist or otherwise; but *The monstrous-feminine* had another, even more important message for me in that moment: just as Barbara Creed discovered that the monstrous women of horror cinema are not necessarily victims, the juxtaposition of Weiss' *Guardian* and *The monstrous-feminine* suggested to me that these marginalised positions of women in Slovenian cinema need not be seen as necessarily disempowering.

Ljubljana

For almost a decade, this remained a brief, passing observation and my interest in Slovenian cinema remained that of a keen, but passive and distant observer, discovering more and more details about the unenviable position of women in Slovenian cinema: about unfinished projects and impossible visions;[13] about the fact that the national film school had never had any women professors and it was only in the twenty-first century that the first woman started teaching film editing there; and most importantly, about the fact that a comprehensive feminist analysis of Slovenian film history and the local film culture is still lacking. This was not the reason for my decision to return to Slovenia in 2008; it was, however, the reason to become involved in 2011 in a research project on *The role of women's migrations and migrants in the construction of the Slovene national identity*.[14] Through work on this project I met Maja Weiss and started studying her work and the work of other Slovenian women directors more closely. Gradually, my initial *monstrous-feminine*-inspired observation started taking a more substantial, more elaborate shape, and I shall outline one such case study below.

If we stay with Slovenian women *directors*, there are only eight women to choose from. This scarcity is hardly unique to Slovenian cinema. Iordanova (2003, p. 119) argues that women have been 'traditionally marginalised' in Eastern European cinemas, whereas Mantziari (2014) documents this absence as a wide-spread phenomenon in global art-house cinema. It would be hard to argue, then, that Slovenian women film-makers are a compelling subject of enquiry simply because of their marginalisation. I want to argue that what makes them fascinating is the way they actively and imaginatively adopt their marginal positions and through their creative process transform them into perfectly enabling and unique positions.

I studied this process in-depth in relation to Maja Weiss' work (Petek 2017). She was the obvious choice for my first case study not only because of her standing as the first woman to have directed a fiction feature-length film in Slovenia, but for number of other reasons, too. Her career spans the entire period of Slovenian national cinema proper;[15] her opus, which contains more than 30 titles, is extremely diverse, and as such appears defiantly 'unauthorial'; yet, it also shows Weiss' peculiar all-encompassing thematic affinity: in all her works, Weiss in one way or another brings into play the issues of borders and border-crossing.[16] She has made documentaries exploring Slovenian border areas; she has made documentaries about the fates of people who were forced into leaving their homes and crossing borders; her directorial debut, *The Guardian of the Frontier*, is a film about exploring, transgressing, and redefining national, sexual, and metaphysical borders; her second feature, *Installation of Love* (2007), is a film about crossing the boundaries between reality and fiction; and Weiss herself crosses professional and geographical borders and blurs genre boundaries. In short, borders and border-crossing pervade Weiss' work not only in a representational, but also in an 'existential' sense; her opus not only thematises these phenomena, but in fact enacts them. They are the enabling *fil rouge* of her creativity.

A similar, yet different process can be observed in the work of Sonja Prosenc. Her directorial curriculum vitae is short, yet, remarkably focussed and consistent. She has directed six titles to date, two of them, *The Tree* (2014) and *History of Love* (2018), are feature-length fiction films. Prosenc is an obvious outsider in Slovenian film culture, not only because she is a woman, but also, even more so, because she has never studied film-making at AGRFT, the national film school, which claims a monopoly, so to speak, on artistically accomplished film-making in Slovenia.[17] Prosenc (b. 1977) studied journalism and cultural studies at the Faculty of Social Sciences, University of Ljubljana, and found her way into film-making via an international path. She took part in Berlinale and Sarajevo Talent Campuses, and was selected for the Script & Pitch postgraduate programme at TorinoFilmLab. She has also completed a Midpoint course in script development and film dramaturgy at FAMU (the renowned Film and TV School of the Academy of Performing Arts in Prague).

Already with her directorial debut, the short film *Free-Spirited Friends* (2005), Prosenc established herself as an unconventional film-maker whose primary interest is certainly not the story, or the action, but rather the psychological states of her characters and the emotional charge of the story, which she uses as a background, a canvas on which she paints her characters' feelings. Nowhere is this more evident than in her latest feature, *History of Love*, a film about a teenage girl (Doroteja Nadrah) whose mother (Zita Fusco) has suddenly died and the girl is now struggling to come to terms with her loss and the discovery that her mother had a secret lover (Kristoffer Joner). The synopsis sounds like a springboard for an emotionally charged drama. Yet, Prosenc hardly develops it in this direction; rather, she uses it as a stage where intense emotions run free, crossing the boundaries between reality and fantasy, anger and sadness, life and death, which the viewers experience through numerous extreme close-ups of human faces and shots of water of all shapes (pools, rivers, streams, ponds, lakes), combined with often completely inarticulate sounds with which the film's mesmerising soundtrack is interspersed.

Yet, it is not crossing the boundaries between reality and fantasy, anger and sadness, or life and death that makes Prosenc stand out in contemporary Slovenian cinema. What has turned her outsider standing into an enabling and empowering stance is her audacious crossing of the tacit boundary separating the turfs of AGRFT and the Ljubljana Academy of Fine Arts and Design (ALUO). The former sees its mission in narrative cinema and claims it as its prerogative, whereas the latter (among other things) cultivates non-narrative screen-based forms of visual art without calling them cinema.[18] Not many Slovenian film-makers have dared to call themselves film-makers and make non-narrative films.[19] By crossing this boundary, Prosenc has succeeded in carving out a unique space for herself as the author of affect-based, almost non-narrative cinematic experiences.

We could go on laying out examples of Slovenian women film-makers' engagement with borders and boundaries. Suffice it to say that this affinity seems to be the common denominator of women who have managed to penetrate the until recently male-dominated world of Slovenian cinema. Where does this come from? What is the fascination, the empowering potential of borders? Barbara Creed would no doubt invoke Julia Kristeva and her notion of abjection here. Since my subject of enquiry is less intimate, less grounded in the body and the psyche, but rather more sociologically constructed, I have turned to social scientists to find a suitable explanation. Dutch scholar Henk van Houtum, professor of political geography and geopolitics, points out that 'border' should be considered primarily a verb: borders are processes rather than objects; the making or the setting up of borders – in short, *bordering* – is a process of ordering as well as 'othering' (van Houtum 2011, pp. 50–51). Yet, he does not suggest that this process is something we should strive to abandon:

> [Borders] are not like eyes that can be shut. [...] By closing the borders, closing the eyes, the fear for the other will not be shut off. The uncertainty will only be greater. [...] It is highly unlikely that the spatial b/ordering of our self-interest to increase our own comfort and to diminish the fear of loss of control will ever end. But that does not mean that we unwillingly and uncritically need to reproduce our own borders or that we are forced to close our eyes obediently. We are not only victims of the border, but also the producers of it.
>
> (van Houtum 2011, pp. 58–60; emphasis added)

And this is what I believe Slovenian women film-makers are acutely aware of. They have been actively recasting the boundaries that had once kept women out. In her book *Cartographies of diaspora*, British sociologist and anthropologist Avtar Brah defines borders as 'arbitrary dividing lines that are simultaneously social, cultural and psychic; [they are] territories to be patrolled against those whom they construct as outsiders, aliens, the Others' (1996, p. 198). Yet, they are also the sites where claims to identity, belonging and ownership are 'staked out, contested, defended, and fought over' (ibid.).

***

It might sound like my interest in Slovenian cinema and its women film-makers has taken me a long way away from *The monstrous-feminine*. I would have to disagree. Indeed, *The monstrous-feminine* is a feminist-inflected psychoanalytic exploration of the horror genre, whereas my work is a feminist-inflected sociological analysis of a national cinema (and one with virtually no horror tradition![20]). Yet, my reading of Slovenian women film-makers' works, which has recently found resonance in sociological and anthropological conceptualisations of borders, is thoroughly indebted to *The monstrous-feminine* – not only for the initial inspiration, but also, more importantly, for the attitude and the intellectual stance cultivated in Barbara Creed's work. I have always read her interpretation of Julia Kristeva and its application to the horror genre as a stance of defiance, the stance of unswerving determination to find something enabling in a situation that seems dismal and disempowering at first sight. Without *The monstrous-feminine*, the position of women in Slovenian cinema would look quite different.

Notes

1 See *Gender equality in the audiovisual sector – a new Council of Europe recommendation* and *Eurimages strategy for gender equality in the film industry 2018*, available at https://www.coe.int/en/web/eurimages/gender-equality-documents (last accessed on 22 September, 2018).

2 The list includes (in chronological order): *The Guardian of the Frontier/Varuh meje* (Weiss dir. 2002), *Blind Spot/Slepa pega* (Slak dir. 2002), *Installation of Love/Instalacija ljubezni* (Weiss dir. 2007), *L… for Love/L kot ljubezen* (Glogovac dir. 2007), *Teah/Tea* (Slak dir. 2007), *Reality/Realnost* (Jemeršić dir. 2008), *For the End of Time/Za konec časa* (Kugler dir. 2009), *Panic/Panika* (Zemljič dir. 2013), *Echoes of Time/Odmevi časa* (Kugler dir. 2014), *The Tree/Drevo* (Prosenc dir. 2014), *The Miner/Rudar* (Slak dir. 2017), *History of Love/Zgodovina ljubezni* (Prosenc dir. 2018), and *My Last Year As a Loser/Ne bom več luzerka* (Menart dir. 2018).

3 *On Our Own Land/Na Svoji Zemlji* (Štiglic dir. 1948) is considered the first Slovenian feature-length sound film. It is worth pointing out that the film was made in Yugoslavia, but the language spoken in the film is Slovenian, the story is set in a small Slovenian village, and the entire crew were Slovenians – the usual criteria for determining retrospectively which Yugoslavian films count as Slovenian.

4 The total number of films in the competition programme was 52. See http://www.fsf.si/2018/en/

5 This is the third time a woman was awarded one of the two most prestigious awards; the first woman to receive the Best Director award was Maja Weiss in 2002 for her directorial debut *The Guardian of the Frontier*, followed by Hanna Slak in 2017 for her third feature *The Miner*.

6 In fact, Melina Pota Koljević received the award for Best Screenplay last year, but she shared the award with Janez Burger, Aleš Čar, and Srdjan Koljević, the co-authors of the screenplay for *Ivan* (Burger dir. 2017).

7 Slovenian film and Slovenian audiences are 'incompatible', argues Veingerl (2016). Rugelj (2007) attributes this to the divide between art-house aspirations of Slovenian film-makers and entertainment-focussed preferences of Slovenian filmgoers.

8 The first film projections in Slovenia (which was then part of the Austro-Hungarian Empire) took place as early as November 1896 and the first films, Lumière style actuality films, were made by lawyer Karol Grossmann in 1905 (Vrdlovec 2013).

9 This may sound surprising, because there had been women before who had graduated from AGRFT (and other European film schools) with formal degrees in film directing. Yet, at best, they ended up making made-for-TV documentaries and TV commercials, or simply doing something completely different. I discuss these issues at length elsewhere (Petek 2017).

10 France Brenk notes that the first book on film in Slovenia, Pavel Debevec's *How to approach film?* (*Kako pridem k filmu?*), was published as early as 1929 (Brenk 1955, p. 7). Zdenko Vrdlovec notes Debevec's book was preceded by two shorter articles published in 1924 (2013, pp. 61–62).

11 Even today, film scholarship is still an 'orphan' in Slovenian academia, an academic discipline with a dispersed and understaffed institutional domicile, with no locally based peer-reviewed journals, and with no recognition as yet as an independent habilitation field.

At the moment, there are three institutions offering programmes and courses on film at the University of Ljubljana, yet, there is no official institutional exchange facilitating or vindicating this situation: AGRFT offers several practice-oriented undergraduate courses and (since 2013) a graduate programme in Film and Television Studies; the Faculty of Social Sciences offers one undergraduate ('Film Studies') and one graduate course ('Aesthetics and Politics of Film'); and the Faculty of Arts offers one undergraduate ('Introduction to Film Studies') and one graduate course ('History of Film Theory').

The term 'habilitation' is derived from the Mediaeval Latin *habilitare*. The academic concept of habilitation developed in Germany in the seventeenth century. Initially, it was synonymous with doctoral and later on with post-doctoral qualification. It is now defined as the qualification to conduct university teaching and it is the prerequisite for lectureship in many European countries including Slovenia.

12 I first studied *The Monstrous Feminine* while working on my Master's thesis (also supervised by Barbara Creed), in which I explored the patriarchal connotations of David Cronenberg's films, particularly in relation to his male protagonists' relationship to women.

13 I am currently writing an article for Slovenian film journal *Kino!* about Polona Sepe's unfinished children's film *Desovila*, which was in production in the early 1980s and could have become the first feature-length film directed by a woman.

14 The full title of the project, funded by the Slovenian Research Agency (ARRS), was *The role of women's migrations and migrants in the construction of the*

Slovene national identity from national to postnational era: Comparative Slovenian, European, and global aspects; project leader: Ksenija Vidmar Horvat; Faculty of Arts, University of Ljubljana.

15 Weiss finished her studies at AGRFT at the end of the 1980s and started making shorts and documentaries for Slovenian national television in the early 1990s.

16 Weiss's thematic interest in these issues has been observed before (Falcinella 2005).

17 See Rugelj (2007) and my own discussion of the peculiar reception of Mitja Okorn in Slovenian film culture (Petek 2017). Okorn is a typical example of a Slovenian film-maker, who remains part of Slovenian film culture, yet, is persistently marginalised by the Slovenian film establishment because he is a self-taught film-maker with a flair for light-hearted genre film-making and a commercially successful transnational career (which has now reached Hollywood). See also Lešničar (2011).

18 The actual programme is called Visual Communications Design; see http://www.aluo.uni-lj.si/studijski-program/oblikovanje-vizualnih-komunikacij/

19 A prominent similar attempt is Jan Cvitkovič's *Archeo* (2011) which critics and the director himself have described as an example of 'pure cinema'. It is worth pointing out that Cvitkovič, too, did not study film-making at AGRFT, but rather archaeology at the Faculty of Arts, University of Ljubljana. On the other hand, Nika Autor, Slovenian representative at the 57th Venice Biennale in 2017, does not describe herself as a film-maker, but rather as a visual artist whose 'practice is primarily based on experimental videos and documentary films, film essays, newsreels and spatial video and film installations' (https://www.autor.si/biography.html). The author obtained her BA degree at ALUO.

20 Many critics have described *Killbillies* (*Idila*, Tomaž Gorkič, 2015, Slovenia), the winner of the Best Film award at the 2015 Slovenian Film Festival, as the first Slovenian horror film.

Bibliography

Brah, A 1996, *Cartographies of diaspora: contesting identities*, Routledge, London.

Brenk, F 1955, *Zapiski o filmu/Notes on film*, Obzorja, Maribor.

Burger, J (dir.) 2017, *Ivan*, motion picture, Staragara, Slovenia.

Creed, B 1993, *The monstrous-feminine: film, feminism, psychoanalysis*, Routledge, London.

Cvitkovič, J (dir.) 2011, *Archeo/Arheo*, motion picture, Staragara, Slovenia.

Falcinella, N 2005, "Films without borders", *Cineuropa*, web interview, 22 August, viewed 1 July 2013, http://cineuropa.org/it.aspx?t=interview&l=en&did=54190

Glogovac, J (dir.) 2007, *L… for Love/L kot ljubezen*, motion picture, Avion Film, Slovenia.

Gorkič, T (dir.) 2015, *Killbillies/Idila*, motion picture, 666 Production, Slovenia.

Gričar, N 2018, *Facts & figures: gender equality*, Slovenski Filmski Center, Ljubljana, viewed 22 September 2018, https://issuu.com/sfilmc/docs/sfc_2018_facts___figures_gender_equ_27512fe95c5704

Iordanova, D, 2003, *Cinema of the other Europe: the industry and artistry of East Central European film*, Wallflower Press, London and New York.

Jemeršić, D (dir.) 2008, *Reality/Realnost*, motion picture, Brigada, Slovenia.

Kugler, E (dir.) 2009, *For the End of Time/Za konec časa*, motion picture, Cinema Epoch, Slovenia.

Kugler, E (dir.) 2014, *Echoes of Time/Odmevi časa*, motion picture, Cinema Epoch, Slovenia.

Lešničar, T 2011, "Velika vrnitev Mitje Okorna", *Delo*, 19 November, viewed 1 March 2019, www.delo.si/kultura/liffe/velika-vrnitev-mitje-okorna.html

Mantziari, D 2014, Women directors in "global' art cinema: negotiating feminism and representation, *Doctoral Thesis*, University of East Anglia, Norwich, unpublished.

Menart, U (dir.) 2018, *My Last Year as a Loser/Ne bom vec luzerka*, motion picture, Vertigo, Slovenia.

Petek, P 2017, "The (m)others of Slovenian cinema? Gender, bordercrossing and the conundrum of national cinema", *Studies in European Cinema*, vol. 14, no. 2, pp. 134–152.

Prosenc, S (dir.) 2005, *Free-Spirited Friends/Nič novega, nič pretiranega*, motion picture, AAC Productions, Slovenia.

Prosenc, S (dir.) 2014, *The Tree/Drevo*, motion picture, Staragara, Slovenia/Italy.

Prosenc, S (dir.) 2018, *History of Love/Zgodovina ljubezni*, motion picture, Monoo, Slovenia/Norway/Italy.

Rugelj, S 2007, *Stranpota slovenskega filma: zapiski o kinematografiji 2000–2007/The Sideways of Slovenian Cinema: Notes on Film 2000–2007*, UMco, Ljubljana.

Slak, H (dir.) 2002, *Blind Spot/Slepa pega*, motion picture, Bindweed Soundvision, Slovenia.

Slak, H (dir.) 2007, *Teah/Tea*, motion picture, Jadran Film Technika Zagreb, Bosnia and Herzegovina/Croatia/Poland/Slovenia.

Slak, H (dir.) 2017, *The Miner/Rudar*, motion picture, Bindweed Soundvision, Slovenia.

Štefančič, M 2005, *Na svoji zemlji: zgodovina slovenskega filma/On our own land: the history of Slovenian cinema*, UMco, Ljubljana.

Štefančič, M 2016, *Slovenski film 2.0: kritična enciklopedija slovenskega celovečernega filma 1991–2016/Slovenian film 2.0: a critical encyclopaedia of Slovenian feature film 1991–2016*, UMco, Ljubljana.

Štiglic, F (dir.) 1948, *On Our Own Land/Na svoji zemlji*, motion picture, Triglav Film, Yugoslavia.

van Houtum, H 2011, "The mask of the border", in D. Wastl-Walter (ed.), *The Ashgate research companion to border studies*, Ashgate Publishing, Surrey, pp. 49–61.

Veingerl, M 2016, "Marcel Štefančič Jr: Slovenski film 2.0: kritična enciklopedija slovenskega celovečernega filma 1991–2016", *Koridor±*, 30. September, viewed 22 September 2018, http://koridor-ku.si/recenzije/marcel-stefancic-jr-slovenski-film-2-0-kriticna-enciklopedija-slovenskega-celovecernega-filma-1991-2016/.

Vrdlovec, Z 2013, *Zgodovina filma na Slovenskem 1896–2011/The history of film in Slovenia 1896–2011*, UMco, Ljubljana.

Weiss, M (dir.) 2002, *The Guardian of the Frontier/Varuh meje*, motion picture, Bela Film, Slovenia/Germany/France.

Weiss, M (dir.) 2007, *Installation of Love/Instalacija ljubezni*, motion picture, Bela Film, Slovenia/Germany.
Zemljič, B (dir.) 2013, *Panic/Panika*, motion picture, Atalanta, Slovenia.
Žižek, S 1989, *The sublime object of ideology*, Verso, London.
Žižek, S 1992a, *Enjoy your symptom!*, Routledge, London.
Žižek, S 1992b, *Everything you always wanted to know about Lacan (but were afraid to ask Hitchcock*, Verso, London.

14 In-Your-Face

The Monstrous-Feminine in Photography, Performance Art, Multimedia, and Painting

Jeanette Hoorn

In recent years, Barbara Creed's concept of the monstrous-feminine has played an increasingly important role in discussions of art and gender. It can be applied to a range of confronting images from those on the plates of Judy Chicago's *Dinner Party* (1974–1979) and Annie Sprinkle's *Public Cervix Announcement* (uncovered 2017), to Cindy Sherman's profoundly abject *Sex Pictures* series (1989–1992) and the chaotic in-your-face images of femininity in Carolee Schneeman's *Eye/Body* (1963–1973) series and *Meat Joy* (dir. Gaisseau 1964) of the 1960s. Frida Kahlo's *My Birth* (1932b) and Mary Kelly's *Post-Partum Document* (1973–1979) both repel yet draw the viewer in their *denouement* of labour and infant excrement. Manifestations of the monstrous-feminine also inspire a diverse range of multi-media works including the profoundly disturbing scenarios of 'female flesh' in Linda Dement's interactive *Cyberflesh Girlmonster* (1995); Destiny Deacon's photographs and installations about rebellious Indigenous women in Australia, *My Boomerang Won't Come Back* (1994), and *Walk & Don't Look Blak* (2004); Maria Abramovic's *Balkan Baroque* performance at the Venice Biennale in 1997; Chrissy Amphlett's shocking stage performances such as *I Touch Myself* (1990) and more recently Lady Gaga's playfully disruptive *Mother Monster Manifesto* (2013) on the birth of 'the eternal mother in the multiverse'. All of these unquestionably tap into *monstrous-feminine* territory.

Although Creed published her major article on the monstrous-feminine in 1986, the concept has proven remarkably relevant to the work of artists from earlier periods, such as Chicago and Schneeman, as well as the contemporary era. Thinking about the work of women artists who explore the monstrous-feminine from the perspective of the abject opens up new ways of understanding how patriarchal ideology continues to construct woman, from earlier centuries to the present, in terms of stereotypes related to female sexuality, reproduction, and the body. Many women artists have taken these stereotypes and recreated them from their own perspectives, often with enormous flair and dark humour, in order to challenge male anxieties and patriarchal myths about women. Gradually, this controversial and challenging figure, the monstrous-feminine, has moved from the margins to the mainstream.

Creed argues: the monstrous-feminine appears in a range of discourses such as 'literature, art, poetry and pornography and other popular fictions' (Creed 1993, p. 166). I would also add bio-art and more recently art that explores human-animal relations. Here I wish to explore ways in which Creed's theory of the monstrous-feminine as abject addresses the work of a range of women artists, as well as, and most importantly, the complex relationship between representations of the abject female body, male power, colonialism, and the position of First Nation Peoples. Race has rarely been interpreted in the context of the monstrous-feminine; however, a number of Australian artists have drawn on this concept to present a critique of white racism and colonial oppression of Indigenous Australians and especially of Black female Australians. Central to this critique is the notion of borders.

Drawing on Kristeva's influential theory, Creed stresses the crucial importance of understanding the emergence of the abject through the erosion of borders. Creed explains:

> [T]he concept of the border is central to the construction of the monstrous ... Although the specific nature of the border changes from film to film, the function of the monstrous remains the same – to bring about an encounter between the symbolic order and that which threatens its stability.
>
> (Creed 1993, p. 11)

Strangely there is pleasure in viewing this struggle between two irreconcilable powers. As Kristeva argues, the abject signifies that which 'disturbs identity, system, order' (Kristeva 1982, p. 4). The irony is that the patriarchal symbolic order has produced a range of feminine stereotypes (witch, vampire, monstrous womb), whose purpose is to shore up that order but which ironically have the power to undermine it. This is because the abject itself, as defined by Kristeva, is profoundly ambiguous. It both attracts yet repels. It lures yet repulses. Its ambiguity relates to its power to undermine borders between the clean and proper self, and the abject, disgusting self: boundaries between the so-called upright masculine and the degraded feminine.

> Horror emerges from the fact that woman has broken with her proper feminine role – she has 'made a spectacle of herself' – put her unsocialized body on display.
>
> (Creed 1993, p. 42)

'There is a pleasure in perversity' (1993, p. 13), Creed writes. Thus, Creed sees the figure of the monstrous-feminine, although inspired by male fears of woman's sexuality and reproductive functions, as having a radical purpose. As Kristeva argues: 'There looms, within, abjection, one of those violent, dark revolts of being' (1982, p. 1). Creed sees this as an ideological struggle. She explores this age-old trope through myth, religious discourses, and surrealist art, but her main focus is on the cinema and the horror film. 'An encounter with the monstrous-feminine of the horror film takes us on an aesthetic and ideological journey' (Creed 1986, p. 166).

What interests me is the work of female artists such as Destiny Deacon who portray the monstrous-feminine as a black woman, thereby extending Creed's argument to explore the borders, and their erosion, between opposing entities: feminine and masculine powers, black and white subjects and between indigenous peoples and colonial invaders. What kind of ideological journey is depicted in artistic works and practices that explore issues of race from the perspective of the monstrous-feminine? How is the monstrous-feminine represented in their works?

Frida Kahlo's remarkable small paintings are now iconic in the history of modernist art and perhaps unique in their revelation of the emotional and physical pain experienced by the artist throughout her life which she places in the context of the colonial history of Mexico. Herself a woman of mixed racial endowment and of indigenous (Mestiza) descent through her maternal grandmother, Kahlo draws from her personal experience in a range of portraits and self-reflexive tableaux in which she speaks from a liminal position that simultaneously attracts and repels the viewer through arresting and confrontational imagery; *My Birth* (1932b), *Henry Ford Hospital* (1932a), and *My Nurse and I* (1937) reveal traumatic narratives of parturition and early life.

My Birth shows a woman (who is the artist's mother), lying upon a bed with the head of her baby (Kahlo herself) fully emerged and bloody from the birth canal. Her mother's head and shoulders are covered in a white sheet in what is a clear reference to the iconography of the surrealists and in particular to some of René Magritte's paintings in which we see the central figure's upper torso draped in a cloth. In *My Nurse and I*, Kahlo is breast-fed by her nurse who wears a black pre-Columbian mask-perhaps a reference to her mother's *mestiza* background. The infant Kahlo is represented with her adult head, and is held by her nurse who is seated in a stormy landscape. These elements combine to present a bleak, indeed horrifying image of the artist's infancy and her own reflections upon it. And in *Henry Ford Hospital*, the artist is lying on a bed, surrounded by the aftermath of a miscarriage connected through umbilical cords to her dead baby, as well as objects of medical paraphernalia associated with the shocking accident she experienced as a young girl as well as her miscarriage.

These abject images are for some viewers too 'monstrous' to countenance, as the bloody reality of parturition and infancy is brought to light and the privacy of what is referred to in English as 'confinement' is overturned. The witnessing of birthing has until relatively recently been almost universally the preserve of women and medical staff, while men kept their distance in hospital waiting rooms, domestic drawing-rooms and outlying spaces. These images make public what has previously remained private, overturning decorum and revealing the real-life trauma of birth.

Frida Kahlo frequently crossed the boundaries of respectability in a range of subject-matter in her work. The numerous self-portraits with small monkeys wrapped around her neck, repeatedly show the artist in closer proximity to tiny primates than is usual in the history of art, revealing the intimate relationship which the artist maintained with her pet animals. Kahlo breaches the boundary between human and animal in these endearing icons. In *Self-Portrait with Cropped Hair* (1940), Kahlo has donned the suit of her husband, Diego Rivera, as she sits on a bright yellow chair drawing attention to her distress. Scattered around her are locks of her luxuriant hair which she has cut in protest over Rivera's infidelity. Once again, Kahlo takes up taboo issues, launching a protest against incest and the philandering of men by self-mutilating and cross-dressing, thus remaking herself as a female/male subject.

> It is through this element of monstrosity that Kahlo resists the patriarchal order...Kahlo steps out of the private sphere of the female artist and into the public... In portraying herself as grotesque, hybrid, and misshapen, Kahlo presents herself as monstrous.
>
> (Gribby 2019)

Kahlo's retablos dealing with violence and death such as *The Suicide of Dorothy Hale* (1938) and *A Few Small Nips* (1935) also take up subjects which breach conventional rules of decorum.

Judy Chicago's *Dinner Party*, is an epic installation of 39 place settings in a range of media, positioned around a triangular table representing women throughout history from the Snake Goddess to Georgia O'Keefe. Each side of the triangle represented women chronologically, with the first wing ranging from Prehistory to Classical Rome; the second the beginning of Christianity to the Reformation and the third, the American Revolution to the Women's Revolution. Fabric, embroidery, china painting, and ceramic sculpture were used to fashion the goblets, cutlery, embroidered runners, and napkins. But what created controversy was the ceramic plate, which consisted of intricate sculptural forms in various subtle glazings, representing the genitals, in particular, the vulva of the woman who was the subject of each place setting, in a truly monumental and spectacular manner. Henry Hopkins, the director of the San Francisco Museum of Modern Art, who had supported the project over many years, presided over the opening in San Francisco on March 14, 1979 to great public enthusiasm. However, controversy immediately erupted and several of the institutions who had booked the exhibition cancelled. A 30-year history of rejections and neglect ensued until in 2007, *Dinner Party* found a donor and was purchased by the Elizabeth A. Sackler Center for Feminist Art at the Brooklyn Museum, New York.

Negative reactions to the installation claimed that Chicago's practice suffered from an overly essentialist view of feminism and that the work is let down by its exclusion of women of colour from its pantheon had some validity. However, suggestions that the work traded in sexual perversion, vulgarity, and pornography and that it was low art masquerading as high art, by prominent critics such as Hilton Kramer and Robert Hughes, reveal the underlining misogyny that informed the reaction to this monumental work of art. Kramer, who was art critic for *The New York Times*, described it as 'an outrageous libel on the female imagination' (1980) and revealing 'an insistence and vulgarity more appropriate perhaps to an advertising campaign' (ibid.). Hughes described it in *Time Magazine* as 'an obsessive feminist pantheon' employing 'colours worthy of a Taiwanese souvenir factory' (1980. It also made headlines for the reaction it created from members of the American parliament with Congressman Robert Dornan from the House of Representatives, calling it 'ceramic 3-D pornography', and fellow California Republican Dana Rohrabacher describing it as 'a spectacle of weird art, weird sexual art at that' (in Beckman 2007). *The Dinner Table* crossed boundaries in terms of both its subject matter and the range of media that it employed. Its liminal nature – the fact that it was accused of being a low art form exhibited in a high art context underlined the general consensus that Chicago's epic work was nothing more than a vulgar display of genitalia ('vaginas on plates') that amounted to a monstrous and abject retelling of history (ibid.).

Laura Mulvey was the first to suggest that Barbara Creed's concept of the monstrous-feminine is helpful in understanding abjection in art using as an example, the photographs of Cindy Sherman. Mulvey points out that while Sherman's 'figures materialise as the stuff of irrational terror, they also have pathos and could easily be understood in terms of 'the monster as victim' (1996, p. 96). Sherman's abject photos such as those of her *Sex Pictures* of 1989–1992 can be collected, Mulvey points out, into a lexicon of horror and the uncanny just like the *Untitled Film Stills*, and are like a lexicon of poses and gestures typical of respectable, but still uncanny femininity (Mulvey 1991, p. 148). Mulvey concludes with an important observation:

> The 1987 series suggests that, although both sexes are subject to abjection, it is woman who can explore and analyse the phenomenon with greater equanimity, as it is the female body that has come, not exclusively but predominantly, to represent the shudder aroused by liquidity and decay.
>
> (Mulvey 1991, p. 148)

Curators of the landmark exhibition, *Abject Art, Repulsion and Desire in American Art,* shown at the Whitney Museum of American Art in 1993, have similarly drawn on Creed's *monstrous-feminine* to interpret the photographs of Cindy Sherman and Kiki Smith that were selected for the exhibition. Simon Taylor in his chapter 'The phobic object: abjection in contemporary art', argued that, as Creed points out:

> the excessive violence and gore in horror films typically produce an ambivalent experience that signals a desire not only for the perverse pleasure (confronting sickening, horrific images, being filled with terror/desire for the undifferentiated) but also a desire, having taken pleasure in perversity, to throw up, throw out, eject the abject (from the safety of the spectator's seat).
>
> (Creed 1986, p. 48)

Taylor also discusses the monstrous-feminine in relation to other important female artists. The abject in Cindy Sherman's and Kiki Smith's work is also characterised by its ambivalence in relation to the monstrous-feminine and Mary Russo's notion of the 'female grotesque' (Taylor 1993, pp. 61–62). Rosemary Betterton has made similar connections between Creed's monstrous-feminine and Cindy Sherman's photographs (Betterton 1996, p. 133).

The performance artist Carolee Schneeman was among the first to represent her body within the framework of the monstrous-feminine in the 1960s and 1970s, which involved appearing naked on stage, alone and as part of a group, being filmed having sex on stage, displaying her pubic hair on stage, and smearing her body and those of others with abject substances. She allowed herself to be photographed in a range of erotic poses covered in toy snakes. In an interview with Steve Rose in *The Guardian* in 2014, Schneeman recalled her own entry into the field of performance art in the UK when she presented a piece at the Institute of Contemporary Arts (ICA) in London in 1968. Schneeman recalls:

> 'I wore farmer's overalls,' she says, 'and I had lots of oranges stuffed everywhere. It was about Cézanne, so I showed slides and talked about his influence – and I kept undressing and dressing. I was naked under my overalls and I'd throw these oranges into the audience, like a still-life escaping. Then I'd do my overalls back up and continue the lecture.' The audience, at the ICA in London, did not appreciate the 29-year-old artist's approach. 'They went a bit nuts,' Schneemann recalls. 'They were outraged, "This is infuriating! What does this mean? How can she be naked and talk about art history?"'.
>
> (Rose 2014)

Schneeman had already broken a great many more taboos four years earlier with *Meat Joy* which she later described as:

> ... an excessive, indulgent celebration of flesh as material: raw fish, chicken, sausages, wet paint, transparent plastic, ropes, brushes, paper scrap. Its propulsion is towards the ecstatic – shifting and turning among tenderness, wildness, precision, abandon; qualities that could at any moment be sensual, comic, joyous, repellent. Physical equivalences are enacted as a psychic imagistic stream, in which the layered elements mesh and gain intensity by the energy complement of the audience. The original performances became notorious and introduced a vision of the 'sacred erotic'.
>
> (in Art Gallery NSW 2007).

She became both subject and object in her own performance 're-enacting a resistant reanimation of the aesthetic/sexual object' (Moton 2017, pp. 134–135). Schneeman recounts having worked with an impressive range of avant-gardists in New York including Yoko Ono, Claes Oldenberg, Robert Morris, Andy Warhol, John Cage, Philip Glass, Robert Rauschenberg, and Stan Brackage. However, Schneemann could not find recognition from her male colleagues and found herself 'excommunicated from the Art Stud Club' (in Schneider 1997, p. 35) stating that she felt like the 'cunt mascot on the men's art team' (in Rose 2014). As a result, she decided to abandon painting – by stepping right into it. In 1963, Schneemann produced her *Eye/Body* series in which she incorporated her own naked, paint-smeared body into tableaux she created out of painted panels, broken mirrors, old umbrellas, and toy snakes in images that are confrontational, primal, unashamedly erotic, and far from passive (ibid.). Recognising the powerful place which the nude occupied in the history of art and also the powerlessness of the models who embodied the nude, Schneeman decided to intervene by becoming an empowered nude. As artist she executed the performance and was simultaneously the nude. What her performance art sought to achieve was to take the authority over depictions of her nudity away from the male artists who were inevitably in control of it – who simply made the model available for the viewer. Instead, she produced an image of the nude over which she as the model was in control and which pleased her as boisterous, vulgar, outrageous, monstrous, abnormal, and obscene (Frank 2017). In other words, by representing herself as monstrous, she gave agency to the concept of the monstrous-feminine as an in-your-face outrageous figure.

Singing from a similar song sheet two decades later, Chrissy Amphlett, the lead singer of the rock group The Divinyls, outraged Australian audiences with on-stage performances and the videos recorded from them.

The band debuted with Chrissy dressed in a school uniform and fishnet stockings performing *Boys in Town* (1982). Amphlett declared:

> I was surrounded by so many men and so the uniform was me giving the finger to everyone. And the audience, as they tried to think that they could have their way with me, I would react and get in first... and become this monster and then I had the power.
>
> (Women's Agenda 2013)

This use of a monstrous identity to 'take the power' continued to manifest in Amphlett's stage performances with The Divinyls over the next decade. *I Touch Myself* (1990) was right off the respectability register and reached no. 1 in Australia, no. 4 in the US, and no. 10 in the UK. Wandering across the stage in a low-cut flouncy black body suit and high heels, Amphlett touched her own body erotically, declaring 'I don't want anybody else when I think about you, I touch myself' (ibid.).

Destiny Deacon (Ku Ku/Erub/Mer) has worked in Melbourne for over 30 years making photographs which celebrate monstrosity through a range of objects, people, and situations that evoke her past and present and which give rise to her memories of being Indigenous (Black) in urban Australia. Central to her evocation of the monstrous-feminine within her practice is the adaptation of a range of kitsch items about Aboriginal cultures produced throughout the Commonwealth and stretching over the twentieth century. These became central to the representation of Australia in art objects manufactured for tourists which were broadly available for purchase by overseas visitors as well as by Australians travelling to holiday destinations in outback Queensland, the Top End, and The Kimberley from the 1930s. These were also prominent in the imagery contained in advertising Australia as an attractive place for British and other European migrants. Today, they are dismissed by many Australians as a kitsch art form whose racist overtones are apparent. They are unwelcome reminders of the pervasiveness of the racism within the community that existed in the recent past and should in the opinion of many Australians be allowed to fade from the communal memory. As Marcia Langton points out:

> The tension between assimilating Aboriginal people by extraordinarily brutal means in reality and yet at the same time depicting them as fascinating primitives reflected the need of the older colonists for security and for emblems of cultural uniqueness and difference from Europe. The meaning at the heart of these depictions was the British conquest and genocide best forgotten.
>
> (Langton 1997, pp. 106–107)

However, many Indigenous Australians value these objects as material markers of their past. Deacon appropriates these into her photographs and installations in a potent satire in which she makes clear the uncertain position which Aboriginal people occupy within white Australia. Perhaps the most defining aspect of her work are her strident interventions into the white art scene in which she undermines 'the proper feminine role' of black women in Australia. But not only does her work challenge the colonial oppression of Indigenous women she also takes on the abuse which women endure at the hands of black men, thereby challenging patriarchal authority through intervening at multiple levels.

This challenging of the 'blak patriarchy' animates her *No Fixed Dress* (1997a) series, the title of which lampoons the name of the black rock group No Fixed Address. The group formed in Adelaide in 1979 and was the first Australian Indigenous rock reggae band to tour the UK and Europe. The band's first recording *We Have Survived* on Rough Diamond Records, a subsidiary of Polygram Records, and launched by the Prime Minister Bob Hawke in 1982, was the first to incorporate the didgeridoo in a rock repertoire. *No Fixed Dress* interrogates the band's reputation in a range of confronting imagery that draws on horror and abjection. In two photographs from the series, a white doll holds a string of beads attached to the decapitated head of a black doll and the other, a white doll holds onto a chain connected to the head of a black doll which floats in the space above the head. These photographs recall Deacon's earlier work in which a black doll lies decapitated on a wooden floor with an axe located between the head and the body of the doll. The images of the dolls who appear as benign and smiling simulacra – there is no blood or evidence of violence – are, nevertheless, gruesome reminders of the axe murders perpetrated by whites and blacks upon each other and of the placing of Indigenous people in chains by whites from the first moments of the arrival of Europeans on Australian shores. The pun on the title *No Fixed Address* produced as *No Fixed Dress* and the alternating of white and black decapitated heads and bodies suggest that both white and black men are complicit in the violence against women.

This undermining of the 'proper role of [blak] women' is also brilliantly achieved in the large photographic *Portrait – Eva Johnson, Writer* (1994) in which a woman of Indigenous descent is depicted with grave intent, pausing with an axe over her shoulder which she is ready to wield at any moment. The photograph is a re-configuration of an iconic image from colonial Australia, the *Portrait of Nannultera, a Young Poonindie Cricketer* (1854) by John Michael Crossland. Poonindie was a mission established close to Adelaide in the mid-nineteenth century, to train Indigenous men in agricultural and pastoral work. Cricket was thought to present 'civilising capacities' to young Indigenous men and Poonindie was famous for its own Black Eleven who played matches against white teams from Port Lincoln and the elite St Peter's college. Here is Nannultera, dressed in his cricketing whites shown displaying his cricket bat which he holds at almost shoulder height, ready for the first ball. He wears a red sweater over his whites and these details are copied in Deacon's darkly parodic *Portrait – Eva Johnson, Writer.* But Crossland's *Portrait of Nannultera* is a profoundly sad image. Alone in the composition, his handsome body dominates the canvas, flanked by a dry South Australian landscape. He is a figure of grace and humility; a saintly figure. In this beautiful and deeply disturbing image, race, colonialism, and the pastoral entwine as the man Nannultera, and the reality of his existence is powerfully conveyed to Crossland's third millennium audience. After their labours in the fields and when the carting of wool was complete, young workers like Nannultera were free to play cricket to participate in the sacred sport of kings. They were allowed this pastoral pleasure as a brief taste of the rewards of white upper-class culture, but when it came to the ownership of a small parcel of their own land, they were refused. (For a discussion of the mission at Poonindie, see Hoorn 2007, pp. 116–119.) In Deacon's portrait, a female Nannultera, now armed with an axe rather than a cricket bat, interrogates the betrayal of civic humanism that the young black cricketer and those like him endured.

As is clear in her *Portrait – Eva Johnson, Writer*, Destiny Deacon's photographs are about liminality, about living on the borders of white Australia disenfranchised and in poverty. Marcia Langton's words, written more than 20 years ago, still hold true:

> To really understand Destiny and her work, it is almost essential to live in a shared household, probably a squat, with a group of Aboriginal, single mothers and or/ black separatists – whether inspired by Sappho or Malcolm X or both – but more relevant, perhaps to have been poor, very poor, to have a big intellectual take on the work and to have been marginalised from the discourses of power.
>
> (Langton 1997, p. 100)

Deacon's work is also defined by its ambiguity – by its power to attract and repel. On the one hand, her most acute interpreters such Langton recognise Deacon's 'brilliant encapsulation of post-colonial anxiety, as a window of understanding for new generations of Australians turning away from the psychosis of the colonial relationship' (Langton 1997, p. 101). On the other hand, and in the same breath, she admits: 'I have often wondered if her work irritates whites in the same way as it irritates me. Or is the message different for them' (Langton 1997, p. 105). Langton explains 'Destiny loves to resurrect the imagery of our oppression, position her favourite dolls or people in her stage sets, and eke out the discomfort' (ibid.).

Occasionally, Deacon's images profoundly horrify, but more often they throw the viewer off-balance, scandalising and unsettling, rather than repulsing. She seems to invite the viewer to engage with the work, to stay with it and to think about it. In this sense, Deacon uses abjection and horror in a subtle and nuanced manner designed to bring in the viewer, often with dark humour prominently in the mix. This is seen in works such as *Trustee* (2001), in which she plays with abjection and masculinity. Here the image of a black man, whose head is represented in sharp focus and who is wearing a baseball cap which announces in prominent lettering TRUST ME: I AM A WITCH DOCTOR. His face melds into folds of orange and yellow fabric in soft focus in the foreground and is located in front of a line of beer cans, a bottle of Jim Beam and knick-knacks containing tropical references. The overall effect is simultaneously charming and unsettling. It brings to mind the life of a slightly seedy bar, yet the barman/witch doctor is sympathetic – even seductive – as he charms the viewer with his soft gaze and appealing visage. *Skid Row* (Deacon 1997b), which engages directly with the monstrous-feminine, is more confrontational; it depicts as three dolls: two black or in blackface, with one female in a free-flowing dress; the other wearing a red cap and tie. These figures are flanked by a young white person of indeterminate gender who seems relaxed or a bit bemused. They make a jolly and sympathetic group of young folk out on the town. However, the title, *Skid Row,* suggests that life may not be as buoyant and light hearted as the imagery contained in the photo appears, pointing in the direction of the black exploitation of popular theatre in the last century and to the struggle of people of colour to represent themselves on stage.

Throughout her career, the image of black femininity presented in her photographs undercuts any ideal of respectability. Her women are not quiet girls brought up in missions who seek integration with white Australia and a subservient role in the patriarchal order, black or white. *Last Laughs* (Deacon 1995a), like Tracey Moffat's *Nice Coloured Girls* (dir. 1987), is a representation of uproar and of female insubordination and monstrosity. *Nice Coloured Girls* is about, what, in the early nineteenth century, pidgin were called *captains*, men who were fooled by adventurous black women into buying them drinks and cigarettes with the aim of easy sex, but who in this contemporary adaptation are hoodwinked by girls looking for a free night out. Similarly, in *Last Laughs*, Deacon appears as part of a trio of lovely ladies who seek out and prefer each other's company, deriving pleasure from their own entertainment and their own bodies, drunk with pleasure, depraved, and disorderly.

In her photograph, *Peach Blossom's Revenge* (Deacon 1995b) the monstrous-feminine is again at work as Deacon pastiches the cover of a cheap video from the era of the Vietnam War. A woman dressed in a *cheongsam* graces the cover in various provocative poses all involving the American flag and the brandishing of a gun. Offensive and satirical quotes, which give the appearance of having been cut from the newspaper with a pair of pinking shears, include 'I spit on your medals' (a reference to the cult rape-revenge exploitation film, *I Spit on Your Grave* [dir. Zarchi 1978]) completes this outrageous penny shocker. Here the artist traverses more controversial territory than much of her other output which often is humorous rather than incendiary. Deacon's exhibition in Adelaide entitled, *My Boomerang Won't Come Back*, satirises through hard-hitting humour, a very racist and offensive song enormously popular in Australia as well as the UK and Canada where it reached number 3 on the hit parade. Every child in Australia of my generation knew the song. It was not banned in Australia until 2015. Deacon's later work, *My Boomerang Did Come Back* (2003) depicts a woman's hand holding a boomerang on high – it is covered in blood that drips down onto her hand. Decapitated dolls, a bloodied boomerang, a black woman brandishing an axe – many of Deacon's images, along with her irreverent word-play, suggest both a relentless attack on the white symbolic order as well as the challenging figure of a black woman seeking justice.

The monstrous-feminine, which began as a concept for understanding female 'monsters' in myth, religion, and film, has over the last three decades become a much more widely used concept for negotiating a range of art forms as well as conceptual entities that come from outside of the visual arts emerging in areas quite distinct from the humanities such as those that have emerged in the social sciences and medicine. Here, I have selected some of the best-known examples from the art of the twentieth century and into the new millennium in which we find the monstrous-feminine appearing in critical writings about artists. Ranging from Freda Kahlo to mid-century feminists such as Judy Chicago and Carolee Schneeman, I have also re-interpreted the photographs of contemporary artists working on race and gender such as Destiny Deacon and Tracey Moffatt whose photography brings to light the connection between female authority and a powerful Indigenous voice within colonial and postcolonial cultures. Drawing on a range of artistic strategies which implicate the monstrous-feminine, from sexual shock to black humour and carnivalesque display, these women artists seek a new culture and a new language to enable and inspire their fight for equality.

References

Abramovic, M 1997, *Balkan Baroque*, multimedia performance, Venice Biennale, Italy.

Amphlett, C 1982, *Boys in Town*, song, Warner-Elektra-Atlantic, Australia.

Amphlett, C 1990, *I Touch Myself*, song, Virgin Records, Australia.

Art Gallery NSW 2007, *Collection*, viewed 7 March 2019, www.artgallery.nsw.gov.au/collection/works/311.2007/

Beckman, R 2007, 'Her table is ready', *Washington Post*, 22 April, viewed 7 March 2019, www.washingtonpost.com/wp-dyn/content/article/2007/04/20/AR2007042000419.html

Betterton, R 1996, *An intimate distance: women, artists and the body*, Routledge, London, pp. 132–135.

Chicago, J 1974–1979, *Dinner Party*, art installation, Brooklyn Museum, New York.

Creed, B 1986, 'Horror and the monstrous-feminine: an imaginary abjection', *Screen*, vol. 27, no. 1, pp. 44–71.

Creed, B 1993, *The monstrous-feminine: film, feminism, psychoanalysis*, London, Routledge.

Crossland, J 1854, *Portrait of Nannultera, a Young Poonindie Cricketer*, online image, viewed 7 March 2019, https://artsearch.nga.gov.au/detail.cfm?irn=62236

Deacon, D 1994, *My Boomerang Won't Come Back*, photographs, Contemporary Art Centre of South Australia, Adelaide.

Destiny, D 1994, *Portrait – Eva Johnson, Writer*, online image, viewed 7 March 2019, https://artsearch.nga.gov.au/detail.cfm?irn=3620

Deacon, D 1995a, *Last Laughs*, photographic exhibition, Ian Potter Museum of Art, Melbourne.

Deacon, D 1995b, *Peach Blossom's Revenge*, online image, viewed 7 March 2019, https://artsearch.nga.gov.au/detail.cfm?irn=8335

Deacon, D 1997a, *No Fixed Dress*, exhibition, Gallery Gabrielle Pizzi, Melbourne.

Deacon, D 1997b, *Skid Row*, online image, viewed 7 March 2019, www.flickr.com/photos/alburycollection/8975556026

Deacon, D 2001, *Trustee*, online image, viewed 7 March 2019, https://possession.blog/post/172645678410/destiny-deacon

Deacon, D 2003, *My Boomerang Did Come Back*, online image, viewed 7 March 2019, www.roslynoxley9.com.au/artists/2/Destiny_Deacon/231/33866/

Deacon, D 2004, *Walk & Don't Look Blak*, exhibition, The Museum of Contemporary Art, Sydney.

Dement, L 1995, *Cyberflesh Girlmonster*, CD-ROM, Adelaide.

Gaisseau, P 1964, *Meat Joy*, Festival de la Libre Expression, Paris.

Gribby, K 2019, 'Frida Kahlo and the monstrous female', *Brigham Young University*, viewed 7 March 2019, http://womensstudies.byu.edu/KristinaGibby_FridaKahlo/

Frank, P 2017, *Huffington Post*, December 7.

Holpuch, A & Rogers, K 2013, 'Lady Gaga's Applause: a look back at mother monster', *The Guardian*, 19 August, viewed 7 March 2019, www.theguardian.com/culture/2013/aug/19/applause-lady-gaga-celebrospective-artpop

Hoorn, J 2007, *Australian pastoral: the making of a white landscape,* Fremantle Art Centre Press, Fremantle.

Hughes, R 1980, 'An Obsessive Feminist Pantheon' *Time Magazine*, Monday December 15.

Kahlo, F 1932a, *Henry Ford Hospital*, online image, viewed 7 March 2019, www.fridakahlo.org/henry-ford-hospital.jsp

Kahlo, F 1932b, *My Birth*, online image, viewed 7 March 2019, www.fridakahlo.org/my-birth.jsp

Kahlo, F 1935, *A Few Small Nips*, online image, viewed 7 March 2019, www.fridakahlo.org/a-few-small-nips-passionately-in-love.jsp
Kahlo, F 1937, *My Nurse and I*, online image, viewed 7 March 2019, www.fridakahlo.org/my-nurse-and-i.jsp
Kahlo, F 1938, *The Suicide of Dorothy Hale*, online image, viewed 7 March 2019, www.fridakahlo.org/the-suicide-of-dorothy-hale.jsp
Kahlo, F 1940, *Self-Portrait with Cropped Hair*, online image, viewed 7 March 2019, www.moma.org/collection/works/78333
Kelly, M 1973–1979, *Post-Partum Document*, art installation, Institute of Contemporary Arts, London.
Kramer, H 1980, 'Art: Judy Chicago's "Dinner Party" comes to Brooklyn Museum; art: Judy Chicago "Dinner Party"', *The New York Times*, 17 October 1980, viewed 8 March 2019, www.nytimes.com/1980/10/17/archives/art-judy-chicagos-dinner-party-comes-to-brooklyn-museum-art-judy.html?module=inline
Kristeva, J 1982, *Powers of horror: an essay on abjection*, Columbia University Press, New York.
Langton, M 1997, 'The valley of the dolls: black humour in the art of Destiny Deacon', *Art and Australia*, vol. 35, no. 1, pp. 100–107.
Moffat, T (dir.) 1987, *Nice Coloured Girls,* motion picture, Ronin Films, Australia.
Moton, F 2017, *Black and blur (consent not to be a single being)*, Duke University Press, Durham.
Mulvey, L 1991, 'A phantasmagoria of the female body: the work of Cindy Sherman', *New Left Review*, vol. 188, pp. 137–150.
Mulvey, L 1996, *Fetishism and curiosity: cinema and the mind's eye*, Bloomsbury, London.
Rose, S 2014, 'Carolee Schneeman: I never thought I was shocking', *The Guardian*, 10 March, viewed 7 March 2019, www.theguardian.com/artanddesign/2014/mar/10/carole-schneemann-naked-art-performance
Schneeman, C 1963–1973, *Eye/Body*, photographs.
Schneider, R 1997, *The explicit body in performance*, Routledge, London.
Sherman, C 1989–1992, *Sex Pictures*, photographs.
Taylor, S 1993, 'The phobic object: abjection in contemporary art', in Houser, C & Jones, L (eds.), *Abject art, repulsion and desire in American art,* Whitney Museum of Art, New York, pp. 59–84.
Uncovered Emotions 2017, *Annie Sprinkle Public Cervix Announcement*, online video, viewed 7 March 2019, https://vimeo.com/184135882
Women's Agenda 2013, 'Chrissy Amphlett: surrounded by men, the uniform was me 'giving the finger'', 22 April, viewed 7 March 2019. https://womensagenda.com.au/latest/chrissy-amphlett-surrounded-by-men-the-uniform-was-me-giving-the-finger/
Zarchi, N (dir.) 1978, *I Spit on Your Grave*, motion picture, Cinemagic Pictures, USA.

List of Contributors

Tara Brabazon is the Dean of Graduate Research and Professor of Cultural Studies at Flinders University, Adelaide. She is the winner of six teaching awards and has published 18 books and over 200 refereed articles and book chapters. She is also a columnist for the Times Higher Education. Her personal website is www.brabazon.net.

Nicholas Chare is Associate Professor in the Department of History of Art and Film Studies at the Université de Montréal. He is the author of *After Francis Bacon* (2012) and *Sportswomen in Cinema* (2015) and the co-editor with Liz Watkins of *Gesture and Film* (2017) and with Katharina Bonzel of *Representations of Sports Coaches in Film* (2017).

Elizabeth Cowie is Professor Emeritus in Film Studies at the University of Kent, Canterbury. She was co-founder and co-editor in the 1970s of *m/f*, a journal of feminist theory, and author of *Representing the Woman: Cinema and Psychoanalysis* (Palgrave Macmillan, 1997). She has subsequently written on film noir, the horror of the horror film, and on the cinematic dream-work. In *Recording Reality, Desiring the Real* (Minnesota University Press, 2011), she addressed documentary film as serious, as spectacle, and as an art of the real. Recent essays include 'Documentary Space, Place, and Landscape', in the online journal *Media Fields* (vol. 1, 2011); 'The Ventriloquism of Documentary First-Person Speech and the Self-Portrait Film', in *Embodied Encounters: New Approaches to Psychoanalysis and Cinema* (Routledge, 2014); 'The World Viewed: Documentary Observing and the Culture of Surveillance', in *A Companion to Contemporary Documentary Film* (Wiley-Blackwell, 2015); *The Time of Gesture in Cinema and Its Ethics*, in *Journal for Cultural Research* (vol. 19, no, 1, 2015); and 'The Difference in Figuring Women Now', in *Moving Image Review & Art Journal* (vol. 4 nos 1 and 2, 2016, special issue on feminism and women's art).

Barbara Creed is Redmond Barry Distinguished Professor at the University of Melbourne. She is the author of six books in feminist film theory, gender, and media, including *The Monstrous-Feminine* (1993) and *Stray* (2017). Her recent research is in animal studies, ethics in the anthropocene, and the inhuman; her articles have appeared in journals such as the Journal for Cultural Research; Necsus: European Journal of Media Studies; and Relations: Beyond Anthropocentrism. She is on the editorial advisory boards of the Animal Studies Journal and the Animal Publics international book series. She is the director of the Human Rights and Animal Ethics Research Network (HRAE).

Brett Farmer is Lecturer in Screen and Design at Deakin University, Australia. He is author of Spectacular Passions: Cinema, Fantasy and Gay Male Spectatorships (Duke 2000) and numerous essays on Thai cinema. Between 2001 and 2016, he developed, established, and headed the cultural studies programme at Chulalongkorn University in Thailand.

Sneja Gunew (FRSC) is Professor Emerita of English and Women's and Gender Studies at the University of British Columbia, Canada. She has edited and co-edited anthologies of Australian women's and multicultural writings including *Feminist Knowledge: Critique and Construct* and *A Reader in Feminist Knowledge* (Routledge 1990–1991). In Australia, she compiled (with others) *A Bibliography of Australian Multicultural Writers* (the first such compilation in Australia) and co-edited *Striking Chords: Multicultural Literary Interpretations* (1992), the first collection of critical essay to deal with ethnic minority writings in the Australian context. Her books include *Framing Marginality: Multicultural Literary Studies* (1994) and *Haunted Nations: The Colonial Dimensions of Multiculturalisms* (Routledge 2004). Her most recent book is titled: *Post-Multicultural Writers as Neo-Cosmopolitan Mediators* (Anthem 2017).

Jeanette Hoorn is Honorary Professorial Fellow and a former Director of Gender Studies and Associate-Dean EO in the Faculty of Arts at the University of Melbourne. In 2014 she designed *Sexing the Canvas*, filmed and taught at National Gallery of Victoria, Museum of Modern Art New York, and Huntington Library in Pasadena on the Coursera platform https://www.coursera.org/course/sexingthecanvas. Her books include *Australian Pastoral, the Making of a White Landscape*, 2007; *Reframing Darwin: Evolution and Art in Australia*, 2009; *Body Trade: Captivity, Cannibalism and Colonialism the Pacific*, 2001; *Idylle Marocaine, Hilda Rix Nicholas et Elsie Rix en Maroc*, due October 2019 with Afrique Orient. Her essays have appeared in *Art and Australia, Screen, Third Text, Continuum, Transnational Cinemas, Hecate, Australian Historical Studies; Photofile*.

E. Ann Kaplan is Distinguished Professor Emerita of English and Cultural Analysis and Theory at Stony Brook University. Kaplan has written many books and articles on topics in cultural studies, media, and women's studies, from diverse theoretical perspectives including psychoanalysis, feminism, postmodernism, and postcolonialism. Kaplan's pioneering research on women in film (see her *Women in Film: Both Sides of the Camera, Women in Film Noir* and *Motherhood and Representation*) continues to be in print. Her *Feminism and Film* (2000) brings together major feminist film theories from 1980 to 2000. Kaplan's more recent research focusses on trauma as evident in her books *Trauma and Cinema: Cross-Cultural Explorations* (co-edited with Ban Wang in 2004), her *Trauma Culture: The Politics of Terror and Loss in Media and Literature* (2005) and her latest book, *Climate Trauma: Foreseeing the Future in Dystopian Film and Fiction* (2015). Her new research project continues her concern with trauma, this time in relation to traumatic memory loss and gender, with a focus on dementia.

Annette Kuhn is Professor and Research Fellow in Film Studies at Queen Mary University of London and a Fellow of the British Academy. As co-editor of *Screen*, she curated the special issue, *Screen and Screen Theorising Today*, in commemoration of the journal's 50th anniversary. Other publications include *Oxford Dictionary of Film Studies* (co-authored with Guy Westwell, 2nd edn, 2020) and *Little Madnesses: Winnicott, Transitional Phenomena and Cultural Experience* (2013).

Laura Mulvey is Professor of Film and Media Studies at Birkbeck, University of London. She is the author of *Visual and Other Pleasures* (1989; second edition 2009), *Fetishism and Curiosity* (1996; second edition 2013), *Citizen Kane* (1992; second edition 2012), and *Death 24x a Second: Stillness and the Moving Image* (2006). She made six films in collaboration with Peter Wollen, including *Riddles of the Sphinx* (1977; DVD publication 2013) and *Frida Kahlo and Tina Modotti* (1980). With artist/filmmaker Mark Lewis, she has made *Disgraced Monuments* (1994) and *23 August 2008* (2013).

Mark Nicholls is Senior Lecturer in Cinema Studies at the University of Melbourne where he has taught film since 1993. He is the author of *Lost Objects of Desire: The Performances of Jeremy Irons*, *Scorsese's Men: Melancholia and the Mob*, and recent articles on Italian Cinema and The Ballets Russes. Mark is a film journalist and worked for many years on ABC Radio and for *The Age* newspaper, for which he wrote a weekly film column between 2007 and 2009. He has an extensive list of credits as a playwright, composer, actor, producer, and director. His ten most recent plays are published as Unconventional Women (Prahran Press).

Polona Petek is Assistant Professor (Film and Television Studies) at the Academy of Theatre, Radio, Film and Television, and Research Fellow at the Faculty of Arts at the University of Ljubljana. She is the author of *Echo and Narcissus: Echolocating the Spectator in the Age of Audience Research* (2008) and co-editor (with Nil Baskar) of *Phenomenology of Film: Traditions and New Approaches* (2014). Her recent research focuses on nationalism, cosmopolitanism, and mobility in cinema; on the intersections of these issues and gender in Slovenian and other European cinemas.

Patricia Pisters is Professor of film at the Department of Media Studies of the University of Amsterdam. She is one of the founding editors of the Open Access journal *NECSUS: European Journal of Media Studies*. Publications include: *The Matrix of Visual Culture* (Stanford University Press, 2003); *The Neuro-Image: A Deleuzian Film-Philosophy of Digital Screen Culture* (Stanford University Press, 2012), and *Filming for the Future* (Amsterdam University Press). In 2019 she is scholar in residence at EYE Film Institute Netherlands and research fellow at Cinepoetic at the Freie Universitat in Berlin. See also www.patriciapisters.com.

Valerie Wee is an Associate Professor in the Department of English Language and Literature at the National University of Singapore and lectures on film and media studies. Her research areas include teen culture and the American culture industries, horror films, and gender representations in the media. Her work has appeared in *Cinema Journal*, *Journal of Film and Video*, *Journal of Popular Film and Television*, and *Feminist Media Studies*. She is the author of two books, *Teen Media: Hollywood and the Youth Market in the Digital Age* and *Japanese Horror Film and their American Remakes: Translating Fear, Adapting Culture*.

Audrey Yue is Professor in Media, Culture and Critical Theory, Head of Communications and New Media, and Convenor of the Cultural Studies in Asia PhD Programme at the National University of Singapore. She is author, co-author, and co-editor of *Sinophone Cinemas* (2014), *Transnational Australian Cinema* (2013), *Queer Singapore* (2012), *Ann Hui's Song of the Exile* (2010), *AsiaPacifiQueer* (2008), and *Mobile Cultures: New Media in Queer Asia* (2003). Her recent essays appear in *Media and Communication*, *International Journal of Communication*, *Inter-Asia Cultural Studies*, and *Urban Studies*.

Index

Note: Page numbers followed by "n" denote endnotes.

Kolibri 360 GmbH
Ferdinand-Jühlke-Straße 7
99095 Erfurt, Deutschland
produktsicherheit@kolibri360.de